AUTISM:
A NEUROLOGICAL DISORDER OF
EARLY BRAIN DEVELOPMENT

Edited by
Roberto Tuchman
Isabelle Rapin

© 2006 Mac Keith Press
30 Furnival Street, London EC4A 1JQ, England

Editor: Hilary Hart
Managing Editor: Michael Pountney
Sub Editor: Pat Chappelle

The views and opinions expressed herein are those of the authors and do not necessarily
represent those of the publisher

First published in this edition 2006

British Library Cataloguing-in-Publication data:
A catalogue record for this book is available from the British Library

ISBN: 1 898683 49 2 (978 1 898683 49 0)

Printed by The Lavenham Press Ltd, Water Street, Lavenham, Suffolk, England
Mac Keith Press is supported by Scope (formerly The Spastics Society)

Distributed to non-members of ICNA by Cambridge University Press

INTERNATIONAL REVIEW OF CHILD NEUROLOGY SERIES

AUTISM:
A NEUROLOGICAL DISORDER OF
EARLY BRAIN DEVELOPMENT

Edited by

ROBERTO TUCHMAN

and

ISABELLE RAPIN

2006
MAC KEITH PRESS
for the
INTERNATIONAL CHILD NEUROLOGY ASSOCIATION

THE INTERNATIONAL REVIEW OF CHILD NEUROLOGY SERIES

CONTENTS

AUTHORS' APPOINTMENTS

Maria T Acosta, MD — Staff Physician, Department of Neurology, Children's National Medical Center, Washington, DC, USA

Michael Alessandri, PhD — Clinical Associate Professor, Department of Psychology; *and* Director, Center for Autism and Related Disabilities, University of Miami, Coral Gables, FL, USA

Evdokia Anagnostou, MD — Assistant Professor, Seaver and NY Autism Center of Excellence, Mount Sinai School of Medicine, New York, NY, USA

Mary E Blue, PhD — Associate Professor, Neurology and Neuroscience, Kennedy Krieger Institute, Johns Hopkins University School of Medicine, Baltimore, MD, USA

Verne S Caviness, Jr, MD, DPhil — Chief Child Neurology Service, Massachusetts General Hospital; *and* Joseph and Rose Kennedy Professor of Child Neurology and Mental Retardation, Harvard Medical School, Boston, MA, USA

Susan L Connors, MD — Research Assistant, Kennedy Krieger Institute, Baltimore, MD, USA

Paolo Curatolo, MD — President, International Child Neurology Association; *and* Professor of Pediatric Neurosciences, Tor Vergata University of Rome, Rome, Italy

Thierry Deonna, MD — Associate Professor, Neuropediatric Unit, Medico-Surgical Department of Pediatrics, Centre Hospitalier Universitaire Vaudois, Lausanne, Switzerland

Jennifer C Gidley Larson, MA — Psychology Associate, Kennedy Krieger Institute, Baltimore, MD, USA

Martha R Herbert, MD, PhD — Assistant Professor, Neurology (Pediatric) and Center for Morphometric Analysis, Massachusetts General Hospital, Harvard Medical School, Charlestown, MA, USA

Michael V Johnston, MD — Chief Medical Officer/Senior VP, Kennedy Krieger Institute; *and* Professor, Neurology and Pediatrics, Johns Hopkins University School of Medicine, Baltimore, MD, USA

Kent R Kelley, MD — Assistant Professor of Pediatrics and Neurology, Feinberg School of Medicine, Northwestern University, Children's Memorial Epilepsy Center, Chicago, IL, USA

Susan K Klein, MD, PhD — Assistant Professor of Pediatrics (Child Neurology), CWRU, UHHS–Rainbow Babies and Children's Hospital, Cleveland, OH, USA

Beth A Malow, MD, MS — Associate Professor, Department of Neurology, *and* Medical Director, Vanderbilt Sleep Disorders Center, Vanderbilt University Medical Center, Nashville, TN, USA

David E Mandelbaum, MD, PhD — Professor of Clinical Neurosciences and Pediatrics, Brown University; *and* Director, Division of Child Neurology, Children's Neurodevelopment Center, Rhode Island and Hasbro Children's Hospitals, Providence, RI, USA

Susan G McGrew, MD — Assistant Professor of Pediatrics, Vanderbilt University Medical Center, Nashville, TN, USA

Jonathan W Mink, MD, PhD — Associate Professor of Neurology, Neurobiology and Anatomy, Brain and Cognitive Sciences, and Pediatrics; *and* Chief, Child Neurology, University of Rochester Medical Center, Rochester, NY, USA

Mark Mintz, MD — President, The Center for Neurological and Neurodevelopmental Health, *and* Clinical Research Center of New Jersey, Voorhees, NJ; *and* Adjunct Associate Professor of Pediatrics and Neurology, University of Pennsylvania School of Medicine, Philadelphia, PA, USA

Solomon L Moshé, MD — Professor of Neurology, Neuroscience and Pediatrics; Vice-Chairman, Department of Neurology; Director, Pediatric Neurology and Clinical Neurophysiology; *and* Martin A and Emily L Fisher Fellow, Department of Neurology, Albert Einstein College of Medicine, Bronx, NY, USA

Stewart H Mostofsky, MD — Assistant Professor of Neurology and Psychiatry, Department of Developmental Cognitive Neurology; *and* Medical Director, Center for Autism and Related Disorders, Kennedy Krieger Institute, Johns Hopkins University School of Medicine, Baltimore, MD, USA

Yoshiko Nomura, MD — Vice-Director, Segawa Neurological Clinic for Children, Tokyo, Japan

Carlos A Pardo-Villamizar, MD — Assistant Professor, Department of Neurology and Pathology, Johns Hopkins University School of Medicine, Baltimore, MD, USA

Phillip L Pearl, MD — Associate Professor of Pediatrics and Neurology, Department of Neurology, Children's National Medical Center, George Washington University School of Medicine and Health Sciences, Washington, DC, USA

Isabelle Rapin, MD

Professor, Saul R Korey Department of Neurology, Department of Pediatrics, and Rose F Kennedy Center for Research in Mental Retardation and Human Development, Albert Einstein College of Medicine, Bronx, NY, USA

Eliane Roulet-Perez, MD

Associate Professor, Head of Neuropediatric Unit, Medico-Surgical Department of Pediatrics, Centre Hospitalier Universitaire Vaudois, Lausanne, Switzerland

Masaya Segawa, MD

Director, Segawa Neurological Clinic for Children, Tokyo, Japan

Michael Shevell, MD, CM, FRCP

Professor, Departments of Neurology/Neurosurgery and Pediatrics, McGill University, *and* Division of Pediatric Neurology, Montreal Children's Hospital–McGill University Health Centre, Montreal, Quebec, Canada

Shlomo Shinnar, MD, PhD

Professor of Neurology and Pediatrics, Hyman Climenko Professor of Neuroscience Research, *and* Director, Comprehensive Epilepsy Management Center, Montefiore Medical Center, Albert Einstein College of Medicine, Bronx, NY, USA

Edwin Trevathan, MD, MPH

Professor of Neurology and Pediatrics, *and* Director, Division of Pediatric and Developmental Neurology, Washington University in St. Louis, School of Medicine; *and* Neurologist-in-Chief, St. Louis Children's Hospital, St. Louis, MO, USA

Roberto F Tuchman, MD

Associate Professor of Neurology, *and* Director, Developmental and Behavioral Neurology, Miami Children's Hospital, University of Miami Miller School of Medicine, Miami, FL, USA

Andrew W Zimmerman, MD

Pediatric Neurologist, Kennedy Krieger Institute, Baltimore, MD, USA

FOREWORD

In the early 1970's Child Neurology was a small but growing speciality. At that time a small group of child neurologists from a number of countries came together and formed the International Child Neurology Association (ICNA) in 1973. In 1975 the First International Child Neurology Congress was held in Toronto, and in 1979 the Second Congress took place in Sydney. Although these Congresses gave child neurologists from around the world the opportunity to meet and exchange ideas, the ICNA Executive, spurred on by John Stobo Prichard from Toronto, believed that something more should be given to its members and to child neurology as a whole. So the idea of the *International Review of Child Neurology* was conceived. The task of editing the series was given to Prichard, with the plan to launch the first book in the series at the Third Congress to be hosted by Copenhagen in 1982. This goal was achieved, and the book *Children with Brain Dysfunction* by Isabelle Rapin was presented to the Congress in mock-up form and formally published later that year.

It is indeed apt that the present volume is co-edited by Isabelle Rapin and will be launched at the Tenth International Child Neurology Congress in Montreal, Canada, the country of John Stobo Prichard, the Founding Editor of this series.

Peter G Procopis
Senior Editor

DEDICATION

To the memory of our colleague and friend, Doris A Allen, Ed D, a pioneer in the diagnosis of children with autism and in research on their language disorders, and in the education of toddlers and preschoolers with high functioning autism and of their parents.

To our families: Medardo, Esther, Laurie, Alexander and Naomi Tuchman; Harold, Anne Louise, Christine, Stephen and Peter Oaklander; Max, Daniel and Maddie Coe Klein; Yeon Sook, Connor and Evan Oaklander.

To child neurologists around the world, in the hopes that this review of what is known in 2006 about the clinical aspects of autism and its neurobiology will encourage them to care for the needs of children of all ages and see to their receiving appropriate interventions, and will stimulate them to advance our scientific knowledge of this challenging developmental disorder of the brain.

ACKNOWLEDGMENTS

The editors thank each of the authors for their scholarly and insightful contributions to this joint enterprise. We are especially grateful for their forbearance and uncomplaining willingness to consider our often many suggestions for revision of their chapters. We are thankful to Dr Martha Bridge Denckla for her incisive preface and to Dr Mark Mehler for his suggestions. We thank Dr Marc Monfort for his elegant illustration and are honored that it graces the front cover of the book. We are grateful to the innumerable children and their parents who taught us most of what we know; without them this book could not have been conceived. Both editors credit the stimulating environment and support of the Saul R Korey Department of Neurology and of the Rose F Kennedy Center for Research in Mental Retardation and Human Development of the Albert Einstein College of Medicine, as well as discussion and collaboration with many colleagues in neurology and other disciplines for fostering the scholarly endeavors which culminated in this monograph.

IR acknowledges the support of NINDS, which funded for 9 years a major longitudinal study of preschool and school-age children with autism and their developmentally impaired controls, a study carried out by many collaborators from many disciplines and their able research assistants. She is especially indebted to Dr Deborah Fein and her graduate students and postdoctoral fellows who continue to report study results and to Dr Michelle Dunn who was the key investigator and manager of the Einstein site – her unflagging and close collaboration over two decades has been enormously enriching, and her innovative approach to social skills training of children on the autism spectrum has had, and will continue to have, a major impact on their lives and on those of their families. Thanks also to the CAN Foundation which supported an investigation of the role of epilepsy in early language/autistic regression, and to the NAAR Foundation currently funding Dr Sylvie Goldman's quantitative analysis of stereotypies as a movement disorder rather than bad habits.

PREFACE

This is a very substantial and comprehensive multi-authored volume on autism; it fills a need for a neurobiological orientation to lead the way into our future understanding of this very seriously impairing, deeply fascinating and equally mysterious spectrum of disordered development. The book reminds us from multiple (yet always neurobiological) perspectives how far the field has come from the days of "refrigerator mothers" or "primal rages". (Younger readers may be amazed and not a little unsettled to learn that when I arrived at Harvard-affiliated Children's Hospital as faculty in the mid-1970's, children with autism were still enrolled in psychoanalytic treatment just down the street.) Overlaps of autism with developmental language disorders, as related to awareness of neurodevelopment within the growing field of learning disabilities, and then the explosion of genetics throughout the medical world, seem to have been the two "hooks" whereby autism was pulled into the sphere of neurobiology. Neuroimaging and neuropsychology became more prominent 25 years ago, and, as applied to autism (and to most of psychiatry), have reinforced the general acceptance of the neurobiological nature of autism. Yet, paradoxically, there have been drawbacks and even conceptual impediments to advances in understanding of autism resulting from the overly conventional, even "classic", approaches within neuropsychology and the functional applications of neuroimaging so closely tied to established neuropsychological frames of reference (even when renamed "cognitive neuroscience"). Explicitly, focus upon cortical association areas and such functional domains as "executive function", "theory of mind", and "dyspraxia" perpetuates a view of autism that is cortical, higher-order, top-down, and later-developing in the maturational timetable. While such studies are for pragmatic reasons limited to older and higher-functioning autistic persons, clinicians rightly comment upon the lack of generalizability of research findings to a disorder that starts early in life and has diverse developmental ramifications that include, but are not specifically limited to, higher integrated functions affiliated with the cerebral cortex. Even the language impairments of classic autism bear scrutiny in terms of basic pathogenesis, since the early aspects of language development of those with Asperger syndrome indicate that core autistic impairments can spare the basic building blocks of this important "higher cortical function". While disordered language was an important clue to the neurobiological nature of autism, it is by now clear that, setting pragmatics and some semantics aside, the phonological–lexical–syntactic aspects of language are neither necessary nor sufficient for normal socioemotional development; a child can be manifestly autistic despite possessing such basic language skills, while many language-impaired children are remarkable in their social relatedness.

Even with preoccupations (so temptingly adaptable to functional magnetic resonance imaging) with presumably socially relevant cognitive elements such as "face processing", this overfocus on the cortical regions diverts researchers from acknowledging what so many of the scientific chapters in this book indicate: namely, "let's talk subcortical and bottom-up influences!" Except for the chapters on epilepsy (again, usually not an early manifestation and thus, like all the cognitive cortical malfunctions, potentially "downstream" of the developmental pathophysiology of autism), the more fundamental scientific chapters point to involvement of important subcortical systems. The glaring gap in our knowledge about the social–emotional brain is like a "black hole" in the book and accurately reflects the field of research it represents. It is not the fault of Roberto Tuchman that his important chapter called "The social deficit in autism" (Chapter 3) falls so short of its title. It reflects the fog and confusion in general surrounding the definition of the social "what" we need to investigate – is it social skills, social competency, social motivation, social orienting, emotional bonding, emotional displaying (the proper meaning of "affect"), or each of these as expected at some specified relevant time in development? Chapter 3 mentions so much that it serves to point us towards all the work we need to do to "zero in on" the social–emotional brain in autism; that will include a lot of comparative biology as well as developmental psychology, because the social–emotional brain is the shared defining neurobiology of mammals. We need to understand the amygdala, the nucleus accumbens, the rest of the limbic system, and those parts of the motor system recently (not classically) in the spotlight, the mirror neurons and the procedural learning system. Much of the basic science data is hinting at vital neighborhoods, systems/circuits "bottom-up" to the cortex; but as Isabelle Rapin reminds us again and again, there are two levels of neurological diagnosis, "what" and "where". The "where" level of localization does not mean pointing to a spot on a map but rather to the developmental dynamics of a system like the social–emotional brain. Rita Rudel warned us 35 years ago to take the sign "Higher Cortical Function Laboratory" off the door of our laboratory at Columbia that was dedicated to research on dyslexia/learning disabilities; how much more compelling for autism research it is to recall Rudel's caution about developmental disabilities. More recently, Antonio Damasio warned us, with the book entitled *Descartes' Error*, that overfocus on "cold cognition" would cause neuropsychology to stagnate; how much more compelling for autism research it is to heed Damasio's message and re-orient our efforts towards understanding the development of the social–emotional brain.

Martha Bridge Denckla
Kennedy Krieger Institute
Baltimore, MD
USA

1
WHERE WE ARE: OVERVIEW AND DEFINITIONS

Isabelle Rapin and Roberto F Tuchman

HISTORICAL BACKGROUND

The term "autism", which was coined by Bleuler to characterize the negative symptoms and social alienation of individuals suffering from schizophrenia, was borrowed by both Kanner (Kanner 1943) and Asperger (Frith 1991) when they independently and almost simultaneously in 1943–44 described developmentally disabled children whose profound deficit in the ability to relate to others marked them as unique. It took close to 40 years for autism to be listed as such in the *Diagnostic and Statistical Manual of Mental Disorders* (DSM). The 3rd edition of the DSM (DSM-III; APA 1980) introduced the term "pervasive developmental disorder" to refer to a group of *behaviorally defined* developmental disorders that share symptomatology with classic autism as described by Kanner, which is labeled "autistic disorder" in both the DSM and the *International Classification of Mental and Behavioural Disorders* (ICD-10; WHO 1992). Over the next quarter century an exponential number of studies were carried out to refine the description of the behaviors that characterize affected individuals and, more recently, to investigate the causes (etiologies) of autism and the neurologic pathophysiology of its many behavioral manifestations.

DEFINITIONS (TABLE 1.1)

In this book, the term autism is used broadly and synonymously with pervasive developmental disorders (PDDs) or the autism spectrum disorders (ASDs), and *not* to refer specifically to autistic disorder (AD) as defined in the DSM and ICD manuals. The term spectrum implies a broad range of severity. We use autism (or ASD) in this book irrespective of the many potential biologic causes of this developmental disorder.

The subcategories under the broader label of PDD introduced in the DSM 4th edition, text revision (DSM-IV-TR; APA 2000) are an attempt to meet scientific (research) needs, as well as to allow for appropriate service development and administrative needs for individuals with autism and related disorders (Rutter and Schopler 1992). Still missing are more specific behavioral criteria to identify homogenous subgroups of individuals within the larger spectrum of autism, both for research and practical purposes.

TABLE 1.1
Definitions*

Term	Abbrev.	Definition
Autism spectrum disorder	ASD	Refers to the entire range of severity of disorders with autistic symptomatology, irrespective of etiology or associated disabilities
Pervasive developmental disorder	PDD	Used synonymously with ASD
Autism, autistic	—	Used as short for ASD/PDD
Autistic disorder	AD	Used narrowly in its DSM-IV definition
Pervasive developmental disorder – not otherwise specified	PDD-NOS	Used narrowly in its DSM-IV definition, refers to the milder end of the ASD spectrum
Asperger syndrome	AS	Used narrowly in its DSM definition
Developmental and Statistical Manual of Mental Disorders	DSM	Refers to any of the editions if unspecified
International Classification of Diseases	ICD	Refers to any of the editions if unspecified
Idiopathic/primary autism	—	Autism without an ascertainable etiology in a non-stigmatized individual
Syndromic/secondary autism	—	Autism with a known or ostensible etiology, whether the individual is stigmatized or not
Non-syndromic autism	—	Autism without stigmata or known etiology

*See Table 1.3 for DSM-IV/ICD-10 correspondences.

CORE DEFICITS AND BEHAVIORAL DESCRIPTORS OF AUTISM IN THE DSM/ICD MANUALS

What makes autism so distinctive that an experienced clinician or educator recognizes classic cases at a glance and rapidly suspects it even in less severely affected persons? Both Kanner and Asperger were impressed by the profound social ineptitude of the children they identified, their rigidity and resistance to change, their repetitive behaviors (stereotypies), and their unusual speech and often bizarre modes of communication – if they communicated at all. Both described children with extremely uneven cognitive abilities, in some of whom extraordinary accomplishments, especially in rote memory and visual skills, coexisted with profound deficits in common sense and reasoning. Psychiatrists and psychologists who spent decades studying affected individuals developed for the

TABLE 1.2
DSM-IV-TR (2000) behavioral descriptors

1. Social interaction domain:
    (a) marked impairment in the use of multiple nonverbal behaviors such as eye-to-eye gaze, facial expression, body postures, and gestures to regulate social interaction
    (b) failure to develop peer relationships appropriate to developmental level
    (c) lack of spontaneous seeking to share enjoyment, interests or achievements (e.g. by lack of showing, bringing, or pointing out of objects of interest)
    (d) lack of social or emotional reciprocity

2. Language, communication and imagination domain:
    (a) delay in, or total lack of, the development of spoken language (not accompanied by an attempt to compensate through alternative modes of communication such as gestures or mime)
    (b) in individuals with adequate speech, marked impairment in the ability to initiate or sustain a conversation with others
    (c) stereotyped and repetitive use of language or idiosyncratic language
    (d) lack of varied, spontaneous make-believe play or social imitative play appropriate to developmental level

3. Behavioral flexibility domain: restricted, repetitive and stereotyped patterns of behavior, interests and activities
    (a) encompassing preoccupation with one or more stereotyped and restricted patterns of interest that is abnormal either in intensity or focus
    (b) apparently inflexible adherence to specific, nonfunctional routines or rituals
    (c) stereotyped and repetitive motor mannerisms (e.g. hand or finger flapping or twisting, or complex whole-body movements)
    (d) persistent preoccupation with parts of objects

DSM/ICD manuals (WHO 1993, APA 2000) a set of operationalized behavioral descriptors to enable investigators and clinicians alike to reach a satisfactory degree of diagnostic consensus.

The first and foremost domain is social skill and the ability to be sufficiently cognizant of others' thinking to enable empathy and insight into what others may be thinking. The second domain is verbal and nonverbal communication, and, in young children, pretend play. The third domain is breadth of interests, behavioral flexibility, and the ability to switch activities and cope with the unexpected. The DSM IV-TR (APA 2000) includes a series of 12 descriptors of deficits, four in each of the three behavioral domains (Table 1.2). We stress that PDD/ASD diagnoses are *behavioral*; neither level of intelligence nor biologic criteria such as epilepsy, motor deficits, visual or auditory impairment, or a specific etiology is an exclusionary criterion for an ASD diagnosis.

DSM/ICD SUBTYPES OF PERVASIVE DEVELOPMENTAL DISORDERS
The ASDs encompass a wide range of symptoms, some or all of which vary greatly in

TABLE 1.3
Correspondence between DSM-IV and ICD-10 subtypes of pervasive developmental disorders (PDDs)

DSM-IV	ICD-10
Autistic disorder	Childhood autism
Asperger's disorder	Asperger syndrome
PDD-NOS	• Atypical autism (by age of onset, symptomatology, or both) • Other pervasive developmental disorder • Pervasive developmental disorder, unspecified
Childhood disintegrative disorder	Childhood disintegrative disorder (Heller syndrome)
Rett's disorder	Rett syndrome

severity. The most recent DSM-IV and ICD-10 systems have adopted parallel and virtually identical names (and criteria) for the subtypes of PDD, as shown in Table 1.3. Diagnostic criteria for these subtypes of autism are based mainly on the number and distribution of behavioral descriptors, therefore on *severity within a continuum*, with some consideration of age of onset (or more realistically age at awareness of the disorder) (Table 1.4). These criteria were arrived at after field trials and international conferences of clinicians and researchers (mostly psychiatrists and psychologists, with little if any input from neurology) whose goals were to create a common language applicable worldwide and to define operational rules or criteria for classification. Achieving a consensus is critical for enabling clinicians and investigators to use a common diagnostic system when referring to individuals of all ages with autistic symptomatology. At least at present, the DSM subtypes, with the exception of Rett syndrome, do not fulfill criteria for any biologically specific disorder.

These behavioral classification systems are very much a work in progress and no doubt will continue to evolve as new information is accrued. It is likely, for example, that Rett syndrome, originally considered an ASD subtype, will be taken off the list in a future DSM-V inasmuch as its diagnostic criteria are no longer strictly behavioral. It is not that girls with Rett syndrome – at least during some phases of their illness – are not autistic, but that there is now a known biologic cause for their behaviorally defined autism. We stress the distinction between biologic and behavioral classifications, a distinction that does not in the least imply that individuals with known biologic etiologies do not have autism when their behavioral criteria put them on the spectrum. Biologic and behavioral classifications are not mutually exclusive but concurrent diagnoses.

TABLE 1.4

DSM-IV-TR criteria for subtypes of PDDs based on the descriptors of Table 1.1*

Criteria for autistic disorder (AD):

(a) Endorsement of a total of 6 (or more) descriptors from (1), (2) and (3), with at least 2 from (1), and one each from (2) and (3)

(b) Onset prior to age 3 years in social interaction, communicative language or imaginative play

(c) The disturbance is not better accounted for by Rett's disorder or childhood disintegrative disorder

Criteria for Asperger's disorder (ASP):

(a) Endorsement of at least 1 (or more) descriptors from (1) and 1 (or more) from (3)

(b) Language not delayed, that is single words by age 2 years, communicative phrases used by age 3 years

(c) No significant delay in cognitive development or in the development of age-approproate self-help skills, adaptive behavior (other than social interaction), and curiosity about the environment in childhood

(d) Criteria are not met for another specific PDD disorder or schizophrenia

Criteria for pervasive developmental disorder–not otherwise specified (PDD-NOS):

(a) Endorsement of at least 1 (or more) descriptor from (1) and at least 1 (or more) from (2) or (3) or both but does not meet criteria for another specific PDD or schizophrenia, schizotypal or avoidant personality disorder, or age of onset. PDD-NOS includes atypical autism

Criteria for childhood disintegrative disorder:

(a) Entirely normal development, including sociability, language, play and adaptive behavior until at least age 2 years

(b) Clinically significant loss (before age 10 years) of previously acquired skills in at least 2 of the following areas:

  (i) expressive or receptive language

  (ii) social skills or adaptive behavior

  (iii) bowel or bladder control

  (iv) play

  (v) motor skills

(c) Endorsement of at least 1 (or more) descriptors from 2 or more of domains (1), (2) or (3)

(d) The disturbance is not better accounted for by another specific PDD or by schizophrenia

Criteria for Rett's disorder:

Such significant progress in defining Rett syndrome has followed the identification of the *MEPCP2* gene on the X chromosome in ~80% of affected girls, in an occasional severely affected boy, and in some older children and women with a broader phenotype that the DSM-IV criteria no longer apply. Postnatal slowing of head growth, postnatal appearance of prominent stereotypies, severe mental retardation with lack of or minimal language, and at least for a time lack of interest in interacting, severely impaired motor skills, development of epilepsy, and other somatic features such as hyperventilation, aerophagia, scoliosis, and cyanosed hands and feet are valid criteria for this diagnosis in girls with classic Rett syndrome. Rett's is but one monogenic etiology of autism

*Numbers in parentheses refer to the behavioral domains listed in Table 1.1.

CAUSES OF AUTISM (ETIOLOGY)

Autism in its very broad spectrum of severity is now known to have many etiologies. The view of inept parenting as its cause, which dominated the first quarter century of its study, has been roundly discredited. It is now established that autism is but one among the (multi)dimensionally defined disorders of brain development that affect complex human behaviors. All are considered to reflect the dysfunction of widely distributed neuronal networks that interconnect widespread functionally disparate groups of neurons in the brain. The complexity of these networks is brought into focus by the fact that individual neurons are likely to be connected to many hundreds of other neurons, and that the strength of their interconnecting synapses is not fixed but varies greatly depending on the history of their functional connections and the influences of other ongoing influences on the brain. The specificity of these connections depends on which of many neuro-transmitters links the neurons in a pathway and on the activity of many more modulators that influence synaptic transmission. The development and functions of these neuro-transmitters, neuromodulators and their specific synaptic receptors are under the control of genes that turn on and off in orchestrated sequences. It is the plasticity of these complex widely distributed brain networks that accounts for the profound effects of the unique environmental influences, including education, to which the individual is exposed from prenatal life to his or her demise that modulates that individual's behavior. The sympto-matology of each developmental disorder depends on which nodes or larger parts of the network are dysfunctional and on the cascading consequences of the dysfunction for other networks, irrespective of the cause or etiology of the dysfunction.

This view of autism (multiple causes converging on a common neuropathogenesis) has a parallel in dementia. Like autism, dementia is defined on the basis of quantitative (dimensional) behavioral criteria, and it too has a broad range (spectrum) of severity. Dementia denotes loss of previously achieved cognitive and, eventually, sensorimotor abilities caused by any one (or more) of many underlying progressive brain degenerations. Dementia, like autism, has a large variety of causes (etiologies), among which Alzheimer disease of the elderly, unlike autism to date, has a well defined neuropathology and bio-chemical basis. Yet even Alzheimer disease has several distinct known – and no doubt other as yet undefined – mostly genetic etiologies, with a phenotype influenced to a greater or lesser degree by environmental contingencies such as prior level of education and current level of brain activity.

The cause of clinically defined autistic phenotypes is thus complex and multifactorial because it is generally both strongly genetic and environmentally influenced, with occasional entirely nongenetic causes as well (Muhle et al. 2004). Its largely multigenic inheritance greatly complicates attempts to link its behaviorally defined phenotype to its causal genes. In an attempt to decrease the complexity of genetic linkage studies, a recently adopted strategy is to use either *biologic endophenotypes* or biologic markers such as hyper-serotonemia or epilepsy, or *behavioral endophenotypes* such as a history of behavioral regression, stereotypies or language disorder, rather than the complex behaviorally defined subtypes of the DSM/ICD systems in order to narrow the search for underlying etiologies (Gottesman and Gould 2003). The most recent, more efficient, strategy is to not search for individually linked genes but to use chip technologies to scan the entire genome for statistically linked groups of genes relevant to autism or autistic subtypes. The hope that drives all of these approaches is that tightly defined phenotypic subtypes will increase the likelihood of linking them to specific pathophysiologic mechanisms, and possibly even to particular etiologies.

"Syndromic" Autism vs "Idiopathic" (Primary) Autism

Autism is a syndrome, not a disease in the sense that measles or sickle cell anemia is a disease, because despite its salient behavioral phenotype it lacks a unique etiology or specific pathology. Coleman (2005) and others use the term "syndromic" autism (others speak of "secondary" autism or autistic comorbidities – see Chapter 2) to refer to autism with a single defined cause or with readily discernible physical or imaging features or epilepsy. "Syndromic" autism is often – but not necessarily – associated with mental retardation. Examples of syndromic autism include tuberous sclerosis, Angelman syndrome, fragile-X syndrome (fra-X), the velo-cardio-facial syndrome resulting from a deletion of chromosome 22q11.2, and congenital rubella, among dozens of others. None of these etiologies is specific to autism because each of them encompasses a variable proportion of individuals with and without autism.

The term "non-syndromic" (or "primary" or "idiopathic") autism, which applies when there are no physical stigmata or readily demonstrable biomarker, is not etiologically specific. "Idiopathic" autism encompasses mainly individuals whose etiologies remain unknown to date. Idiopathic autism might also include, at least transiently, individuals with a potentially definable but undiscovered etiology who have no physical stigmata, for example a young boy in whom fra-X or some metabolic disorder still lacks systemic signs, or even autism in a toddler with a history of regression without epilepsy (although the term "regressive autism" has recently been used to indicate a potential subgroup among children with ASD). Coleman (2005) and others use "idiopathic" autism with full awareness that it is no less organic or multifactorial because its cause(s) is (are) unknown. As etiologies are discovered one by one, the number of individuals with idiopathic autism will shrink. Clearly this nomenclature, like the behavioral nomenclature of the DSM/ICD systems, is a work in progress and will change as research advances.

Comorbid and Coexisting Disorders

Etiology is defined as the biologic cause of diseases and disorders. Causality is generally considered satisfied by the identification of a specific disorder known to produce some or most of the individual patient's signs and symptoms if corroborated by a specific test such as the mutation of a gene, an image, or by the documented past history of a relevant illness. For example, the correlation between autism and intrauterine rubella or tuberous sclerosis is so well established that looking further for a causal explanation for the autism would be considered superfluous, even though neither causes autism in the majority of affected individuals. The attribution is less convincing when the putative etiology is, for example, a history of uncomplicated preterm birth or of bacterial meningitis without discernable brain lesion, cognitive deficit or epilepsy as sequela. Might the condition be coincidental rather than causal, or only causal in a child with a pre-existing genetic vulnerability to autism, i.e. in such cases have a multifactorial etiology?

In addition to the core descriptors of the DSM/ICD systems, individuals with autism have a variety of other symptoms and signs. Some of them, like toe-walking and motor clumsiness, or sleep problems, or enhanced anxiety and deficient joint attention, are so frequent that they have come to be viewed as *coexisting* parts of the autistic phenotype even though they are not listed among the DSM/ICD descriptors of autism. Other neurologic deficits like epilepsy, Tourette syndrome, attention deficit disorder and, for that matter, mental retardation coexist too often with autism to be plausibly considered coincidental. Should they be thought of as separate comorbid disorders – on the grounds that each is considered a disorder in its own right in the DSM/ICD manuals – or are they but other manifestations of the underlying, more often than not multidetermined, cause of the individual's autism?

Comorbidity implies that a complex phenotype results from the joint or independent expression of several *independent* genetic or nongenetic causes interacting on the developing brain. Comorbidity thus implies etiologic heterogeneity, in contrast to phenotypically coexisting symptoms which bespeak pathogenetic – but not necessarily etiologic – complexity. Coexistent social ineptitude with inadequate language and stereotypies signal a common, albeit most often polygenic or, more realistically, an environmentally influenced polygenic common cause. This common causation in no way implies that the phenotypic manifestations have a common pathogenesis in the brain, because there is incontrovertible evidence that the programming of motor movements, language and social skills engages distinct distributed networks.

The conceptual differences between comorbidity and coexistence are not as clear as we make them out to be. Take depression in an intelligent person with autism: depression might be comorbid with autism and be the consequence of co-inherited independent genes concerned with disordered oxytocin and serotonin metabolism affecting distinct cortico-subcortical networks; but an equally likely explanation is that the depression is the expected emotional consequence of inability to secure stable employment because of the inept social skills that characterize autism. But note that only a fraction of individuals with autism will become depressed in response to environmental adversity, therefore those who do may have inherited enhanced vulnerability to stresses, an environmentally modulated comorbidity. The possibility of genetically enhanced susceptibility to environmental insults that most persons would tolerate without persistent damage is being considered increasingly seriously with regard to immunologic, metabolic, toxic, infectious or stress contributors to the cause of autism.

There are two types of comorbidity: coincidental (unrelated, stochastic) and related.

The same phenotype, for example congenital deafness in an unstigmatized child with autism, might represent either a comorbid or a coexistent situation. Uncomplicated congenital deafness no more causes autism than autism causes deafness. If the deafness in this ASD child is due to homozygosity for connexin-26 mutation, this is an example of coincidental comorbidity of deafness with autism, but if the deafness is due to intrauterine cytomegalovirus infection, whose association with hearing loss and with autism is well documented, we are probably faced with coexisting symptomatology arising from a common etiology. Another clear example of coincidental comorbidity would be that of a child with Asperger syndrome and a congenital hemiplegia attributable to an intrauterine middle cerebral artery branch occlusion, because a unilateral focal brain lesion is most unlikely to be responsible for the ASD. The situation is much less clear in the examples of Tourette syndrome, bipolar disease, or attention deficit disorder with hyperactivity. It is even more controversial in the rather frequent situation of a child with autism who has non-autistic family members with developmental language disorders, given that impaired language is a core deficit of autism. The *FOXP2* gene, which is mutated in at least one large family with a severe developmental language disorder (Lai et al. 2003), is considered by some investigators to be a susceptibility gene for autism in families in which the affected child and nonautistic family members have impaired phonologic skills (Wassink et al. 2001), an interpretation disputed by others (Newbury et al. 2002).

From a practical point of view, whether clinically distinct problems are coincidental or related is irrelevant. Each needs to be treated as such, but the possibility, as in the earlier example of depression, that one is the consequence of the other must be kept in mind. Even if they have unrelated causes, the existence of both in one person means that there will inevitably be interactions to be taken into account in planning intervention.

COMPLEXITIES OF GENETIC ETIOLOGIES

Clinical, neuropsychologic, electrophysiologic, imaging and other biologic research supports the view of autism (and other developmental disorders) as the expression of atypical brain development resulting in more or less widespread (and not necessarily etiologically specific) dysfunction of a complex widely distributed neural network. This *pathophysiologic view of developmental disorders* is the antithesis of a "disease" in the sense of a unique genetic or nongenetic biologic condition or of "brain damage" as a frequent cause of autism. Current genetic research, together with the strikingly skewed gender distribution to males (Baron-Cohen et al. 2005) and a less than 10% recurrence risk within sibships, points to a strongly gender-influenced polygenic etiology in the great majority of cases of "idiopathic" (primary) autism. The less than 100% concordance in both diagnosis and severity among monozygotic (MZ or single egg) twins who share 100% of their genes indicates that there are postconceptional epigenetic or environmental influences on the phenotype (Jiang et al. 2004).

Half of the human genome is involved in brain development and function. The growth of the brain and its size, which depends on the differential growth of its different parts and their connectivity, including the many component parts of different neocortical and white matter areas and their subcortical relays, are under the control of specific gene cascades that are turned on and off in appropriate sequences. There are epigenetic regulatory networks, some of them controlled by genes like the *MECP2* gene whose mutations are responsible for Rett syndrome, that influence the widely distributed neuronal networks and the growth of the synapses that interconnect them (Zoghbi 2003). More recently the focus has turned to unraveling the implications of normal and dysregulated components of a newly defined "second genome" (i.e. non-coding or microRNAs), whose role is to orchestrate genome-wide alterations in complex gene profiles and associated gene functional networks at play during neural development in both health and disease (Du and Zamore 2005). It has been known for several years that neurons, in addition to their classic action potentials, also have much slower integrative effects operating on gene expression on a time scale of minutes or even hours, and that these play a role in learning in response to environmental stimulation (Clayton 2000). Hormones exert effects on neuronal expression, some of which potentiate slow transcriptional responses (Vasudevan et al. 2005). The point of these few examples is that this vast array of continuous epigenetic regulatory systems is particularly malleable by environmental influences and will likely become amenable to currently evolving therapeutic interventions. It is also likely that these systems will provide insights into the gene–environment underpinnings of complex and previously intractable neurological disorders.

A host of cytogenetic abnormalities, single mendelian gene defects and mitochondrial abnormalities have been identified in occasional children with autism but, as not all carriers of these genetic abnormalities are autistic, other as yet unidentified interacting factors must come into play. For example, in tuberous sclerosis, one of the more common and better studied monogenic disorders with a high association with autism, it is probably not the gene defect per se but the burden and location of tubers (which is random as far as we know) that determine whether a carrier of a tuberous sclerosis mutation will or will not be autistic (Asano et al. 2001, Bolton 2004). As mentioned earlier, the fact that many blood relatives of individuals with autism are burdened by a variety of developmental non-autistic but related disorders also supports polygenic causation. In each individual the consequences of the mutation of one or multiple genes (or brain insults) are modulated by both the unique genetic background and the environmental experiences of the person, which goes far toward accounting for the wide variability of autistic phenotypes.

LEVELS OF CLASSIFICATION

Determining how various etiologies give rise to particular behavioral symptomatologies requires an understanding of the nature and location of their impacts on the brain. It is research not at the etiologic level but at the level of *neurologic pathogenesis* and its interface with behavior that will illuminate the phenotype of autism. It is critical to keep these three levels (symptomatology, pathophysiology, etiology) firmly in mind and not to jump from one to the other in discussing diagnosis. In other words, the cause (etiology) of the brain dysfunction does not provide a direct explanation for the behavioral phenotype; it is through their consequences for brain function that the many etiologies of autism cause deficiencies in behavior or other skills.

This may sound self-evident but it is common for these levels not to be kept separate. This results in incoherent hybrid classifications. For example, it makes no sense to speak of the differential diagnosis between autism (a behaviorally defined disorder with many different causes) and Rett or fra-X syndromes (diseases due to single gene defects), or to state that autism was mistakenly diagnosed in a child who turns out to have fra-X, when fra-X is a well documented etiology of ASD in some *but not all* the children carriers of expanded trinucleotide CGG repeats on the X chromosome. On the other hand it makes perfect sense to compare "idiopathic" autism (a behaviorally defined disorder with many different causes) to Rett or fra-X syndromes (single gene defects) or to compare commonalities in the behavioral phenotypes, MRIs or neurotransmitter levels in two distinct genetic disorders like Angelman and Williams syndromes.

CLASSIFICATION: CATEGORICAL VERSUS DIMENSIONAL DIAGNOSES

The DSM/ICD classifications are behavioral; they define disorders, not diseases in the medical sense. Many medical diseases are defined categorically: a person does or does not have the disease on the basis of a biologic criterion like an X-ray showing a fracture or a tumor, immunologic evidence or isolation of a virus, or a blood test revealing type I diabetes or sickle cell anemia. Categorical diagnoses remain dichotomous even though the severity of the disease may vary dimensionally depending on host factors, the intensity of the insult, or the degree to which different mutations inactivate a particular gene and variably decrease its product, with resultant variation in the phenotype. Other medical conditions like obesity or arterial hypertension are defined dimensionally on the basis of a measure like body mass index or blood pressure. As in the case of autism, diagnosis in these dimensionally defined morbid conditions is stipulated by an *arbitrary cut in a continuum* based on an agreed-upon distance of the measure from its norm. Like autism, they are also likely to be multiply determined conditions.

DSM/ICD diagnoses are designed to be categorical or mutually exclusive, in the sense that they attempt to separate behaviorally defined disorders as cleanly as possible from one another and from normality based on characteristic clusters of symptoms. In reality they are not categorical because a "diagnosis" of PDD versus not-PDD, which sounds dichotomous, rests on the presence of *qualitative* impairments in three behavioral domains – sociability, communication, and cognitive flexibility – and the term qualitative implies a subjective, graded – thus quantitative – judgment rather than a categorical yes/no criterion.

Not just the autistic vs not autistic diagnosis, but also the subtypes under the PDD umbrella such as autistic vs Asperger vs PDD-NOS (PDD–not otherwise specified) are designed to be mutually exclusive or categorical. They are defined by the *number* of DSM/ICD qualitative behavioral descriptors endorsed on parent teacher, or clinician questionnaires, or by direct observation of the child, or both (Table 1.4), validated by the evaluation of an experienced clinician cognizant of the DSM/ICD criteria. The descriptors themselves are largely dimensional (e.g. how little interest in pretend play must a child display to endorse that criterion?). The *distribution* of responses to the descriptors brings in still another source of dimensional variability. For example, 6 endorsements, with at least 2 relating to sociability, 1 to language and play, and 1 to rigidity, together with symptom onset before age 3 years define DSM-IV autistic disorder (AD), but so might a total of 8 or 12 endorsements. A total of just 5 endorsements excludes AD but might mean either PDD-NOS or Asperger disorder depending on whether language was delayed or not; but so might 2 or 3, or even 6 or more endorsements if they were not distributed as required for a diagnosis of AD.

The consequence is that there is a range of both kind and severity of dysfunctions within PDD subtypes. One child might have a greater degree of social deficit and fewer repetitive behaviors, and the reverse might be the case with another child, yet both might fulfill criteria for AD. Such differences may reflect not just differences in severity of the underlying brain dysfunction but differences in what brain networks are affected. Consequently it is critical not to be satisfied with a DSM/ICD subtype diagnosis for research but to select rigorously homogeneous behaviorally defined groups of subjects or a specific endophenotype for studies like imaging or electrophysiology designed to elucidate the neurologic basis of ASD symptoms.

Extensive questionnaires like the Autism Diagnostic Interview-Revised (ADI-R) (Lord et al. 1994) , or brief screening questionnaires (Robins et al. 2001), or standardized observation schedules like the Autism Diagnostic Observation Schedule – Generic (ADOS-G) (Lord et al. 2000) or Childhood Autism Rating Scale (CARS) (Schopler et al. 1986) yield quantitative criteria for separating autistic disorder from less severe subtypes like Asperger and PDD-NOS and from a diagnosis of non-ASD. Major efforts were expended when the DSM/ICD and these other diagnostic instruments were developed to make the behavioral ratings or observations as objective as possible. All were field tested and standardized on a variety of clinically defined populations, yet agreement between behaviorally defined subtypes remains suboptimal (Zwaigenbaum et al. 2000) because behavior is inherently dimensional, which precludes an entirely sharply defined classification.

Individuals on the autism spectrum are distributed along a bell shaped (Gaussian) curve of severity, with prototypic AD cases most numerous in the center of the distribution. Diagnosis in the lowest, most severe tail of the curve overlaps with severe mental retardation (Berument et al. 2005), and diagnosis in the highest (non-retarded) tail is likely to overlap with other disorders like some developmental language disorders, obsessive–compulsive disorder, Tourette syndrome, schizoid personality, and even with normality. Indeed, there may be no sharp cut between a socially gauche, eccentric solitary scientist and a gifted Asperger individual (Baron-Cohen et al. 2001). It is the degree to which the personality characteristics of the individual interfere with functioning in everyday life that decides whether the person is given a clinical diagnosis or dismissed as normal. The dimensionality of ASD diagnoses has become a big issue as school systems and insurance companies struggle to decide whether or not they will provide benefits to particular individuals. Diagnosis based on changing behavioral criteria, together with greater awareness of the ASDs by both professionals and the public, and heightened awareness that there are efficacious interventions for the ASDs have no doubt played a major role in the so-called autism epidemic (Fombonne 2003).

CLINICAL COURSE OF AUTISM

The behavioral manifestations of the ASDs change and generally improve with age. For example, as individuals enter into adulthood there is frequently an amelioration of the social isolation, although the poverty of social skills and impaired ability to make peer friendships is lasting (Howlin et al. 2000, 2004). Language and communication deficits too often endure into adulthood, and verbal skills in those who acquire speech may have permanent inadequacies in conversational skills such as turn taking, understanding the subtleties of language like jokes or sarcasm, and interpreting body language, intonation and facial expression. Stereotypies may decrease over time or become "miniaturized", whereas abnormal body posture and gait abnormalities often persist. We know very little about the long-term effects of early intervention on many of the manifestations of autism and on outcome. Among the less severely affected individuals with autism there are a number who improve with little or no intervention, whereas progress in others is extremely limited despite intensive behavioral, educational and pharmacological intervention.

About a third of parents report an *early regression* of language and behavior, most often between 18 and 24 months, or later in the rare previously entirely normally developing child with *disintegrative disorder* in whom regression may occur as late as 10 years. There is no accepted definition of regression, and most studies documenting regression have been based on parent reports of their children losing single words or phrases, together with loss of sociability and of interest in playing with toys, and the appearance of behavioral rigidity and stereotypies. Investigators who examined family videotapes made prior to the identification of symptoms of autism often find signs of preexisting developmental differences (Osterling et al. 2002, Werner and Dawson 2005). There is some preliminary evidence that cognitive impairment is more likely in individuals with ASD who experienced a regression, although this is disputed (Kobayashi and Murata 1998, Kurita et al. 2004, Lord et al. 2004). There is also controversy regarding whether disintegrative disorder and autistic regression are discrete entities. There are almost no prospective studies on autistic regression, and its cause or causes remain unexplained. Regression is more profound in disintegrative disorder as the children regress in adaptive behaviors like toilet training and in overall cognitive ability; its prognosis for improvement is poor (Volkmar et al. 1997).

Overall, prognosis in autism is variable and depends most directly on its severity and underlying causes (Ballaban-Gil et al. 1996, Howlin 2003, Howlin et al. 2004). Early intervention programs for the child – but equally important, training of parents in how to deal more effectively with such difficult children – may make a difference and may produce long-lasting gains, as may the provision of social skills training as the need arises throughout childhood (Dunn 2005). We have very little empirical evidence to support any particular type of intervention, and no intervention fits universal needs, although the most effective behavioral and educational interventions share the common characteristics of intensity, frequency, structure, and being provided to toddlers and preschoolers (National Research Council 2001). We stress that our ability to predict outcome in very early childhood is limited. There are no systematic accounts or epidemiological studies to provide data regarding longevity or long term prognosis of older individuals with autism.

THE ROLE OF THE CHILD NEUROLOGIST IN THE ASSESSMENT AND TREATMENT OF CHILDREN WITH ASDs

There is no biologic test to validate the diagnosis of an ASD. The goal of the neurological examination is to assess what, if any, tests are needed, depending of course on the history and neurological examination. The initial work-up of an individual with autism should have a clear clinical goal. It will differ from the evaluation and tests required for a research protocol. There are evidence-based guidelines established for the diagnosis and evaluation of children with autism and related disorders (Volkmar et al. 1999a,b; Filipek et al. 2000; Committee on Children with Disabilities 2001). As is the case for children with mental retardation or dementia, a detailed developmental evaluation is always required. Other tests like a formal speech and language evaluation and neuropsychological assessment need to be carried out in selected children with autism in order to define their individual educational plans (IEPs) more precisely. The history and neurologic evaluation may mandate tests such as neuroimaging or neurophysiologic investigations, or referral to a geneticist for cytogenetic studies, DNA tests for fra-X, Rett syndrome, and other known genetic conditions highly associated with autism, in the hopes of being able to provide a target medical treatment or genetic counseling. We stress that there is no such thing as a routine test battery for autism except in the context of a formal research protocol. Rigorous behavioral subgrouping for research is required if we hope to gain an understanding of the pathophysiology of the ASDs and make progress toward providing more specific biologically targeted interventions and prognosis.

Early identification of children with an ASD is essential for enhancing the efficacy of early intervention at a time when the brain is most plastic. No one treatment fits all. Subgrouping is required for management, which needs to be individualized and multidisciplinary. Besides specially trained educators it may involve a variety of therapists, a psychopharmacologist, and a social worker/child/family advocate.

The child neurologist plays a unique role in providing or interpreting genetic information to parents, educating families, primary care physicians, other allied health professionals, and educators on the early signs of autism, what it is and is not, and what investigations and interventions are optimal. As child neurologists we have an understanding of the neurologic basis of autism, as well as being trained in the coordination of the multiple disciplines and individualized interventions that each child with ASD deserves. Because we are used to dealing with chronic diseases that affect the quality of the life of the affected individuals, and equally that of their families, we have not discharged our duty unless we have made sure that the family, as well as the child, have access to practical help and emotional support. We have organized this book from this perspective, emphasizing the need to understand both the neurobiological and clinical heterogeneity of autism, and have emphasized both medical and behavioral/educational interventions.

OUTLINE OF THE BOOK

In organizing this book by neurologists for neurologists, we have in this first chapter provided some general definitions, and discussed the terminology and concepts that have placed autism at the forefront of behaviorally defined complex disorders of the developing brain. There follows a discussion of the epidemiology of autism, pointing out how important it is to use a common language to determine the frequency of a problem. It is clear that autism is no longer considered a rare disorder, and clinicians are recognizing and making this diagnosis much more often than even 10 years ago. What is more controversial is the possibility that specific and yet unidentified risk factors may be accounting for the increased number of children diagnosed with ASDs. The next three chapters discuss what are considered the core symptoms of autism; they provide the clinical material that needs to be understood from the perspective of both the clinician managing a child with an ASD and the researcher trying to understand its neurobiologic basis. These chapters are followed by a review of the evidence that suggests that autism is a disorder of neuronal development, followed by discussions of the genetics, neuroanatomy and neuroradiology, neurochemistry, immunology, and neurophysiology of autism. Reviews of problems commonly associated with autism such as epilepsy, sleep disturbances, and sensory and motor deficits come next. Consideration is then given to the neuropsychological assessment of children with ASDs, medical and psychopharmacologic management, educational and behavioral interventions, and outcome. The concluding chapter briefly summarizes where we are now in our understanding of the neurology of autism, but more importantly it proposes a research agenda that ensures that child neurologists continue to have a positive impact on the lives of children and families coping with this complex disorder of neurodevelopment.

REFERENCES

Committee on Children with Disabilities (2001) American Academy of Pediatrics: The pediatrician's role in the diagnosis and management of autistic spectrum disorder in children. *Pediatrics* 107: 1221–6.

APA (1980) *Diagnostic and Statistical Manual of Mental Disorders, 3rd edn (DSM-III)*. Washington, DC: American Psychiatric Association.

APA (2000) *Diagnostic and Statistical Manual of Mental Disorders, 4th edn, text revision (DSM IV-TR)*. Washington, DC: American Psychiatric Association.

Asano E, Chugani DC, Muzik O, Behen M, Janisse J, Rothermel R, Mangner TJ, Chakraborty PK, Chugani HT (2001) Autism in tuberous sclerosis complex is related to both cortical and subcortical dysfunction. *Neurology* 57: 1269–77.

Ballaban-Gil K, Rapin I, Tuchman RF, Shinnar S (1996) Longitudinal examination of the behavioral, language, and social changes in a population of adolescents and young adults with autistic disorder. *Pediatr Neurol* 15: 217–23.

Baron-Cohen S, Wheelwright S, Skinner R, Martin J, Clubley E (2001) The Autism-Spectrum Quotient (AQ): evidence from Asperger syndrome/high-functioning autism, males and females, scientists and mathematicians. *J Autism Dev Disord* 31: 5–17.

Baron-Cohen S, Knickmeyer RC, Belmonte MK (2005) Sex differences in the brain: implications for explaining autism. *Science* 310: 819–23.

Berument SK, Starr E, Pickles A, Tomlins M, Papanikolaouou K, Lord C, Rutter M (2005) Pre-Linguistic Autism Diagnostic Observation Schedule adapted for older individuals with severe to profound mental retardation: a pilot study. *J Autism Dev Disord* 35: 821–9.

Bolton PF (2004) Neuroepileptic correlates of autistic symptomatology in tuberous sclerosis. *Ment Retard Dev Disabil Res Rev* 10: 126–31.

Clayton DF (2000) The genomic action potential. *Neurobiol Learn Mem* 74: 185–216.

Coleman ME (2005) *The Neurology of Autism*. New York: Oxford University Press.

Du T, Zamore PD (2005) microPrimer: the biogenesis and function of microRNA. *Development* 132: 4645–52.

Dunn M (2005) *S.O.S.: Social Skills in our Schools (A Social Skills Program for Children with Pervasive Developmental Disorders and their Typical Peers)*. Shawnee Mission, KS: Autism & Asperger Publishing.

Filipek PA, Accardo PJ, Ashwal S, Baranek GT, Cook EH, Dawson G, Gordon B, Gravel JS, Johnson CP, Kallen RJ, Levy SE, Minshew NJ, Ozonoff S, Prizant B, Rapin I, Rogers SJ, Stone WL, Teplin S, Tuchman RF, Volkmar FR (2000) Practice parameter: screening and diagnosis of autism: report of the Quality Standards Subcommittee of the American Academy of Neurology and the Child Neurology Society. *Neurology* 55: 468–79.

Fombonne E (2003) Epidemiological surveys of autism and other pervasive developmental disorders: an update. *J Autism Dev Disord* 33: 365–82.

Frith U (1991) *Autism and Asperger Syndrome*. Cambridge: Cambridge University Press.

Gottesman II, Gould TD (2003) The endophenotype concept in psychiatry: etymology and strategic intentions. *Am J Psychiatry* 160: 636–45.

Howlin P (2003) Outcome in high-functioning adults with autism with and without early language delays: implications for the differentiation beween autism and Asperger syndrome. *J Autism Dev Disord* 33: 3–13.

Howlin P, Mawhood L, Rutter M (2000) Autism and developmental receptive language disorder—a follow-up comparison in early adult life. II: Social, behavioural, and psychiatric outcomes. *J Child Psychol Psychiatry* 41: 561–78.

Howlin P, Goode S, Hutton J, Rutter M (2004) Adult outcome for children with autism. *J Child Psychol Psychiatry* 45: 212–29.

Jiang YH, Bressler J, Beaudet AL (2004) Epigenetics and human disease. *Ann Rev Genom Hum Genet* 5: 479–510.

Kanner L (1943) Autistic disturbances of affective contact. *Nerv Child* 2: 217–50.

Kobayashi R, Murata T (1998) Setback phenomenon in autism and long-term prognosis. *Acta Psychiatr Scand* 98: 296–303.

Kurita H, Osada H, Miyake Y (2004) External validity of childhood disintegrative disorder in comparison with autistic disorder. *J Autism Dev Disord* 34: 355–62.

Lai CS, Gerrelli D, Monaco AP, Fisher SE, Copp AJ (2003) FOXP2 expression during brain development coincides with adult sites of pathology in a severe speech and language disorder. *Brain* 126: 2455–62.

Lord C, Risi S, Lambrecht L, Cook EH, Leventhal BL, DiLavore PC, Pickles A, Rutter M (2000) The Autism Observation Schedule-Generic: A standard measure of social and communication deficits associated with the spectrum of autism. *J Autism Dev Disord* 30: 205–23.

Lord C, Rutter M, Le Couteur A (1994) Autism Diagnostic Interview-Revised: A revised version of a diagnostic interview for caregivers of individuals with possible pervasive developmental disorders. *J Autism Dev Disord* 24: 659–85.

Lord C, Shulman C, DiLavore P (2004) Regression and word loss in autistic spectrum disorders. *J Child Psychol Psychiatry* 45: 936–55.

Muhle R, Trentacoste SV, Rapin I (2004) The genetics of autism. *Pediatrics* 113: e472–86.

National Research Council (2001) *Educating Children with Autism.* Washington, DC: National Academy Press.

Newbury DF, Bonora E, Lamb JA, Fisher SE, Lai CS, Baird G, Jannoun L, Slonims V, Stott CM, Merricks MJ, Bolton PF, Bailey AJ, Monaco AP; International Molecular Genetic Study of Autism Consortium (2002) FOXP2 is not a major susceptibility gene for autism or specific language impairment. *Am J Hum Genet* 70: 1318–27.

Osterling JA, Dawson G, Munson JA (2002) Early recognition of 1-year-old infants with autism spectrum disorder versus mental retardation. *Dev Psychopathol* 14: 239–51.

Robins DL, Fein D, Barton ML, Green JA (2001) The Modified Checklist for Autism in Toddlers: an initial study investigating the early detection of autism and pervasive developmental disorders. *J Autism Dev Disord* 31: 131–44.

Rutter M, Schopler E (1992) Classification of pervasive developmental disorders: some concepts and practical considerations. *J Autism Dev Disord* 22: 459–82.

Schopler E, Reichler RJ, Renner BR (1986) *The Childhood Autism Rating Scale (CARS) for Diagnostic Screening and Classification in Autism.* New York: Irvington.

Vasudevan N, Kow LM, Pfaff D (2005) Integration of steroid hormone initiated membrane action to genomic function in the brain. *Steroids* 70: 388–96.

Volkmar FR, Klin A, Marans W, Cohen DJ (1997) Childhood disintegrative disorder. In: Cohen DJ, Volkmar FR, eds. *Handbook of Autism and Pervasive Developmental Disorders, 2nd edn.* New York: John Wiley, pp. 47–59.

Volkmar F, Cook EH, Pomeroy J, Realmuto G, Tanguay P (1999a) Practice parameters for the assessment and treatment of children, adolescents, and adults with autism and other pervasive developmental disorders. American Academy of Child and Adolescent Psychiatry Working Group on Quality Issues. *J Am Acad Child Adolesc Psychiatry* 38 suppl: 32S–54S [erratum in *J Am Acad Child Adolesc Psychiatry* 2000 39: 938].

Volkmar F, Cook EH, Pomeroy J, Realmuto G, Tanguay P (1999b) Summary of the Practice Parameters for the Assessment and Treatment of Children, Adolescents, and Adults with Autism and other Pervasive Developmental Disorders. American Academy of Child and Adolescent Psychiatry. *J Am Acad Child Adolesc Psychiatry* 38: 1611–6.

Wassink TH, Piven J, Vieland VJ, Huang J, Swiderski RE, Pietila J, Braun T, Beck G, Folstein SE,

Haines JL, Sheffield VC (2001) Evidence supporting WNT2 as an autism susceptibility gene. *Am J Med Genet* 105: 406–13.

Werner E, Dawson G (2005) Validation of the phenomenon of autistic regression using home videotapes. *Arch Gen Psychiatry* 62: 889–95.

WHO (1992) *International Classification of Mental and Behavioural Disorders. Clinical Descriptions and Diagnostic Guidelines, 10th edn (ICD-10).* Geneva: World Health Organization.

WHO (1993) *Mental Disorders: Glossary and Guide to their Classification in Accordance with the Tenth Revision of the International Classification of Diseases.* Geneva: World Health Organization.

Zoghbi HY (2003) Postnatal neurodevelopmental disorders: meeting at the synapse? *Science* 302: 826–30.

Zwaigenbaum L, Szatmari P, Mahoney W, Bryson S, Bartolucci G, MacLean J (2000) High functioning autism and childhood disintegrative disorder in half brothers. *J Autism Dev Disord* 30: 121–6.

2

EPIDEMIOLOGY OF AUTISM SPECTRUM DISORDERS

Edwin Trevathan and Shlomo Shinnar

Epidemiology is the study of the distribution and determinants of disease frequency (MacMahon and Pugh 1970). This includes studying how the prevalence of disorders varies in populations (descriptive epidemiology); monitoring trends in disease over time (epidemiologic surveillance); and carrying out special investigations to try to understand risk and protective factors associated with disease occurrence (analytic epidemiology). The tools of epidemiology are just beginning to be used in the study of autism and autism spectrum disorders.

ANALYTIC TOOLS

There are two primary measures of disease occurrence used in epidemiologic studies, disease incidence and disease prevalence (Fig. 2.1) (Rothman 2002). Disease incidence refers to the rate of new cases in a defined population per unit of time, and is typically defined as:

$$\text{Incidence rate} = \frac{\text{Number of new cases in a defined population per year}}{\text{Person-years from the at-risk population}}$$

Incidence rates are usually reported as number of new cases per 100,000 at-risk people per year. Individuals in the defined population can only contribute to the person-time in the denominator for the period that they are known to be at risk for the disease, but have not (yet) acquired the disease of interest. For relatively large populations and relatively rare disorders, the incidence rate denominator can be estimated by the person-years from the population.

Disease prevalence is the burden or status of a disease in a defined population at a specified time and includes all cases of disease in the population regardless of the time of diagnosis (Gordis 1996, Rothman 2002).

$$\text{Prevalence} = \frac{\text{Number of people in a defined population with disease at prevalence date}}{\text{Number of people in the population during prevalence date}}$$

Prevalence is usually expressed as the number of cases per 1000 population. Prevalence for a defined period of time is referred to as a *period prevalence* (e.g. prevalence for 2005)

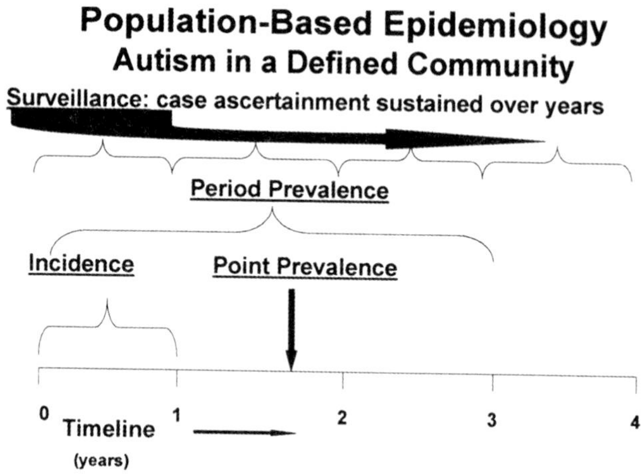

Population-Based Epidemiology
Autism in a Defined Community
Surveillance: case ascertainment sustained over years

Fig. 2.1. Types of frequency measures of autism in the community. *Incidence measures* are rates of new cases among the at-risk population per unit time (usually 1 year). *Prevalence measures* typically include all cases measured either over a period of years (period prevalence) or at a specific date (point prevalence). Surveillance systems identify cases over a period of several years in order to determine trends in the same population.

or, for a single point in time (e.g. June 1, 2005), as a *point prevalence*. Prevalence is a function of the incidence of the disease in the population and the duration of disease. Prevalence has been used for health and policy planning related activities (Armstrong et al. 1992, Gordis 1996).

Incidence rates are often used in etiologic studies, but calculation of the incidence rates of autism is challenging if not impossible because the initial manifestations of autism are often insidious and difficult to define in time. Although many children exhibit recognized abnormalities in development in the first and second year of life, the average age of autism diagnosis is often quite delayed (Rogers and DiLalla 1990, Stanley et al. 2000, Yeargin-Allsopp et al. 2003). As a result of these challenges, most epidemiologic studies of autism have used period prevalence as the measure of disease occurrence.

MEASURES OF DISEASE ASSOCIATION
One of the primary objectives of epidemiology is to identify causal risk factors for disease. When a child develops a disorder following an exposure, the exposure should not be assumed to be causal just because the exposure is associated with the disorder. In determining whether the exposure is causal, the epidemiologist compares the disease occurrence among children with the exposure to those without the exposure (Armstrong et al. 1992, Gordis 1996, Rothman 2002). In comparing the disease occurrence in the two groups, there are standard measures of association (or effect) to describe and quantify the strength of the association between a risk factor and disease outcome. The *risk ratio* or *rate*

ratio is used to describe the risk (or rate) of disease in the exposed group relative to that in the unexposed group and is calculated as:

$$\text{Risk ratio} = \frac{\text{Incidence risk (or rate) of disease in the exposed group}}{\text{Incidence risk (or rate) of disease in the unexposed group}}$$

Similarly, the prevalence rate ratio is used to describe the association between the prevalence of disease and the exposure of interest and is defined as:

$$\text{Prevalence rate ratio} = \frac{\text{Incidence risk (or rate) of disease in the exposed group}}{\text{Incidence risk (or rate) of disease in the unexposed group}}$$

STUDY DESIGNS

The major epidemiologic study designs are the *cohort* and *case–control* designs. In a cohort study the epidemiologist selects a group of exposed individuals and a group of non-exposed individuals and follows both groups together with the same methods of data collection to compare the incidence of disease in the two groups (Armstrong et al. 1992, Gordis 1996). The "population at risk" within the cohort includes those who do not yet have the disease and are therefore still at risk of developing the disease of interest. A birth cohort includes all live-born children in a specified geographic region during a defined period of time. A cohort study design involves measuring disease occurrence among individuals by whether or not they are exposed to a factor of interest. For example, a very high rate of autism (4%) was reported among women in Sweden who were exposed very early in pregnancy to thalidomide (an anti-nausea drug), a rate much higher than was found in the general Swedish population (Stromland et al. 2002). A clinical trial is a modification of the cohort design in which exposures (e.g. to a treatment or a diagnostic test) are randomized to members of a cohort and the cohort is then followed for various outcome measures.

Cohort studies can be either *retrospective* or *prospective* in nature; prospective means defining the population at risk of disease and following it concurrently in time; retrospective refers to going back in time to historically assemble the cohort (population at risk) and ascertain exposure status and disease occurrence. A retrospective study requires the use of historical records that are relatively complete (e.g. hospital labor and delivery records, vital birth records); retrospective studies are considerably less costly than prospective studies and usually, depending on the nature of the research question, take much less time to conduct.

In contrast to a cohort study, which begins with the population at risk, the *case–control study* begins with identifying disease in a defined population and then looking retrospectively among those with the disease and a comparison group of individuals without the disease to determine prior exposure. A case–control study is most often used for the study of relatively rare disorders, or of disorders in which there is a prolonged time between exposure and development of the disease of interest.

Cohort and case–control studies are both considered *longitudinal* studies in that the exposure is clearly separated in time from the onset of disease. In contrast, *cross-sectional* studies measure both exposure and disease outcomes simultaneously for each subject at a particular point in time. Cross-sectional studies yield period prevalence data describing the burden or status of disease for various subgroups of the population (Gordis 1996).

EPIDEMIOLOGIC SURVEILLANCE

Surveillance is the ongoing monitoring of disease in the population (Fig. 2.1). Surveillance data are used to detect clusters of disease in space and time, and to provide information on the natural history of diseases, describe the size and scope of health problems, and evaluate the impact of health interventions (Stroup et al. 2004). Cases identified from surveillance activities can be used as the basis for analytic studies to investigate risk factors and causes of developmental disabilities. Surveillance of developmental disabilities has been an ongoing activity of the Centers for Disease Control and Prevention (CDC) in the USA (Yeargin-Allsopp et al. 1992) and in several other countries (Surman et al. 2003). Surveillance can be done using a period prevalence rate (e.g. prevalence of 8-year-old children in St Louis with autism) or using a birth cohort perspective (e.g. prevalence of autism from age 2 to 10 years in children born in St Louis in 1996, 1997, 1998, etc.) (Armstrong et al. 1992, Gordis 1996).

CASE ASCERTAINMENT

Epidemiologic studies (including surveillance) have used primarily three methods to identify children with autism: (1) questionnaires that ask parents or care providers information on children's functioning; (2) reviews of administrative medical and school records for children with autism and related developmental problems; and (3) screening of population samples (either total population or high risk subgroups). Questionnaire surveys are dependent on the parent or primary caretaker's understanding of the specific aspects of the child's diagnosis, as well as the ability of the survey questions to elicit such information correctly. The validity of using administrative records (medical and educational) to identify case children is dependent on the child's coming to the attention of a health care provider and/or educator, on the appropriate testing and the recording of that information, and on obtaining appropriate access to such records. Administrative record surveillance yields reasonably complete ascertainment for children with moderate to severe disabilities, but will miss children with milder disabilities. The evolution of the autism (autism spectrum disorder) case definitions over time makes it very difficult, if not impossible, to use consistent case definitions applied in a uniform fashion over time in surveillance projects. The gold standard for autism surveillance in terms of validity of diagnostic assessment is population screening followed by clinical assessment of the child, yet this methodology is not only expensive, but it also has challenges in terms of obtaining complete ascertainment or obtaining a large, representative sample (Yeargin-Allsopp 2002).

CHALLENGES IN THE DESIGN AND CONDUCT OF EPIDEMIOLOGIC STUDIES OF AUTISM

The major challenges in conducting epidemiologic studies of autism include:

- Insidious onset of the clinical features of autism and delayed autism diagnosis
- Change (broadening) of diagnostic criteria over time, making it difficult to compare rates of occurrence when they were determined on the basis of different case definitions
- Apparent long time lag (measured in months to years) between exposure and onset of diagnosed autism – obtaining accurate exposure information retrospectively (biologic confirmation of exposure, record confirmation, or recall by parent or caretaker) is difficult and prone to bias
- Heterogeneity of autism spectrum disorder phenotypes and presumed significant etiologic heterogeneity.

Children with autism have impairments in three neurodevelopmental areas: (1) reciprocal social interaction, (2) communication and language, and (3) behavior and interests (Volkmar et al. 1992, APA 1994) (for a full discussion of diagnostic criteria, see Chapter 1). Rett syndrome, which is due to mutations in the *MECP2* gene found on the X chromosome, occurs almost exclusively among girls, and is characterized by loss of language skills, loss of functional hand use, gait abnormalities, seizures, mental retardation, and deceleration of head growth after an initial period of normal development (Rett Syndrome Diagnostic Criteria Work Group 1988). Although autistic-like behaviors are seen in the early stages of Rett syndrome, many epidemiologic studies of autism spectrum disorders have excluded children with Rett syndrome (Yeargin-Allsopp 2002). According to the DSM-IV, the features of autism must be clinically apparent before the age of 3 years. However, population studies have reported that the mean age of diagnosis of the disorder is later, at 4–10 years of age (Charman 2003, Tidmarsh and Volkmar 2003, Yeargin-Allsopp et al. 2003).

PREVALENCE OF ASD – METHODS

Studies of ASD prevalence have typically used a case ascertainment protocol for case finding followed by one of case confirmation (Fombonne 1999, Yeargin-Allsopp 2002, Yeargin-Allsopp et al. 2003). The most comprehensive method of case finding involves *total population screening* using schools, early intervention programs and/or pediatric well-child clinics. The advantage of total population screening is that it allows identification of previously undiagnosed children, especially those who are relatively high functioning. The high cost and intensive nature of total population screening has limited this method to studies of relatively small populations. Prevalence studies in larger populations tend to *target at-risk populations* by focusing on programs and clinics specifically for children with autism and developmental disabilities, including special education programs, specialty diagnostic clinics, early intervention programs, and other service programs for special needs children. Complete and accurate ascertainment of ASD using an *at-risk* approach is dependent on the quality and comprehensiveness of diagnostic and treatment services in the community, as well as the degree of detailed data in the individual records. Successful community surveillance of ASDs requires education and outreach programs that encourage community involvement with the surveillance system.

Various methods of case confirmation have been used in population-based studies (Fombonne 1999). One method has been the clinical evaluation of the child using a "gold standard" instrument for diagnosing ASD. Earlier studies used autism-specific instruments such as the Childhood Autism Rating Scale (CARS) (Schopler et al. 1998), while recent studies have used the ADOS-G (Lord et al. 2000) or ADI-R (Lord et al. 1994), or both, to assess the presence of various behaviors associated with autism. As with case finding techniques, the complexity and costs of this approach have generally limited its use in large population studies. Another approach has been to use expert clinician review based on available diagnostic record information on the child (Yeargin-Allsopp et al. 2003). While the expert clinician review approach has advantages, it is dependent on the quality of the records, the expertise of the reviewers, and the rigor of the expert review protocols. Some investigators have relied solely on a diagnosis as provided by a service provider. However, because the diagnosis of autism varies widely between and within communities, surveillance relying solely on the diagnosis provided by service providers is prone to bias. Surveillance systems that rely on the diagnoses provided by service providers should include diagnostic validation by examination of a sample of the cases identified from records.

PREVALENCE OF ASD – A REPORTED INCREASE

Whether the prevalence of autism and ASDs has increased over the past 20 years has been the topic of lively debate in recent years. Since the first prevalence studies of autism were published in the late 1960s and 1970s (Lotter 1966, Treffert 1970, Wing and Gould 1979), there have been multiple population-based prevalence studies from different countries (Hoshino et al. 1982, Bohman 1983, Ishii and Takahashi 1983, Gillberg 1984, McCarthy et al. 1984, Steffenburg and Gillberg 1986, Steinhausen et al. 1986, Burd et al. 1987, Matsuishi et al. 1987, Bryson et al. 1988, Tanoue et al. 1988, Cialdella and Mamelle 1989, Ritvo et al. 1989, Sugiyama and Abe 1989, Gillberg et al. 1991, Fombonne and du Mazaubrun 1992, Honda et al. 1996, Arvidsson et al. 1997, Fombonne et al. 1997, Webb et al. 1997, Sponheim and Skjeldal 1998, Kadesjo et al. 1999, Baird et al. 2000, Kielinen et al. 2000, Powell et al. 2000, Bertrand et al. 2001, Chakrabarti and Fombonne 2001, Croen et al. 2001, Magnusson and Saemundsen 2001). The studies published since the early 1980s vary in their methods, use different case definitions, and have been performed in different populations. Therefore comparisons of temporal trends in rates of autism must be viewed with caution.

The first population-based prevalence study of autism reported a prevalence of 4.5 per 10,000. Other studies using the same (Kanner) criteria, with the exception of one US study, reported similar prevalence rates (Lotter 1966, Treffert 1970, Wing and Gould 1979, Hoshino et al. 1982, McCarthy et al. 1984). Three studies used the Rutter criteria, similar to the Kanner criteria, but the prevalence rates differed considerably (1.9, 3.0, and 16 per 10,000 children) (Ishii and Takahashi 1983, Bohman 1983, Steinhausen et al. 1986). The DSM-III (APA 1980) was the first to use the term "pervasive developmental disorder", which broadened the autism diagnostic criteria, to differentiate between autism and childhood schizophrenia, and describe the onset of autism as occurring before age 30 months. Studies using DSM-III criteria yielded rates from 1.2 to 15.5 per 10,000 children (Gillberg 1984, Steffenburg and Gillberg 1986, Burd et al. 1987, Matsuishi et al. 1987, Bryson et al. 1988, Tanoue et al. 1988, Cialdella and Mamelle 1989, Ritvo et al. 1989, Sugiyama and Abe 1989). Three studies using the DSM-III-R criteria (APA 1987) reported rates of 7.0, 9.6 and 11.0 per 10,000 children (Gillberg et al. 1991, Powell et al. 2000, Croen et al. 2001). DSM-IV (APA 1994) and ICD-10 (WHO 1992) criteria are very similar (Volkmar et al. 1992), yet studies using either criteria have reported prevalence rates ranging from 0.4 per 1000 in Norway to 6.0 per 1000 in Sweden (Fombonne and du Mazaubrun 1992, Honda et al. 1996, Arvidsson et al. 1997, Fombonne et al. 1997, Webb et al. 1997, Sponheim and Skjeldal 1998, Kadesjo et al. 1999, Baird et al. 2000, Kielinen et al. 2000, Powell et al. 2000, Bertrand 2001, Chakrabarti and Fombonne 2001, Croen et al. 2001, Magnusson and Saemundsen 2001, Yeargin-Allsopp et al. 2003).

There have been only a few studies of trends in the prevalence of "autism"[1] within a single population. The prevalence of "autism" in two French birth cohorts (children born in 1972 and 1976) demonstrated no significant change in prevalence (5.1 and 4.9 per 10,000 children) (Fombonne and du Mazaubrun 1992). In the most comprehensive analysis of the French surveys, multiple birth cohorts were surveyed between 1972 and the 1980s and the prevalence rate was 5.35/10,000 or 16.3/10,000 if other pervasive developmental disorders are included (Fombonne et al. 1997).

The prevalence of "autism" was determined in Sweden for 1962 through 1976 and later for 1975 through 1984 and was reported to increase from 4.0 to 11.6 per 10,000 children (Gillberg 1984, Gillberg et al. 1991). The rates of "autism" in Swedish children with mild mental retardation remained relatively stable, while the rates increased in children with severe mental retardation (IQ <50) and in children with normal intelligence (IQ >70). The Swedish investigators suggested that changes in the overall prevalence are influenced by the improved ability to identify children with autism who have very low as well as normal to high levels of functioning. One report on the trends in autistic disorder prevalence in preschool children in the UK from 1991 thru 1996 reported an increase in "autism" by 18% per year; there was a much larger increase for the other ASDs (Powell et al. 2000). The British investigators attributed their reported increase to improved awareness among clinicians rather than to true changes in the occurrence of

---

[1]Inverted commas added because it is likely that autism in most studies refers to DSM/ICD autistic disorder or classic autism rather than to autism as short for PDD or ASD as used in this book. It is also very likely that stringent criteria were not applied in every study.

"autism". Recently investigators from the Mayo Clinic using the Mayo record linkage system in Olmstead County, Minnesota reported that the incidence of "autism", defined as having indications in records of DSM-IV criteria for "autism", increased from 5.5 per 100,000 children from 1980 to 1983 to 44.9 per 100,000 from 1995 to 1997 (Barbaresi et al. 2005). The increased rates of "autism" in Olmstead County were confined to the subgroup of children who were less than 10 years of age (born after 1987), prompting the authors to hypothesize that the increase was due to changes in diagnostic criteria, service availability and improved awareness.

While many other investigators have also attributed the recently reported increases in prevalence to greater recognition and expansion of diagnostic criteria for ASD (Gill-berg et al. 1991; Fombonne 1996, 1999, 2003; Wing and Potter 2002; Lingam et al. 2003; Blaxill 2004), some authors question this assumption. For example, Blaxill (2004) evaluated the published data from the 1970s up to 1990 on "autism" and ASD prevalence, and attempted to account for changes in nomenclature and in diagnostic criteria. Although Blaxill acknowledged that the shift away from the Kanner criteria for an autism diagnosis and the use of either ICD-10 or DSM-IV diagnostic criteria have broadened the scope and likely increased the number of children who meet diagnostic criteria for an ASD, he also suggests that the 10-fold increase in reported prevalence rates for "autism" cannot be explained solely by changes in diagnostic criteria and by improved ascertain-ment. While attempting to apply criteria in use today to individuals identified in the past is fraught with many assumptions, Wing and Potter (2002) estimated that only about 30–50% of children meeting ICD-10 diagnostic criteria for ASD would satisfy Kanner's original requirements for the diagnosis of classic autism (Kanner 1943).

Until recently, because of the lack of current prevalence data for the USA, there had been considerable attention paid to trends in service provider data which have shown an increase in the numbers of children receiving services for "autism" (Fig. 2.2). However, these data are limited because (1) the diagnosis of "autism" has not been applied consis-tently over time, and (2) the numbers of individuals receiving services do not represent a true prevalence rate. In addition, such data depend on other sources of services within a community and are community-specific for a range of factors. Data from the California Department of Developmental Services (CADDS) from 1987 to 1998 showed a 273% increase in the number of individuals receiving autism services (2778 to 10,360), whereas the number receiving services related to a diagnosis of other developmental dis-abilities increased only 44% (CADDS 1999). During the same time period, the number of individuals with a diagnosis of other pervasive developmental disorders receiving services increased by 1966%. Furthermore those diagnosed in 1998 with "autism" were younger and higher functioning than those receiving services in 1987. An updated CADDS report in 2003 showed an increase from 10,360 cases of "autism" in 1998 to 20,377 in 2002, a 97% increase in just 4 years (CADDS 1999, 2003). US Department of Education data also indicate that the number of children with "autism" served under the Individuals with Disabilities Education Act (IDEA), Part B (children aged 6 through

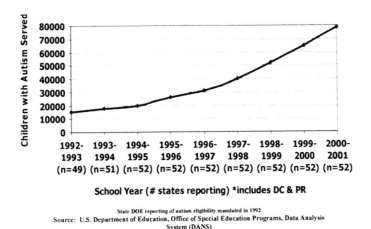

Fig. 2.2. Number of children with autism aged 6–21 years served under the Individuals with Disabilities Education Act (IDEA), Part B, 1992–93 to 2000–01. Reproduced by permission from Trevathan (2004).

21 years), increased 6-fold, from 22,664 in 1994 to 141,022 in 2003 (IDEA 2004). Of note is that autism is not the only category of special education classification that has experienced significant increase during the 1990s; attention deficit hyperactivity disorder (ADHD) has experienced a similar increase (US Department of Education 2003).

Newschaffer et al. (2005) used reporting data on special education designations for children 6–17 years of age receiving special education services between 1992 and 2001 and found that the "autism" prevalence increase was higher in younger cohorts, with a suggestion of a recent slowing of the rate of increase. Under the category of "other health impairment", which is often the category used to provide services for many children with ADHD, there was a pattern of increased prevalence very similar to that for autism.

The Centers for Disease Control and Prevention (CDC) initiated several prevalence studies in the 1990s to address this lack of prevalence data for ASDs in the USA. A study conducted in Brick Township, New Jersey, included an intensive case identification phase using schools and service providers and case verification (clinical examinations, psychological examinations, and administration of the Autism Diagnostic Observation Schedule–Generic [ADOS-G; Lord et al. 2000]). The prevalence of autistic disorder was found to be 4 per 1000 children (95% confidence interval [CI]: 28–56) and the prevalence for ASD was 6.7 per 1000 children (95% CI: 51–87) (Bertrand et al. 2001). The prevalence of autism in Brick Township was higher than most prevalence rates reported from studies in the 1980s and early 1990s. The CDC next conducted a population-based study to determine the prevalence of autism in five counties of metropolitan Atlanta, a large study with a base population of 290,000 children (Yeargin-Allsopp et al. 2003). Children with ASD were identified through screening and abstraction of records at multiple medical and educational sources, with expert review to determine autism case status. A total of 987 children who displayed behaviors consistent with the DSM-IV criteria for autistic disorder, PDD-NOS or Asperger's disorder were identified. The prevalence for autistic disorder was 3.4 per 1000 children. Overall, the prevalence was similar for black and white children. A total of 68% of children had cognitive impairment. As severity of cognitive impairment increased, the male to female ratio decreased from 4.4 to 1.3. About 40% of children with autism were identified only at school sources. Schools were the most important source for information on black children, children of younger mothers, and children of mothers with less than 12 years of education. Clearly, the rate of autism found in this study was higher than the rates from studies conducted in the USA during the 1980s and early 1990s, but the rate is consistent with the Brick investigation and several recent non-US studies that used intensive case finding (Arvidsson et al. 1997, Kadesjo et al. 1999, Baird et al. 2000). Based on the data from these studies, the CDC investigators concluded that autism is not a rare condition and is an extremely important public health problem.

Although improved recognition of autism, facilitated by greater public awareness of autism and greater availability of services, is partially responsible for the higher reported prevalence rates, the relative contribution of improved recognition to the reported increase in the prevalence of autism is not known. Methodological issues related to conduct of the studies may also play a role in the increased reported prevalence rates, or the increased prevalence may reflect a true increase in occurrence of the disorder. Regardless, there seem to be more children with ASDs today than in the past, and continued monitoring of the prevalence of autism might shed some light on the contribution of each of these factors.

GENDER

All studies have found more boys than girls with autism, with sex ratios ranging from 2:1 to 4:1, with a few exceptions (Fombonne 1999, Gillberg and Wing 1999). When considering the sex ratio by IQ level, there is a decreasing male to female ratio with decreasing IQ, i.e. the sex ratio is close to 1:1 for children with IQ <50, while for higher functioning children (IQs >50) the sex ratio is around 3:1 to 4:1 (Lord and Schopler 1985, Nordin and Gillberg 1996, Fombonne 1999, Yeargin-Allsopp et al. 2003). The ratio of males to females is even higher for children with Asperger syndrome and very high functioning children with autism.

SOCIODEMOGRAPHIC FACTORS

There are very limited data on the differences in autism prevalence by race. A recent study in metropolitan Atlanta reported that the rates were the same in black and white children (3.4 per 1000 among 3- to 10-year-old children), although black children had a much higher prevalence of non-isolated autism than white children (Yeargin-Allsopp et al. 2003).

Early studies of autism reported an association with higher socioeconomic status

(SES) (Kanner 1943, Treffert 1970, Cox et al. 1975), but these reports may be confounded by the improved recognition of autism among more affluent families. Schopler et al. (1979) reported that higher SES families were more able to travel longer distances for services and gave more detailed responses to questions about their children's development. Wing and Potter (2002) also supported the idea of a possible SES bias in autism due to differences in referral and diagnosis. The perception and experience of diagnosticians may impact reports of autism by race and SES. A study by Cuccaro et al. (1996) found that diagnoses made by clinicians differed for children of different racial backgrounds and the diagnosis of autism was more reliant on the experience of the clinician examining the child, with psychiatrists (assumed to be more experienced with autism) recognizing the behaviors associated with autism more often than school psychologists. Regardless of whether there are methodologic and ascertainment biases that affect the results of studies examining SES factors in autism, a few epidemiologic studies recently have shown an increased risk for autism among higher SES families and in mothers with higher education levels (see Croen et al. 2002).

Some studies have also shown increased maternal age to be associated with autism (Gillberg 1980, Hoshino et al. 1982), whereas others have shown no effect (Steinhausen et al. 1986, Lotter 1967). Croen et al. (2002) found that there was a 4-fold increased risk for autism in children born to mothers aged 35 years or older compared to mothers 20 years of age.

GENETIC RISK FACTORS AND ETIOLOGIES

Several studies have concluded that genetic factors are important in the etiology of autism (see Chapter 7). The reports of twin studies have provided much of the empirical basis for the belief that there is a strong genetic component to the etiology of autism. Folstein and Rutter (1988) reported a significant difference in the concordance of autism between monozygotic (MZ) and dizygotic (DZ) twins, 36% and 0%, respectively. Additional twin studies by other investigators with larger sample sizes provided even higher concordance rates ranging from 60% to 96% for MZ twins compared with a consistently low concordance of autism among DZ twins (0–24%) (Ritvo et al. 1985, Steffenburg et al. 1989, Bailey et al. 1995). That MZ twins do not have 100% concordance has been discussed as evidence consistent with genetic–environmental interactions in the etiology of autism (Piven and Folstein 1994) or infrequent nongenetic etiologies of autism.

Folstein and Rutter (1977) also reported that within MZ twin pairs the concordance for autism extended to behavioral and cognitive characteristics beyond classic autism, suggesting genetic factors in a broader phenotype and the possibility of genetic heterogeneity. These findings have been supported and extended by more recent reports (Bailey et al. 1995, Le Couteur et al. 1996). Greenberg et al. (2001) hypothesized that MZ twins are at higher risk of autism not only because of their shared genetic traits, but also as a result of the shared physical environment and the competition for limited intrauterine resources.

Family studies have consistently shown that the rate of autism in siblings ranges from 2% to 6%, similar to that among DZ twins. The recurrence risk estimates range from 10 to 30 times greater than the population prevalence (Smalley et al. 1988, Newschaffer et al. 2002).

Twin and family based studies, molecular and chromosomal findings, and the association of autism with other known genetic disorders have provided convincing support for genetic susceptibility in the etiology of autism. Conceptual advances in genetic epidemiologic methods have made it possible to discuss options for future research to elucidate the specific roles of genetic and nongenetic factors and their interactions.

NONGENETIC RISK FACTORS

In utero exposure to thalidomide at 20-24 weeks gestation is one of the very few well documented prenatal risk factors for development of autism. In a group of 15 adults prenatally exposed to thalidomide at 20-24 weeks gestation, 4 of the 15 were found to have autism (Stromland et al. 1994). This association between thalidomide and autism and exposure at 20-24 weeks of fetal brain development document when an exposure responsible for autism may occur; therefore a systematic search for other exposures during this time of gestation is indicated (Rodier et al. 1996).

The earliest evidence for the role of viruses in autism comes from a report in the early 1970s in which 12 of 243 preschool children with congenital rubella were found to have ASD (Chess 1971). There have also been reports suggesting a role for herpes simplex, rubeola, syphilis and varicella (Libbey et al. 2005). Despite reports of an association between maternal autoimmune diseases and autism, a recent report failed to document maternal autoimmune disease, asthma, allergies and psoriasis and ASD in their offspring (Croen et al. 2005). (See Chapter 9 for further consideration of the potential role of immunologic factors in autism.)

Parents of children with autism may have a history of more reproductive problems, including infertility, maternal menstrual irregularities and spontaneous abortions, compared to parents of normally developing children (Harper and Williams 1974, Campbell et al. 1978, Dykens and MacMahon 1979, Gillberg and Gillberg 1983). There is also increasing interest in looking at the potential adverse effects of assisted reproductive technologies on a range of developmental outcomes, including autism, and birth defects (Hansen et al. 2002, Schieve et al. 2002, Stromberg et al. 2002). Several perinatal risk factors have also been examined as possible causes for ASD, singly and in combination to produce an "optimality score" for pregnancy and delivery. However, whereas some researchers have found that children with autism have lower optimality scores that controls (Gillberg and Gillberg 1983, Bryson et al. 1988, Bolton et al. 1997), others have found no difference in optimality scores between children with ASD and typically developing controls (Lord et al. 1991, Piven et al. 1993, Cryan et al. 1996).

The possible increase in prevalence of autism and ASD has prompted parents and investigators alike to search for an explanation. The question of whether the measles, mumps and rubella (MMR) vaccine is causally associated with autism was initially raised by a case series of children with autistic regression and colitis with the onset of autistic behavior occurring shortly after receipt of the MMR vaccination (Wakefield et al. 1998). However, the American Academy of Pediatrics (Halsey and Hyman 2001) and the British Medical Research Council (MRC 2001) have reviewed the available scientific information on the proposed relationship between the MMR vaccine and autism and have concluded that there is no evidence of a causal association at the population level. Their conclusion is based on the fact that several population-based epidemiological studies have not shown any relationship between the MMR vaccine and autism. The available evidence to date indicates that the MMR vaccine does not cause autistic disorder or any of the other ASD subtypes and does not cause the unique syndrome of developmental regression and gastroenterological disorders (DeStefano and Thompson 2004). In a retrospective cohort study from Denmark, 537,303 children in a birth cohort from January 1991 thru December 1998, 82% of whom received the MMR vaccine, were studied. Within this very large birth cohort 316 children were identified with a diagnosis of autistic disorder and 422 children with a diagnosis of other ASDs. The authors did a detailed evaluation of the risk of autistic disorder in the group of vaccinated children compared to those who were not vaccinated, controlling for potential confounding variables. There was no relationship between MMR vaccination and autism. There was no relationship between age at the time of vaccination, the time since vaccination, date of the vaccination, and the development of either autistic disorder or other ASDs (Madsen et al. 2002). More recent studies have also supported the lack of an association between MMR and ASDs (Smeeth et al. 2004, Honda et al. 2005).

In addition to this conjecture about MMR vaccine, questions have also been raised about the safety of mercury-containing vaccines and whether these vaccines are related to the increased prevalence of ASD. To date, no consistent association has been found between thimerosal-containing vaccines and neurodevelopmental outcomes using large datasets from the USA, Sweden and Denmark (Stehr-Green et al. 2003), and to date, none of the studies from these countries support a causal relationship between thimerosal-containing vaccine exposure in the general population and, specifically, the prevalence of autism (Stehr-Green et al. 2003, Parker et al. 2004).

Regardless of the reasons for the higher prevalence of autism reported today, the higher prevalence means more individuals affected by this serious life-long disability, making autism a major public health problem (Newschaffer and Curran 2003, Rice et al. 2004). Autism is not preventable today, but early diagnosis and intensive behavioral and educational intervention may improve functional outcomes in some children (Dawson and Osterling 1997, Volkmar et al. 1999, Lord and McGee 2001).

REFERENCES

APA (1980) *Diagnostic and Statistical Manual of Mental Disorders, 3rd edn (DSM-III).* Washington, DC: American Psychiatric Association.

APA (1987) *Diagnostic and Statistical Manual of Mental Disorders, 3rd edn, revised (DSM-III-R)*. Washington, DC: American Psychiatric Association.

APA (1994) *Diagnostic and Statistical Manual of Mental Disorders, 4th edn (DSM-IV)*. Washington, DC: American Psychiatric Association.

Armstrong BK, White E, Saracci R (1992) *Principles of Exposure Measurement in Epidemiology*. Oxford: Oxford University Press.

Arvidsson T, Danielsson B, Forsberg P, Gillberg C, Johansson M, Kjellgren G (1997) Autism in 3–6 year-old children in a suburb of Goteborg, Sweden. *Autism* 1: 163–73.

Bailey A, Le Couteur A, Gottesman I, Bolton P, Simmonoff E, Rutter M (1995) Autism is a strongly genetic disorder: evidence from a British twin study. *Psychol Med* 25: 63–77.

Baird G, Charman T, Baron-Cohen S, Cox A, Swettenham J, Wheelwright S, Drew A (2000) A screening instrument for autism at 18 months of age: a 6-year follow-up study. *J Am Acad Child Adolesc Psychiatry* 39: 694–702.

Barbaresi WJ, Katusic SK, Colligan RC, Weaver AL, Jacobsen SJ (2005) The incidence of autism in Olmsted County, Minnesota, 1976–1997: results from a population-based study. *Arch Pediatr Adolesc Med* 159: 37–44.

Bertrand J, Mars A, Boyle C, Bove F, Yeargin-Allsopp M, Decoufle P (2001) Prevalence of autism in a United States population: the Brick Township, New Jersey investigation. *Pediatrics* 108: 1155–61.

Blaxill MF (2004) What's going on? The question of time trends in autism. *Public Health Rep* 119: 536–51.

Bohman M (1983) Childhood psychosis in a northern Swedish county: some preliminary findings from an epidemiological survey. In: Schmidt M, Remschmidt H, eds. *Epidemiological Approach in Child Psychiatry*. New York: Thieme-Stratton, pp. 164–73.

Bolton PF, Murphy M, Macdonald H, Whitlock B, Pickles A, Rutter M (1997) Obstetric complications in autism: consequences or causes of the condition? *J Am Acad Child Adolesc Psychiatry* 36: 272–81.

Bryson SE, Clark BS, Smith IM (1988) First report of a Canadian epidemiological study of autistic syndromes. *J Child Psychol Psychiatry* 29: 433–45.

Burd L, Fisher W, Kerbeshian J (1987) A prevalence study of pervasive developmental disorders in North Dakota. *J Am Acad Child Adolesc Psychiatry* 26: 700–3.

CADDS (1999) *Changes in the Population of Persons with Autism and Pervasive Developmental Disorders in California's Developmental Services System: 1987–1998. A Report of the Legislature*. Sacramento, CA.: California Department of Developmental Services.

CADDS (2003) *Autistic Spectrum Disorders: Changes in the California Caseload; An Update: 1999 through 2002*. Sacramento, CA.: California Department of Developmental Services.

Campbell M, Hardesty AS, Burdock EI (1978) Demographic and perinatal profile of 105 autistic children: a preliminary report [proceedings]. *Psychopharmacol Bull* 14: 36–9.

Chakrabarti S, Fombonne E (2001) Pervasive developmental disorders in preschool children. *JAMA* 285: 3093–9.

Charman T (2003) Epidemiology and early identification of autism: research challenges and opportunities. *Novartis Found Symp* 251: 10–9; discussion 19–25, 109–11, 281–97.

Chess S (1971) Autism in children with congenital rubella. *J Autism Child Schizophr* 1: 33–47.

Cialdella P, Mamelle N (1989) An epidemiological study of infantile autism in a French department (Rhone): a research note. *J Child Psychol Psychiatry* 30: 165–75.

Cox A, Rutter M, Newman S, Martak L (1975) A comparative study of infantile autism and specific developmental receptive language disorder. II. Parental characteristics. *Br J Psychiatry* 126: 146–59.

Croen LA, Grether JK, Selvin S (2001) The epidemiology of mental retardation of unknown cause. *Pediatrics* 107: E86.

Croen LA, Grether JK, Selvin S (2002) Descriptive epidemiology of autism in a California population: who is at risk? *J Autism Dev Disord* 32: 217–24.

Croen LA, Grether JK, Yoshida CK, Odouli R, Van de Water J (2005) Maternal autoimmune diseases, asthma and allergies, and childhood autism spectrum disorders: a case–control study. *Arch Pediatr Adolesc Med* 159: 151–7.

Cryan E, Byrne M, O'Donovan A, O'Callaghan E (1996) Brief report: a case-control study of obstetric complications and later autistic disorder. *J Autism Dev Disord* 26: 453–60.

Cuccaro ML, Wright HH, Rownd CV, Abramson RK, Waller J, Fender D (1996) Professional perceptions of children with developmental difficulties: the influence of race and socioeconomic status. *J Autism Dev Disord* 26: 461–9.

Dawson G, Osterling J (1997) Early intervention in autism. In: Guralnick MJ, ed. *The Effectiveness of Early Intervention.* Baltimore: Brookes, pp. 307–26.

DeStefano F, Thompson WW (2004) MMR vaccine and autism: an update of the scientific evidence. *Expert Rev Vaccines* 3: 19–22.

Dykens E, MacMahon G (1979) Viral exposure and autism. *Am J Epidemiology* 109: 628–38.

Folstein S, Rutter M (1977) Infantile autism: a genetic study of 21 twin pairs. *J Child Psychol Psychiatry* 18: 291–321.

Folstein SE, Rutter ML (1988) Autism: familial aggregation and genetic implications. *J Autism Dev Dis* 18: 3–30.

Fombonne E (1996) Is the prevalence of autism increasing? *J Autism Dev Disord* 26: 673–6.

Fombonne E (1999) The epidemiology of autism: a review. *Psychol Med* 29: 769–86.

Fombonne E (2003) Epidemiological surveys of autism and other pervasive developmental disorders: an update. *J Autism Dev Disord* 33: 365–82.

Fombonne E, du Mazaubrun C (1992) Prevalence of infantile autism in four French regions. *Soc Psychiatry Psychiatr Epidemiol* 27: 203–10.

Fombonne E, Du Mazaubrun C, Cans C, Grandjean H (1997) Autism and associated medical disorders in a French epidemiological survey. *J Am Acad Child Adolesc Psychiatry* 36: 1561–9.

Gillberg C (1980) Maternal age and infantile autism. *J Autism Dev Disord* 10: 293–7.

Gillberg C (1984) Infantile autism and other childhood psychoses in a Swedish urban region. Epidemiological aspects. *J Child Psychol Psychiatry* 25: 35–43.

Gillberg C, Gillberg IC (1983) Infantile autism: a total population study of reduced optimality in the pre-, peri-, and neonatal period. *J Autism Dev Disord* 13: 153–66.

Gillberg C, Wing L (1999) Autism: not an extremely rare disorder. *Acta Psychiatr Scand* 99: 399–406.

Gillberg C, Steffenburg S, Schaumann H (1991) Is autism more common now than ten years ago? *Br J Psychiatry* 158: 403–9.

Gordis L (1996) *Epidemiology.* Philadelphia: WB Saunders.

Greenberg GA, Hodge SE, Sowinski J, Nicoll D (2001) Excess of twins among affected sibling pairs with autism: implication for the etiology of autism. *Am J Hum Genet* 69: 1062–7.

Halsey NA, Hyman SL (2001) Measles-mumps-rubella vaccine and autistic spectrum disorder: report from the New Challenges in Childhood Immunizations Conference convened in Oak Brook, Illinois, June 12–13, 2000. *Pediatrics* 107: E84.

Hansen M, Kurinczuk J, Bower C, Webb S (2002) The risk of major birth defects after intracytoplasmic sperm injection and in vitro fertilization. *N Engl J Med* 346: 725–30.

Harper J, Williams S (1974) Early environmental stress and infantile autism. *Med J Aust* 1: 341–6.

Honda H, Shimizu Y, Misumi K, Niimi M, Ohashi Y (1996) Cumulative incidence and prevalence of childhood autism in children in Japan. *Br J Psychiatry* 169: 228–35.

Honda H, Shimizu Y, Rutter M (2005) No effect of MMR withdrawal on the incidence of autism: a total population study. *J Child Psychol Psychiatry* 46: 572–9.

Hoshino Y, Kumashiro H, Yashima Y, Tachibana R, Watanabe M (1982) The epidemiological study of autism in Fukushima-ken. *Folia Psychiatr Neurol Jpn* 36: 115–24.

Ishii T, Takahashi O (1983) The epidemiology of autistic children in Toyota, Japan. *Jpn J Child Adolesc Psychiatry* 24: 311–21.

Kadesjo B, Gillberg C, Hagberg B (1999) Brief report: autism and Asperger syndrome in seven-year-old children: a total population study. *J Autism Dev Disord* 29: 327–31.

Kanner L (1943) Autistic disturbances of affective contact. *Nervous Child* 2: 217–50.

Kielinen M, Linna SL, Moilanen I (2000) Autism in Northern Finland. *Eur Child Adolesc Psychiatry* 9: 162–7.

Le Couteur A, Bailey A, Goode S, Pickles A, Robertson S, Gottesman I, Rutter M (1996) A broader phenotype of autism: the clinical spectrum in twins. *J Child Psychol Psychiatry* 36: 785–801.

Libbey JE, Sweeten TL, McMahon WM, Fujinami RS (2005) Autistic disorder and viral infections. *J Neurovirol* 11: 1–10.

Lingam R, Simmons A, Andrews N, Miller E, Stowe J, Taylor,B.(2003) Prevalence of autism and parentally reported triggers in a north east London population. *Arch Dis Child* 88: 666–70.

Lord C, McGee JP (eds.) (2001) *Committee on Educational Interventions for Children with Autism. Educating Children with Autism.* Washington, DC: National Academy Press.

Lord C, Schopler E (1985) Differences in sex ratios in autism as a function of measured intelligence. *J Autism Dev Disord* 15: 185–93.

Lord C, Mulloy C, Wendelboe M, Schopler E (1991) Pre- and perinatal factors in high-functioning females and males with autism. *J Autism Dev Disord* 21: 197–209.

Lord C, Rutter M, Le Couteur A (1994) Autism Diagnostic Interview-Revised: a revised version of a diagnostic interview for caregivers of individuals with possible pervasive developmental disorders. *J Autism Dev Disord* 24: 659–85.

Lord C, Risi S, Lambrecht L, Cook EH, Leventhal BL, DiLavore PC, Pickles A, Rutter M (2000) The Autism Diagnostic Observation Schedule-Generic: a standard measure of social and communication deficits associated with the spectrum of autism. *J Autism Dev Disord* 30: 205–23.

Lotter V (1966) Epidemiology of autistic conditions in young children. I: Prevalence. *Soc Psychiatry* 1: 124–37.

Lotter V (1967) Epidemiology of autistic conditions in young children. II: Some characteristics of the parent and children. *Soc Psychiatry* 1: 163–73.

MacMahon B, Pugh TF (1970) *Epidemiology: Principles and Methods.* Boston: Little, Brown.

Madsen KM, Hviid A, Vertergaard M, Schendel D, Wohlfahrt J, Thorsen P, Olsen J, Melbye M (2002) A population-based study of measles, mumps, and rubella vaccination and autism. *N Engl J Med* 347: 1477–82.

Magnusson P, Saemundsen E (2001) Prevalence of autism in Iceland. *J Autism Dev Disord* 31: 153–63.

Matsuishi T, Shiotsuki Y, Yoshimura K, Shoji H, Imuta F, Yamashita F (1987) High prevalence of infantile autism in Kurume City, Japan. *J Child Neurol* 2: 268–71.

McCarthy P, Fitzgerald M, Smith MA (1984) Prevalence of childhood autism in Ireland. *Ir Med J* 77: 129–30.

MRC (2001) *Review of Autism Research: Epidemiology and Causes.* London: Medical Research Council.

Newschaffer CJ, Curran LK (2003) Autism: an emerging public health problem. *Public Health Rep* 118: 393–9.

Newschaffer CJ, Fallin D, Lee NL (2002) Heritable and nonheritable risk factors for autism spectrum disorders. *Epidemiol Rev* 24: 137–53.

Newschaffer CJ, Falb MD, Gurney JG (2005) National autism prevalence trends from United States special education data. *Pediatrics* 115: e277–82.

Nordin V, Gillberg C (1996) Autism spectrum disorders in children with physical or mental disability or both. II: Screening aspects. *Dev Med Child Neurol* 38: 314–24.

Parker SK, Schwartz B, Todd J, Pickering LK (2004) Thimerosal-containing vaccines and autistic spectrum disorder: a critical review of published original data. *Pediatrics* 114: 793–804.

Piven J, Folstein S (1994) The genetics of autism. In: Baumann ML, Kemper TL, eds. *The Neurobiology of Autism*. Baltimore: Johns Hopkins University Press, pp. 18–44.

Piven J, Simon J, Chase GA, Wzorek M, Landa R, Gayle J, Folstein S (1993) The etiology of autism: pre-, peri- and neonatal factors. *J Am Acad Child Adolesc Psychiatry* 32: 1256–63.

Powell JE, Edwards A, Edwards M, Pandit BS, Sungum-Paliwal SR, Whitehouse W (2000) Changes in the incidence of childhood autism and other autistic spectrum disorders in preschool children from two areas of the West Midlands, UK. *Dev Med Child Neurol* 42: 624–8.

Rett Syndrome Diagnostic Criteria Work Group (1988) Diagnostic criteria for Rett syndrome. *Ann Neurol* 23: 425–8.

Rice C, Schendel D, Cunniff C, Doernberg N (2004) Public health monitoring of developmental disabilities with a focus on the autism spectrum disorders. *Am J Med Genet C Semin Med Genet* 125: 22–7.

Ritvo EG, Freeman BJ, Mason-Brothers A, Mo A, Ritvo AM (1985) Concordance for the syndrome of autism in 40 pairs of afflicted twins. *Am J Psychiatry* 142: 74–7.

Ritvo ER, Freeman BJ, Pingree C, Mason-Brothers A, Jorde L, Jenson WR, McMahon WM, Petersen PB, Mo A, Ritvo A (1989) The UCLA–University of Utah epidemiologic survey of autism: Prevalence. *Am J Psychiatry* 146: 194–9.

Rodier PM, Ingram JL, Tisdale B, Nelson S, Romano J (1996) Embryological origin for autism: developmental anomalies of the cranial nerve motor nuclei. *J Comparative Neurol* 370: 247–61.

Rogers SJ, DiLalla DL (1990) Age of symptom onset in young children with pervasive developmental disorders. *J Am Acad Child Adolesc Psychiatry* 29: 863–72.

Rothman KJ (2002) *Epidemiology: An Introduction*. Philadelphia: Lippencott-Raven.

Schieve LA, Meikle SF, Ferre C, Peterson HB, Jeng G, Wilcox LS (2002) Low and very low birth weight in infants conceived with use of assisted reproductive technology. *N Engl J Med* 346: 731–7.

Schopler E, Andrews CE, Strupp K (1979) Do autistic children come from upper-middle-class parents? *J Autism Dev Disord* 9: 139–52.

Schopler E, Reichler R, Rochen RB (1998) *The Childhood Autism Rating Scale (CARS)*. Los Angeles: Western Psychological Services.

Smalley SL, Asarnow RF, Spence MA (1988) Autism and genetics. A decade of research. *Arch Gen Psychiatry* 45: 953–61.

Smeeth L, Cook C, Fombonne E, Heavey L, Rodrigues LC, Smith PG, Hall AJ (2004) MMR vaccination and pervasive developmental disorders: a case–control study. *Lancet* 364: 963–9.

Sponheim E, Skjeldal O (1998) Autism and related disorders: epidemiological findings in a Norwegian study using ICD-10 diagnostic criteria. *J Autism Dev Disord* 28: 217–27.

Stanley FJ, Blair E, Alberman E (2000) *Cerebral Palsies: Epidemiology and Causal Pathways. Clinics in Developmental Medicine No. 151*. London: Mac Keith Press.

Steffenburg S, Gillberg C (1986) Autism and autistic-like conditions in Swedish rural and urban areas: a population study. *Br J Psychiatry* 149: 81–7.

Steffenburg S, Gillberg C, Hellgren L, Anderssson L, Gillberg IC, Jakobsson G, Bohman M (1989) A twin study of autism in Denmark, Finland, Iceland, Norway, and Sweden. *J Child Psychol Psychiatry* 30: 405–16.

Stehr-Green P, Tull P, Stellfeld M, Mortenson PB, Simpson D (2003) Autism and thimerosal-containing vaccines: lack of consistent evidence for an association. *Am J Prev Med* 25: 101–6.

Steinhausen HC, Gobel D, Breinlinger M, Wohlleben B (1986) A community survey of infantile autism. *J Am Acad Child Psychiatry* 25: 186–9.

Stromberg B, Dahlquist G, Ericson A, Finnstrom O, Koster M, Stjernqvist K (2002) Neurological sequelae in children born after in vitro fertilization: a population based study. *Lancet* 359: 461–5.

Stromland K, Nordin V, Miller M, Akerstrom B, Gillberg C (1994) Autism in thalidomide embryopathy: a population study. *Dev Med Child Neurol* 36: 351–6.

Stromland K, Philipson E, Andersson Gronlund M (2002) Offspring of male and female parents with thalidomide embryopathy: birth defects and functional anomalies. *Teratology* 66: 115–21.

Stroup DF, Brookmeyer R, Kalsbeek D (2004) Public health surveillance in action: a framework. In: Brookmeyer R, Stroup DF, eds. *Monitoring the Health of Populations: Statistical Principles and Methods for Public Health Surveillance.* Oxford: Oxford University Press, pp. 5–12.

Sugiyama T, Abe T (1989) The prevalence of autism in Nagoya, Japan: a total population study. *J Autism Dev Disord* 19: 87–96.

Surman G, Newdick H, Johnson A (2003) Cerebral palsy rates among low-birthweight infants in the 1990's. *Dev Med Child Neurol* 45: 456–62.

Tanoue Y, Oda S, Asano F, Kawashima K (1988) Epidemiology of infantile autism in southern Ibaraki, Japan: differences in prevalence in birth cohorts. *J Autism Dev Disord* 18: 155–66.

Tidmarsh L, Volkmar FR (2003) Diagnosis and epidemiology of autism spectrum disorders. *Can J Psychiatry* 48: 517–25.

Treffert DA (1970) Epidemiology of infantile autism. *Arch Gen Psychiatry* 22: 431–8.

Trevathan E (2004) Seizures and epilepsy among children with language regression and autistic spectrum disorders. *J Child Neurol* 19 Suppl 1: S49–57.

US Department of Education (2003) Children ages 3 through 21 served under IDEA, Part B. In: *25th Annual Report to Congress on the Implementation of the Individuals with Disabilities Education Act, vol 1.* Washington, DC: US Department of Education. Office of Special Education and Rehabilitative Services, pp. 13–76.

Volkmar FR, Cicchetti DV, Bregman J, Cohen DJ (1992) Three diagnostic systems for autism: DSM-III, DSM-III-R, and ICD-10. *J Autism Dev Disord* 22: 483–92.

Volkmar FR, Cook EH, Pomeroy J, Realmuto G, Tanguay P (1999) Practice parameters for the assessment and treatment of children, adolescents, and adults with autism and other pervasive developmental disorders. *J Am Acad Child Adolesc Psychiatry* 38: 32S–54S.

Wakefield AJ, Murch SH, Anthony A, Linnell J, Casson DM, Malik M, Berelowitz M, Dhillon AP, Thomson MA, Harvey P, Valentine A, Davies SE, Walker-Smith JA (1998) Ileal–lymphoid–nodular hyperplasia, non-specific colitis, and pervasive developmental disorder in children. *Lancet* 351: 637–41.

Webb EV, Lobo S, Hervas A, Scourfield J, Fraser WI (1997) The changing prevalence of autistic disorder in a Welsh health district. *Dev Med Child Neurol* 39: 150–2.

Wing L, Gould J (1979) Severe impairments of social interaction and associated abnormalities in children: epidemiology and classification. *J Autism Dev Disord* 9: 11–29.

Wing L, Potter D (2002) The epidemiology of autistic spectrum disorders: is the prevalence rising? *Ment Retard Dev Disabil Res Rev* 8: 151–61.

Yeargin-Allsopp M (2002) Past and future perspectives in autism epidemiology. *Mol Psychiatry* 7 Suppl 2: S9–11.

Yeargin-Allsopp M, Murphy CC, Oakley GP, Sikes K (1992) A multiple-source method for studying prevalence of developmental disabilities in children: the Metropolitan Atlanta Developmental Disabilities Study. *Pediatrics* 89: 624–30.

Yeargin-Allsopp M, Rice C, Karapurkar T, Doernberg N, Boyle C, Murphy C (2003) Prevalence of autism in a US metropolitan area. *JAMA* 289: 49–55.

3

THE SOCIAL DEFICIT IN AUTISM

Roberto F Tuchman

The characteristic clinical features that set autism apart from other disorders of communication and behavior are the impairments in reciprocal social interaction (Walters et al. 1990). Constantino and colleagues (Constantino and Todd 2003; Constantino et al. 2000, 2004) have demonstrated in a series of studies that social interaction is under strong genetic influence, with a continuous distribution of abilities and deficits of social interaction in the general population. In addition, there is recent evidence for a genetic basis and strong heritability for the quantitative trait of social motivation in autism (Sung et al. 2005).

The criteria for determining who is and who is not affected by autism are based on arbitrary clinical cut-offs, and the DSM-IV (see Table 1.1, p. 2) uses four types of behaviors to define the social domain of autism. These behaviors range from impairments in the use of nonverbal communication such as eye gaze and body posture to a lack of social or emotional reciprocity. The other two groups of behaviors include a failure to develop peer relationships appropriate to developmental level, and a lack of spontaneous seeking to share enjoyment, interests or achievements. All four of these groups of behaviors are defined by the type and quality and not by the quantity of the behaviors. This approach does not capture the broad dimensional spectrum of social skill that exists in the general population and among those diagnosed with autism. In addition, defining autism as a categorical diagnosis makes it extremely difficult to understand and define the neural basis of this heterogenous disorder. From a neurological perspective, it is much more instructive to delineate the basic constructs that allow us to determine an individual's distinctive social phenotype. The questions then become: how does social cognition in autism differ from the general population, how do early deficits in social communication lead to the clinical phenotype of social cognitive disorders and specifically autism, and, more interestingly to the neurologist, what are the cellular and neural mechanisms that define the social constructs that determine social cognition?

CONSTRUCTS OF SOCIAL COGNITION

Impairment in social interaction may present as social isolation or inappropriate social behavior, with a wide range of reciprocal social impairments represented by a variety of behaviors that include gaze avoidance, failure to respond when called, failure to participate in group activities, lack of awareness of others, indifference to affection or inappropriate affection, and a lack of social or emotional empathy. The clinical differences in the phenotypic expression of social impairments in autism reflect variables that include developmental age and cognitive ability. In addition, the type of social environment, for example structured versus unstructured, in which the evaluation takes place can influence the phenotypic expression of social skills (Lord 1991). As such, playing with developmentally appropriate toys, carrying out age-appropriate conversations, and observing or obtaining a history of how an individual functions in diverse social environments are essential features to assess the social competency of a child, adolescent or adult in whom one suspects a diagnosis of autism.

An admittedly simplistic view of complex social development would include three accepted social constructs that are defective in autism: affective reciprocity, joint attention, and "theory of mind" (Robertson et al. 1999). Affective reciprocity represents the initial phase of social communication and is evident before 6 months of age. It is characterized by the reciprocal orienting and exchange of emotional signals between caregiver and child (Bakeman et al. 1990). Affective reciprocity is manifest in infancy by the use of eye contact and gestures to focus attention on the object or event of interest and progresses in toddlers to eye gaze and pointing to draw attention to an object or event of interest. Later in childhood, affective reciprocity becomes part of the pragmatic level of language (see Chapter 4), and is reflected in the ability to carry out age-appropriate conversations and interpret emotional expressions and behavior in other people (Wellman et al. 1996).

Joint attention refers to the capacity of individuals to coordinate attention with a social partner in relation to some object or event. Joint attention begins to emerge by 6 months of age and is one of the earliest and critical foundations for the establishment of social communication and social cognition in children (Mundy et al. 1986). Impairments in joint attention and social orienting differentiate infants with autism from those who are typically developing and from those with mental retardation without autism (Osterling et al. 2002). The development of joint attention is a fundamental prerequisite for much of early language acquisition (Mundy et al. 1987), and joint attention appears to be a reliable predictor of concurrent language ability (Tomasello and Farrar 1986, Dawson et al. 2004).

Theory of mind (ToM) or metacognition refers to an individual's ability to understand that others possess covert mental intentions. Understanding another person's inner state requires that an individual be able to interpret emotional expressions and behavior. The high functioning individual with autism may understand that people think but they lack the ability to infer subtle social cues from a person's emotional expressions and behavior. Difficulty understanding that others have beliefs, intentions and desires is a crucial skill that, when deficient, leads to impairments in reciprocal social interaction (Baron-Cohen et al. 1985). ToM is a complex neuropsychological construct, and individuals with autism, especially those with adequate cognitive skills, may perform well on basic ToM tasks but still have difficulty with more naturalistic tasks such as interpretation of complex stories (Happe 1994). Several investigators have suggested strong links between joint attention and ToM (Buitelaar et al. 1991, Tager-Flusberg 1992, Charman 1997, Morgan et al. 2003, Mundy 2003). However, despite research linking ToM to joint-attention and social deficits in autism, there are studies that question the specificity of this relationship, as well as pointing out that there is a strong link between language ability and ToM (Happe 1993, Sparrevohn and Howie 1995, Shields et al. 1996, Yirmiya et al. 1996).

All of the key social constructs of early childhood have strong links to language, especially to the social use of language or what is referred to as the semantics and pragmatics of language. In addition to the links between language abilities and social cognition there are a variety of developmental functions that may not be specific to social skills but which may contribute to the ultimate social deficit. These broader phenotype autistic traits include face processing, specifically the structural encoding of facial features and face movements such as eye gaze, social motivational impairments, the ability to imitate gestures and other motor activities, memory systems, and executive function (Dawson et al. 2002). In autism, perceptual processes, for example reading facial expressions, are impaired, so that individuals with autism have difficulty linking socially relevant information perceived visually with social knowledge and appropriate social responses (Adolphs et al. 2001, Barton et al. 2004, Brosnan et al. 2004). It has also been suggested that children who later develop autism, as infants may shift their attention to non-social stimuli as opposed to social stimuli (Maestro et al. 2002).

The role and contribution to the social deficit in autism of specific developmental processes such as inadequate executive functions like working memory, inhibitory control and planning is an area of active research and controversy (McEvoy et al. 1993, Hill 2004, Ozonoff et al. 2004). The concept of weak central coherence, which has been offered as an indirect contributor to the social deficit in autism, proposes that individuals with autism have difficulty integrating different sources of information into a coherent whole (Frith and Happe 1994, Happe 1999). It has also been suggested that the contribution that executive control skills and ToM make to the cognitive–language aspects of autism is distinct from the more fundamental social–perceptual information conveyed through the eyes, face and voice, implying that this information, which is used in comprehending mental states, may be more closely linked to autism's deficient social reciprocity (Joseph and Tager-Flusberg 2004). Furthermore the role of cognitive–affective functions in determining the social deficit of autism has led to the extreme male brain theory of autism (Baron-Cohen 2004). In this theory proposed by Baron-Cohen (Bayliss et al. 2005, Kanazawa and Vandermassen 2005), empathy, which includes both the ability to attribute mental states to oneself and others and having an emotional reaction that is appropriate to another's mental state, is not only deficient in individuals with autism but is an extreme example of a male brain (Baron-Cohen and Wheelwright 2004). That is, according to this theory, the male brain in general has less capacity for "emphathizing", that is a relatively diminished drive to identify another's mental state and to respond with an appropriate emotion to this state, as compared to the female brain.

Screening instruments like the CHAT and the CHAT-M (Baron-Cohen et al. 1992, 2000; Robins et al. 2001) use social behaviors to identify children at risk for autism and distinguish it from other developmental disorders. The Autism Diagnostic Observation Schedule (ADOS-G; Lord et al. 2000), currently considered the "gold standard" for the observational diagnosis of autism, includes joint attention measures, as well as the more complex constructs and concepts just discussed.

There are many unanswered questions regarding the role of developmental processes such as attention, perception and language, and of neuropsychological constructs such as executive function and central coherence to the core symptom of reciprocal social interaction. Although they no doubt play a role in the social deficit in autism, their specificity is uncertain and we have much more to learn about their contribution to autism's social deficit. From a developmental neurology point of view, the focus has to be on what are the basic building blocks of reciprocal social interaction and also to develop tools that can measure these constructs in a manner that would allow for mapping these discreet aspects of social cognition onto neural networks.

CLINICAL PHENOTYPES OF SOCIAL DEFICITS

In very general terms, the social spectrum of autism can be divided into the three subtypes delineated by Wing and Gould (1979): aloof, passive, and active-but-odd. These subtypes are strongly related to IQ (Volkmar et al. 1989). Castelloe and Dawson (1993) developed and validated a questionnaire (the Wing Subgroups Questionnaire, or WSQ) for assigning children with autism to one of Wing's three hypothesized subgroups; the WSQ is a useful tool for subclassifying individuals with autism. The two aloof and active-but-odd subtypes seem to be predictors of behaviors across the language/communication, reciprocal social interaction, and stereotyped behavior/restricted interest domains; individuals assigned to these subtypes differ in a number of important ways (e.g. severity of autism, IQ, adaptive behavior). There is less support for an intermediate, passive subtype (Borden and Ollendick 1994).

Clinical experience suggests that the social communication spectrum encompasses individuals with what are conventionally considered distinct disorders. These include attention deficit disorders, or in the Gillberg terminology deficits in attention, motor control and perception (DAMP; Gillberg 2003); the semantic–pragmatic language deficit disorders (see Chapter 4); the learning disorders with social deficits, or what Rourke has termed the syndrome of nonverbal learning disability (Rourke and Finlayson 1978, Rourke 1988); Asperger syndrome (Wing 1981); atypical autism, or what has been termed pervasive developmental disorder–not otherwise specified (PDD-NOS); autistic disorder; and children with severe mental retardation and the triad of autistic behaviors encountered, for example, in Rett syndrome (Percy et al. 1988). A current hypothesis is that there is a spectrum of social reciprocal deficits that can be found in a wide variety of neurodevelopmental disorders, and that the effects of cognition, age and affect may modulate the social phenotype.

Despite the fact that adequacy of cognitive function, specifically intelligence as measured by standard IQ testing, is not part of the definition of autism, it is an important variable that affects the social phenotype. Two common neurodevelopmental disorders associated with mental retardation and autism are Rett syndrome and fragile-X syndrome (Amir et al. 1999, Kaufmann et al. 2004). Although both are almost always associated with significant levels of cognitive impairment, the social deficits in these disorders are variable. In addition, when a social deficit coexists with mental retardation, it may be distinct from the social deficit found in autism with less or no mental retardation, although how to make this distinction is still controversial. There are distinct mental retardation syndromes that are not necessarily, or even usually, associated with autism, such as Cockayne and Down syndromes; consequently it is unlikely that mental retardation per se is responsible for the social deficit in Rett syndrome and fragile-X. It is probable that the variability in severity of the social deficits in mental retardation syndromes is indirectly linked to the level of expression of the gene defect and directly related to the consequences for brain structure or function of more or less severe curtailment of the gene product (Beckel-Mitchener and Greenough 2004, Kau et al. 2004, Samaco et al. 2004). The hypothesis is that the phenotypic expressions of the malfunctioning genes reflect variable curtailments in the proteins they code and their effects, in most cases, on multiple networks in the developing brain. These effects in turn are modulated by the individual genetic background of the carrier of the gene defect, or even possibly by random environmental effects, and this determines the social phenotype of these mental retardation syndromes.

There are several groups of children in whom level of intelligence as measured by IQ testing is relatively spared but in whom social cognition is nevertheless impaired (Sturm et al. 2004). How one goes about classifying disorders of social communication, especially in individuals with relatively spared intelligence, is controversial and has been discussed in detail in Chapter 1. An excellent example of how age, cognition and affect contribute to the social deficit can be seen in individuals with Asperger syndrome. In Asperger syndrome the impairment in social communication may be subtle and difficult to identify in early childhood and continue to be difficult to detect in adulthood, inasmuch as many of these individuals learn to interact socially through compensatory learning (Frith 2004). Adults with Asperger syndrome may share with other disorders of social cognition such as Rourke's syndrome of nonverbal learning disabilities, deficits in empathy and in their ability to talk about their own emotions; these difficulties may be attributable to depression and anxiety (Baron-Cohen and Wheelwright 2004, Frith 2004).

Although making the diagnosis of a mood disorder in autism is difficult, there is evidence to suggest that individuals with autism, especially adolescents and adults with autism, are at greater risk for having affective disorders than the general population (Lainhart and Folstein 1994). From another perspective, it is becoming increasingly clear that deficits in social cognition are related to mood disorders and schizophrenia (Smalley et al. 1995, Bolton et al. 1998, Horan and Blanchard 2003, Tse and Bond 2004).

Furthermore, there are numerous studies suggesting an increased frequency of mood disorders, obsessive-compulsive disorders and social phobia in relatives of individuals with autism (DeLong and Nohria 1994, Smalley et al. 1995, Bolton et al. 1998, DeLong 2004).

CELLULAR AND NEURAL CORRELATES OF SOCIAL COGNITION

The cellular and neural mechanisms of social cognition are complex, and the lack of animal models limits research in this area. Nevertheless, there is evidence to suggest that two related neuropeptides, oxytocin and vasopressin, may influence complex social behavior (Insel 1997). Animal studies have implicated oxytocin and oxytocin receptors in the mediation of social cognition and behavior (Winslow and Insel 2002, Bielsky et al. 2004). Oxytocin and vasopressin influence social behavior through the arginine–vasopressin (AVP) system mediated through the AVP receptor 1a (AVPR1a) (Keverne and Curley 2004). The adult prairie vole is a good model for studying social bonds (Wang and Aragona 2004): in this monogamous group of rodents vasopressin neurotransmission has been demonstrated in the ventral pallidum during mating, and V1a receptor subtype (V1aR) activation in this region is required for the formation of a pair bond (Lim and Young 2004). The role of oxytocin in autism has been suggested by studies that indicate that children with autistic disorder have alterations in the endocrine oxytocin system and that these alterations may be greater in the subset of children with autism who are aloof (Modahl et al. 1998, Green et al. 2001). There are also preliminary data suggesting the *AVPR1a* gene may play a role in autism susceptibility (Wassink et al. 2004) and that in animal models these effects may be specific to social motivation (Wersinger et al. 2004).

Studies in adults suggest that impairments of emotion and social behavior are correlated with abnormal function of the ventromedial region of the prefrontal cortex and that this abnormality is demonstrable prior to age 16 months (Anderson et al. 1999, Bechara 2002, Bar-On et al. 2003). Other studies suggest that "mirror neurons", which are found in the frontal cortex and which are activited in relation both to specific actions performed by self and matching actions performed by others, play a role in the development of early social cognitive functions (Williams et al. 2001). The mirror neuron system has been linked to important functions of early social development such as imitation and language development (Rizzolatti and Craighero 2004), as well as to emotional processing and, specifically, to empathy (Leslie et al. 2004).

An increasing number of neuroimaging studies indicate that face recognition and the interpretation of social cues on the face are impaired in autism (Schultz et al. 2000, 2003; Pierce et al. 2001, 2004; Ida Gobbini et al. 2004). Supportive neurophysiological data suggest that speed of face processing is slow in adults with autism (McPartland et al. 2004). Innovative work by Klin and colleagues at Yale uses eye-tracking technology to demonstrate that the difficulty in tasks such as face perception in autism is correlated with subjects' focus on the wrong parts of the face when trying to derive social information (Klin et al. 2002a). Individuals with autism spend more time looking at the mouth rather than the eyes when trying to obtain social information and pay preferential attention to physical over social cues (Klin et al. 2002b).

Neuroimaging research investigating specific social constructs such as theory of mind suggests that brain activity in the dorsal medial frontal cortex (Brodmann's areas 8/9) and superior temporal gyrus are the most consistent correlates of ToM task performance (Fletcher et al. 1995, Frith 2003). Language based ToM tasks activate an extensive neural network that includes the medial frontal cortex, the superior frontal cortex, the anterior and retrosplenial cingulate, the anterior temporal pole and the contralateral right cerebellum, as well as the anterior vermis (Calarge et al. 2003). In addition, there is evidence to suggest a role for the amygdala in ToM tasks, judging from cases in which the amygdala was damaged early in development (Shaw et al. 2004).

There are very preliminary EEG coherence studies in young children with autism which suggest that asymmetries in resting electroencephalogram (EEG) alpha power in the frontal regions of the brain correlate with measures of joint-attention (Mundy et al. 2000, Henderson et al. 2002). The study of initiation typically requires an interactive paradigm that provides individuals with a framework that motivates them to generate social goals and behaviors. The lack of such paradigms has limited the exploration of the neural correlates of self-initiated social behaviors.

OUTCOME – CLINICAL IMPLICATIONS OF SOCIAL DEFICIT FOR INTERVENTION

Interventions that attempt to ameliorate the social deficits of autism are focused on early correction of joint-attention deficits and teaching reciprocal social interaction skills. Early intervention for the social deficit is based on the hypothesis that a lack of social orienting and joint attention in infancy and early childhood leads to atypical social neurodevelopment by attenuating the types of experiences which a typically developing child has with his or her environment and which lead to the positive reinforcement of reciprocal social interaction skills (Mundy and Crowson 1997, Mundy and Neal 2001). In other words, if combined impairments in joint attention and social orienting distinguish young children with autism from those without autism, targeting interventions to correct these deficits early on may be crucial to preventing a cycle of inadequate interactions with the environment which may hinder the development of appropriate social skills (Dawson et al. 2004).

Recent work on interventions for social deficit has made it clear that the clinical heterogeneity of this disorder requires tailored strategies. One pilot randomized study taught parents how to communicate effectively with their child; the children of parents who received the training did better than the controls (Aldred et al. 2004). Another small study used video modeling to teach three children appropriate social behaviors (Nikopoulos and Keenan 2004). Although social skills groups are commonly used to teach social skills, there is a paucity of data regarding the effectiveness of these programs. A group of investigators designed a program to teach specific social skills such as greeting, conversation and play skills in a brief therapy format that included eight training sessions. Greeting and play skills, and to a lesser extent conversation skills improved during the sessions but did not generalize to settings outside of the clinic (Barry et al. 2003). Another study combined aspects of behavior therapy, peer modeling and naturalistic communication strategies and assessed efficacy of a social skills intervention for children with autism. It focused on individual and group play with LEGO® blocks that allow children to build different projects, and was used to teach specific reciprocal social skills. Results revealed significant improvement in motivation to initiate social contact with peers, and in the ability to sustain interaction with peers for a period of time, and lessening of autistic symptoms of aloofness and rigidity (LeGoff 2004). The problems with all of these intervention studies for sociability are the same problems that plague any intervention in autism and are reviewed in more detail in Chapter 17.

In general, as individuals enter into adulthood there is an amelioration of the social isolation, but the poverty of social skills and the impaired ability to make peer friendships persist (Ballaban-Gil et al. 1996, Howlin et al. 2004). Adolescents and adults with autism have significant misapprehensions of how others perceive them. The adult with autism and adequate cognitive skills is in general a loner. We do not know if there are specific variables that influence social cognitive outcome distinct from those reviewed in Chapter 18. It may be that environmental effects have a greater influence on social outcome than they have on language or repetitive behaviors, but there are no data to determine this. The hope is that early intervention strategies that are just becoming available to young children with autism will have a positive impact on social outcome, but as discussed the effectiveness of these interventions is still largely unknown.

REFERENCES

Adolphs R, Sears L, Piven J (2001) Abnormal processing of social information from faces in autism. *J Cogn Neurosci* 13: 232–40.

Aldred C, Green J, Adams C (2004) A new social communication intervention for children with autism: pilot randomised controlled treatment study suggesting effectiveness. *J Child Psychol Psychiatry* 45: 1420–30.

Amir RE, Van den Veyver IB, Wan M, Tran CQ, Francke U, Zoghbi HY (1999) Rett syndrome is caused by mutations in X-linked MECP2, encoding methyl-CpG-binding protein 2. *Nat Genet* 23: 185–8.

Anderson SW, Bechara A, Damasio H, Tranel D, Damasio AR (1999) Impairment of social and moral behavior related to early damage in human prefrontal cortex. *Nat Neurosci* 2: 1032–7.

Bakeman R, Adamson LB, Konner M, Barr RG (1990) Kung infancy: the social context of object exploration. *Child Dev* 61: 794–809.

Ballaban-Gil K, Rapin I, Tuchman R, Shinnar S (1996) Longitudinal examination of the behavioral, language, and social changes in a population of adolescents and young adults with autistic disorder. *Pediatr Neurol* 15: 217–23.

Bar-On R, Tranel D, Denburg NL, Bechara A (2003) Exploring the neurological substrate of emotional and social intelligence. *Brain* 126: 1790–800.

Baron-Cohen S (2004) The cognitive neuroscience of autism. *J Neurol Neurosurg Psychiatry* 75: 945–8.

Baron-Cohen S, Wheelwright S (2004) The empathy quotient: an investigation of adults with Asperger syndrome or high functioning autism, and normal sex differences. *J Autism Dev Disord* 34: 163–75.

Baron-Cohen S, Leslie AM, Frith U (1985) Does the autistic child have a "theory of mind"? *Cognition* 21: 37–46.

Baron-Cohen S, Allen J, Gillberg C (1992) Can autism be detected at 18 months? The needle, the haystack, and the CHAT. *Br J Psychiatry* 161: 839–43.

Baron-Cohen S, Wheelwright S, Cox A, Baird G, Charman T, Swettenham J, Drew A, Doehring P (2000) Early identification of autism by the CHecklist for Autism in Toddlers (CHAT). *J R Soc Med* 93: 521–5.

Barry TD, Klinger LG, Lee JM, Palardy N, Gilmore T, Bodin SD (2003) Examining the effectiveness of an outpatient clinic-based social skills group for high-functioning children with autism. *J Autism Dev Disord* 33: 685–701.

Barton JJ, Cherkasova MV, Hefter R, Cox TA, O'Connor M, Manoach DS (2004) Are patients with social developmental disorders prosopagnosic? Perceptual heterogeneity in the Asperger and socio-emotional processing disorders. *Brain* 127: 1706–16.

Bayliss AP, di Pellegrino G, Tipper SP (2005) Sex differences in eye gaze and symbolic cueing of attention. *Q J Exp Psychol A* 58: 631–50.

Bechara A (2002) The neurology of social cognition. *Brain* 125: 1673–5.

Beckel-Mitchener A, Greenough WT (2004) Correlates across the structural, functional, and molecular phenotypes of fragile X syndrome. *Ment Retard Dev Disabil Res Rev* 10: 53–9.

Bielsky IF, Hu SB, Szegda KL, Westphal H, Young LJ (2004) Profound impairment in social recognition and reduction in anxiety-like behavior in vasopressin V1a receptor knockout mice. *Neuropsychopharmacology* 29: 483–93.

Bolton PF, Pickles A, Murphy M, Rutter M (1998) Autism, affective and other psychiatric disorders: patterns of familial aggregation. *Psychol Med* 28: 385–95.

Borden MC, Ollendick TH (1994) An examination of the validity of social subtypes in autism. *J Autism Dev Disord* 24: 23–37.

Brosnan MJ, Scott FJ, Fox S, Pye J (2004) Gestalt processing in autism: failure to process perceptual relationships and the implications for contextual understanding. *J Child Psychol Psychiatry* 45: 459–69.

Buitelaar JK, van Engeland H, de Kogel KH, de Vries H, van Hooff JA (1991) Differences in the structure of social behaviour of autistic children and non-autistic retarded controls. *J Child Psychol Psychiatry* 32: 995–1015.

Calarge C, Andreasen NC, O'Leary DS (2003) Visualizing how one brain understands another: a PET study of theory of mind. *Am J Psychiatry* 160: 1954–64.

Castelloe P, Dawson G (1993) Subclassification of children with autism and pervasive developmental disorder: a questionnaire based on Wing's subgrouping scheme. *J Autism Dev Disord* 23: 229–41.

Charman T (1997) The relationship between joint attention and pretend play in autism. *Dev Psychopathol* 9: 1–16.

Constantino JN, Todd RD (2003) Autistic traits in the general population: a twin study. *Arch Gen Psychiatry* 60: 524–30.

Constantino JN, Przybeck T, Friesen D, Todd RD (2000) Reciprocal social behavior in children with and without pervasive developmental disorders. *J Dev Behav Pediatr* 21: 2–11.

Constantino JN, Gruber CP, Davis S, Hayes S, Passanante N, Przybeck T (2004) The factor structure of autistic traits. *J Child Psychol Psychiatry* 45: 719–26.

Dawson G, Toth K, Abbott R, Osterling J, Munson J, Estes A, Liaw J (2004) Early social attention impairments in autism: social orienting, joint attention, and attention to distress. *Dev Psychol* 40: 271–83.

Dawson G, Webb S, Schellenberg GD, Dager S, Friedman S, Aylward E, Richards T (2002) Defining the broader phenotype of autism: genetic, brain, and behavioral perspectives. *Dev Psychopathol* 14: 581–611.

DeLong R (2004) Autism and familial major mood disorder: are they related? *J Neuropsychiatry Clin Neurosci* 16: 199–213.

DeLong R, Nohria C (1994) Psychiatric family history and neurological disease in autistic spectrum disorders. *Dev Med Child Neurol* 36: 441–8.

Fletcher PC, Happe F, Frith U, Baker SC, Dolan RJ, Frackowiak RS, Frith CD (1995) Other minds in the brain: a functional imaging study of "theory of mind" in story comprehension. *Cognition* 57: 109–28.

Frith C (2003) What do imaging studies tell us about the neural basis of autism? *Novartis Found Symp* 251: 149–66; discussion 166–76, 281–97.

Frith U (2004) Emanuel Miller lecture: confusions and controversies about Asperger syndrome. *J Child Psychol Psychiatry* 45: 672–86.

Frith U, Happe F (1994) Autism: beyond "theory of mind". *Cognition* 50: 115–32.

Gillberg C (2003) Deficits in attention, motor control, and perception: a brief review. *Arch Dis Child* 88: 904–10.

Green L, Fein D, Modahl C, Feinstein C, Waterhouse L, Morris M (2001) Oxytocin and autistic disorder: alterations in peptide forms. *Biol Psychiatry* 50: 609–13.

Happe FG (1993) Communicative competence and theory of mind in autism: a test of relevance theory. *Cognition* 48: 101–19.

Happe FG (1994) An advanced test of theory of mind: understanding of story characters' thoughts and feelings by able autistic, mentally handicapped, and normal children and adults. *J Autism Dev Disord* 24: 129–54.

Happe F (1999) Autism: cognitive deficit or cognitive style? *Trends Cogn Sci* 3: 216–22.

Henderson LM, Yoder PJ, Yale ME, McDuffie A (2002) Getting the point: electrophysiological correlates of protodeclarative pointing. *Int J Dev Neurosci* 20: 449–58.

Hill EL (2004) Executive dysfunction in autism. *Trends Cogn Sci* 8: 26–32.

Horan WP, Blanchard JJ (2003) Neurocognitive, social, and emotional dysfunction in deficit syndrome schizophrenia. *Schizophr Res* 65: 125–37.

Howlin P, Goode S, Hutton J, Rutter M (2004) Adult outcome for children with autism. *J Child Psychol Psychiatry* 45: 212–29.

Ida Gobbini M, Leibenluft E, Santiago N, Haxby JV (2004) Social and emotional attachment in the neural representation of faces. *Neuroimage* 22: 1628–35.

Insel TR (1997) A neurobiological basis of social attachment. *Am J Psychiatry* 154: 726–35.

Joseph RM, Tager-Flusberg H (2004) The relationship of theory of mind and executive functions to symptom type and severity in children with autism. *Dev Psychopathol* 16: 137–55.

Kanazawa S, Vandermassen G (2005) Engineers have more sons, nurses have more daughters: an evolutionary psychological extension of Baron-Cohen's extreme male brain theory of autism. *J Theor Biol* 233: 589–99.

Kau AS, Tierney E, Bukelis I, Stump MH, Kates WR, Trescher WH, Kaufmann WE (2004) Social behavior profile in young males with fragile X syndrome: characteristics and specificity. *Am J Med Genet* 126A: 9–17.

Kaufmann WE, Cortell R, Kau AS, Bukelis I, Tierney E, Gray RM, Cox C, Capone GT, Stanard

P (2004) Autism spectrum disorder in fragile X syndrome: communication, social interaction, and specific behaviors. *Am J Med Genet* 129A: 225–34.

Keverne EB, Curley JP (2004) Vasopressin, oxytocin and social behaviour. *Curr Opin Neurobiol* 14: 777–83.

Klin A, Jones W, Schultz R, Volkmar F, Cohen D (2002a) Defining and quantifying the social phenotype in autism. *Am J Psychiatry* 159: 895–908.

Klin A, Jones W, Schultz R, Volkmar F, Cohen D (2002b) Visual fixation patterns during viewing of naturalistic social situations as predictors of social competence in individuals with autism. *Arch Gen Psychiatry* 59: 809–16.

Lainhart JE, Folstein SE (1994) Affective disorders in people with autism: a review of published cases. *J Autism Dev Disord* 24: 587–601.

LeGoff DB (2004) Use of LEGO as a therapeutic medium for improving social competence. *J Autism Dev Disord* 34: 557–71.

Leslie KR, Johnson-Frey SH, Grafton ST (2004) Functional imaging of face and hand imitation: towards a motor theory of empathy. *Neuroimage* 21: 601–7.

Lim MM, Young LJ (2004) Vasopressin-dependent neural circuits underlying pair bond formation in the monogamous prairie vole. *Neuroscience* 125: 35–45.

Lord C (1991) Methods and measures of behavior in the diagnosis of autism and related disorders. *Psychiatr Clin North Am* 14: 69–80.

Lord C, Risi S, Lambrecht L, Cook EH, Leventhal BL, DiLavore PC, Pickles A, Rutter M (2000) The Autism Diagnostic Observation Schedule–Generic: a standard measure of social and communication deficits associated with the spectrum of autism. *J Autism Dev Disord* 30: 205–23.

Maestro S, Muratori F, Cavallaro MC, Pei F, Stern D, Golse B, Palacio-Espasa F (2002) Attentional skills during the first 6 months of age in autism spectrum disorder. *J Am Acad Child Adolesc Psychiatry* 41: 1239–45.

McEvoy RE, Rogers SJ, Pennington BF (1993) Executive function and social communication deficits in young autistic children. *J Child Psychol Psychiatry* 34: 563–78.

McPartland J, Dawson G, Webb SJ, Panagiotides H, Carver LJ (2004) Event-related brain potentials reveal anomalies in temporal processing of faces in autism spectrum disorder. *J Child Psychol Psychiatry* 45: 1235–45.

Modahl C, Green L, Fein D, Morris M, Waterhouse L, Feinstein C, Levin H (1998) Plasma oxytocin levels in autistic children. *Biol Psychiatry* 43: 270–7.

Morgan B, Maybery M, Durkin K (2003) Weak central coherence, poor joint attention, and low verbal ability: independent deficits in early autism. *Dev Psychol* 39: 646–56.

Mundy P (2003) The neural basis of social impairments in autism: the role of the dorsal medial–frontal cortex and anterior cingulate system. *J Child Psychol Psychiatry* 44: 793–809.

Mundy P, Crowson M (1997) Joint attention and early social communication: implications for research on intervention with autism. *J Autism Dev Disord* 27: 653–76.

Mundy P, Neal R (2001) Neural plasticity, joint attention and a transactional social-orienting model of autism. *Int Rev Ment Retard* 23: 139–68.

Mundy P, Sigman M, Ungerer J, Sherman T (1986) Defining the social deficits of autism: the contribution of non-verbal communication measures. *J Child Psychol Psychiatry* 27: 657–69.

Mundy P, Sigman M, Ungerer J, Sherman T (1987) Nonverbal communication and play correlates of language development in autistic children. *J Autism Dev Disord* 17: 349–64.

Mundy P, Card J, Fox N (2000) EEG correlates of the development of infant joint attention skills. *Dev Psychobiol* 36: 325–38.

Nikopoulos CK, Keenan M (2004) Effects of video modeling on social initiations by children with autism. *J Appl Behav Anal* 37: 93–6.

Osterling JA, Dawson G, Munson JA (2002) Early recognition of 1-year-old infants with autism spectrum disorder versus mental retardation. *Dev Psychopathol* 14: 239–51.

Ozonoff S, Cook I, Coon H, Dawson G, Joseph RM, Klin A, McMahon WM, Minshew N, Munson JA, Pennington BF, Rogers SJ, Spence MA, Tager-Flusberg H, Volkmar FR, Wrathall D (2004) Performance on Cambridge Neuropsychological Test Automated Battery subtests sensitive to frontal lobe function in people with autistic disorder: evidence from the Collaborative Programs of Excellence in Autism network. *J Autism Dev Disord* 34: 139–50.

Percy AK, Zoghbi HY, Lewis KR, Jankovic J (1988) Rett syndrome: qualitative and quantitative differentiation from autism. *J Child Neurol* 3 suppl: S65–7.

Pierce K, Muller RA, Ambrose J, Allen G, Courchesne E (2001) Face processing occurs outside the fusiform 'face area' in autism: evidence from functional MRI. *Brain* 124: 2059–73.

Pierce K, Haist F, Sedaghat F, Courchesne E (2004) The brain response to personally familiar faces in autism: findings of fusiform activity and beyond. *Brain* 127: 2703–16.

Rizzolatti G, Craighero L (2004) The mirror-neuron system. *Annu Rev Neurosci* 27: 169–92.

Robertson JM, Tanguay PE, L'Ecuyer S, Sims A, Waltrip C (1999) Domains of social communication handicap in autism spectrum disorder. *J Am Acad Child Adolesc Psychiatry* 38: 738–45.

Robins DL, Fein D, Barton ML, Green JA (2001) The Modified Checklist for Autism in Toddlers: an initial study investigating the early detection of autism and pervasive developmental disorders. *J Autism Dev Disord* 31: 131–44.

Rourke BP (1988) Socioemotional disturbances of learning disabled children. *J Consult Clin Psychol* 56: 801–10.

Rourke BP, Finlayson MA (1978) Neuropsychological significance of variations in patterns of academic performance: verbal and visual-spatial abilities. *J Abnorm Child Psychol* 6: 121–33.

Samaco RC, Nagarajan RP, Braunschweig D, LaSalle JM (2004) Multiple pathways regulate MeCP2 expression in normal brain development and exhibit defects in autism-spectrum disorders. *Hum Mol Genet* 13: 629–39.

Schultz RT, Gauthier I, Klin A, Fulbright RK, Anderson AW, Volkmar F, Skudlarski P, Lacadie C, Cohen DJ, Gore JC (2000) Abnormal ventral temporal cortical activity during face discrimination among individuals with autism and Asperger syndrome. *Arch Gen Psychiatry* 57: 331–40.

Schultz RT, Grelotti DJ, Klin A, Kleinman J, Van der Gaag C, Marois R, Skudlarski P (2003) The role of the fusiform face area in social cognition: implications for the pathobiology of autism. *Philos Trans R Soc Lond B Biol Sci* 358: 415–27.

Shaw P, Lawrence EJ, Radbourne C, Bramham J, Polkey CE, David AS (2004) The impact of early and late damage to the human amygdala on 'theory of mind' reasoning. *Brain* 127: 1535–48.

Shields J, Varley R, Broks P, Simpson A (1996) Social cognition in developmental language disorders and high-level autism. *Dev Med Child Neurol* 38: 487–95.

Smalley SL, McCracken J, Tanguay P (1995) Autism, affective disorders, and social phobia. *Am J Med Genet* 60: 19–26.

Sparrevohn R, Howie PM (1995) Theory of mind in children with autistic disorder: evidence of developmental progression and the role of verbal ability. *J Child Psychol Psychiatry* 36: 249–63.

Sturm H, Fernell E, Gillberg C (2004) Autism spectrum disorders in children with normal intellectual levels: associated impairments and subgroups. *Dev Med Child Neurol* 46: 444–7.

Sung YJ, Dawson G, Munson J, Estes A, Schellenberg GD, Wijsman EM (2005) Genetic investigation of quantitative traits related to autism: use of multivariate polygenic models with ascertainment adjustment. *Am J Hum Genet* 76: 68–81.

Tager-Flusberg H (1992) Autistic children's talk about psychological states: deficits in the early acquisition of a theory of mind. *Child Dev* 63: 161–72.

Tomasello M, Farrar MJ (1986) Joint attention and early language. *Child Dev* 57: 1454–63.

Tse WS, Bond AJ (2004) The impact of depression on social skills. *J Nerv Ment Dis* 192: 260–8.

Volkmar FR, Cohen DJ, Bregman JD, Hooks MY, Stevenson JM (1989) An examination of social typologies in autism. *J Am Acad Child Adolesc Psychiatry* 28: 82–6.

Walters AS, Barrett RP, Feinstein C (1990) Social relatedness and autism: current research, issues, directions. *Res Dev Disabil* 11: 303–26.

Wang Z, Aragona BJ (2004) Neurochemical regulation of pair bonding in male prairie voles. *Physiol Behav* 83: 319–28.

Wassink TH, Piven J, Vieland VJ, Pietila J, Goedken RJ, Folstein SE, Sheffield VC (2004) Examination of AVPR1a as an autism susceptibility gene. *Mol Psychiatry* 9: 968–72.

Wellman HM, Hollander M, Schult CA (1996) Young children's understanding of thought bubbles and of thoughts. *Child Dev* 67: 768–88.

Wersinger SR, Kelliher KR, Zufall F, Lolait SJ, O'Carroll AM, Young WS (2004) Social motivation is reduced in vasopressin 1b receptor null mice despite normal performance in an olfactory discrimination task. *Horm Behav* 46: 638–45.

Williams JH, Whiten A, Suddendorf T, Perrett DI (2001) Imitation, mirror neurons and autism. *Neurosci Biobehav Rev* 25: 287–95.

Wing L (1981) Asperger's syndrome: a clinical account. *Psychol Med* 11: 115–29.

Wing L, Gould J (1979) Severe impairments of social interaction and associated abnormalities in children: epidemiology and classification. *J Autism Dev Disord* 9: 11–29.

Winslow JT, Insel TR (2002) The social deficits of the oxytocin knockout mouse. *Neuropeptides* 36: 221–9.

Yirmiya N, Solomonica-Levi D, Shulman C, Pilowsky T (1996) Theory of mind abilities in individuals with autism, Down syndrome, and mental retardation of unknown etiology: the role of age and intelligence. *J Child Psychol Psychiatry* 37: 1003–14.

4

LANGUAGE AND COMMUNICATION: CLINICAL ASSESSMENT AND DIFFERENTIAL DIAGNOSIS

Isabelle Rapin

One of the most frequent ways in which toddlers with autism spectrum disorders (ASDs; autism) present to the physician is lack of, delayed, or inadequate speech or, less frequently, regression of early language and communication. Among 551 consecutive children with either a developmental language disorder (DLD) or autism, the chief complaint of 80% of the parents of those with autism was inadequate language development (Tuchman et al. 1991).

There is a short list of items to consider in the differential diagnosis of a toddler with inadequate language. *Hearing loss* is always the first consideration because of the specific management it mandates, and therefore hearing must be tested definitively in every single child with an inadequate amount of speech or poorly intelligible speech. Besides hearing loss and autism, the other two items in the differential diagnosis are *overall mental retardation* (referred to as developmental delay in some countries) and a *developmental language disorder* (DLD), now often labeled specific language impairment (SLI), a term that implies the absence of an associated deficit of any kind, which is by no means always the case in the clinic. *Selective mutism*, a diagnosis that requires recorded documentation of entirely appropriate speech in some situation, usually the home, is rarely a consideration, although it is sometimes associated with DLD or ASD.

DSM-IV (APA 2000) lists qualitative impairments in communication as manifested by at least one of the following:
(1) delay in, or total lack of, the development of spoken language not accompanied by an attempt to compensate through alternative modes of communication such as gestures or mime
(2) in individuals with adequate speech, marked impairment in the ability to initiate or sustain a conversation with others
(3) stereotyped and repetitive use of language or idiosyncratic language
(4) lack of varied, spontaneous make-believe play or social imitative play appropriate to developmental level. (Perhaps inadequate pretend play, a suggestive marker for autism in preschoolers, was included with language in DSM-IV because even solitary play calls for inner language which is largely verbal.)

BRIEF REVIEW OF THE LEVELS OF LANGUAGE

Language is an arbitrary set of encoded auditory or gestural signals that any group of humans develops in order to facilitate complex and unambiguous communication within the group. Language also plays a critical role in thought. Language is encoded at four levels: (1) *phonology* (individual speech sounds – assessed clinically by speech intelligibility and accuracy of speech sounds – and melody of sentences [prosody]); (2) *grammar* (rules for producing unambiguous sentences, including markers on words [morphology] and word order [syntax]); (3) *semantics* (the lexicon or dictionary of words in the brain, and the meaning of longer utterances); and (4) *pragmatics* (rules that govern communicative speech). For each of these levels, speech/language pathologists and neuropsychologists have devised the batteries of standardized tests they use to provide a detailed quantitative analysis of children's communicative skills.

The *input–processing–output model of language* applies and needs to be considered at each of the four levels of language, keeping in mind that at the language-learning age input disorders will always impair subsequent language operations. Consequently input disorders will present in young children as mixed receptive/expressive disorders, in contrast to output disorders which may exist in isolation. This sequential input–processing–output or bottom-up model is the one familiar to neurologists and the one they use clinically in most diagnostic contexts. It is of course grossly oversimplified because top-down operations are brought on-line as soon as the brain of a verbal individual detects that a sensory input is language. Top-down processing greatly speeds up decoding and decision-making in order to prepare an appropriate response. In short, there are many feedback and feedforward loops at each level of language processing: these will not be considered here.

ASSESSMENT OF LANGUAGE BY THE CHILD NEUROLOGIST

In order to consider the types of language disorders of the toddlers in their offices, child neurologists need to learn to pay attention to the characteristics and quality of children's communication skills (Table 4.1). In particular, does the child use communicative gestures (e.g. point to request or draw attention, head shake to signify "No", nod to mean "Yes"), turn reliably when called, initiate communication, or chatter to no one in particular? It is important to keep in mind that elicited language in children who have been trained with applied behavior analysis (ABA) (an approach based on operant conditioning) may be much superior to their spontaneous language, or their ability to converse which may be dominated by overlearned phrases. In addition, the adequacy of spontaneous language is strongly correlated with the quantitative tests of language abilities that require the expertise of a speech–language pathologist (speech therapist) (Condouris et al. 2003). Results of formal language tests must be interpreted in the context of other cognitive abilities (see Chapter 16).

It will help neurologists to think of language in terms of the familiar input–processing–output model of nervous system disorders. In order to differentiate autism from DLD and mental retardation, they must take into account the *levels of language* involved,

TABLE 4.1
Aspects of language to which the neurologist needs to pay attention

A. Production
  • Amount of speech
  • Communicative use of language (both speech and gestures) - i.e. pragmatics
  • Intelligibility of words - i.e. phonology
  • Complexity and correctness of utterances - i.e. grammar
  • Size and richness of the vocabulary, appropriateness of the words produced, i.e. semantics
  • Abnormal features, e.g. echolalia, scripts, unusual intonation, jargon

B. Comprehension (without visual clues, in and out of context)
  • Words, simple commands
  • Questions (yes/no, either/or, what's/who's that, who, what, where [with referent out of view], when, why, how)
  • Connected speech (discourse)
  • Jokes, metaphors, irony, etc.

C. Conversational use (pragmatics)
  1. Nonverbal pragmatics
     • Orientation to speaker
     • Gaze maintenance
     • Use of gestures to supplement speech
     • Tone of voice
     • Facial expression, etc.
  2. Verbal pragmatics
     • Appropriateness of utterances
     • Intent of utterances (e.g. request, draw attention, comment)
     • Topic maintenance
     • Turn taking
     • Choice of words, etc.

as well as the way in which toddlers use language. They need to be sensitive to *unusual features or frank abnormalities* such as speaking without communicative intent or the need for a communication partner, the use of esoteric words, language that consists mostly of echoes of what was just said or of overlearned formulaic scripts, perseveration, incessant questioning, a wooden rhythm, and a singsong, high pitched or rising tone of voice. Physicians should assess language in a naturalist way, not by asking questions that require only pointing or single word responses, but by brief observation in the office of how the child gestures and uses language conversationally with a parent or themselves, notably during play with representational toys. Therefore child neurologists need to have *in their office* a variety of representational toys, puzzles and books appropriate to the child's age. They need to try to engage the child in conversation and play, which will provide information on the various levels of language, on affect and social skills, and also yield a rough estimate of cognitive level.

I find that I can do this and observe language skills efficiently while reviewing the history with the parents, and later as part of my brief mental status evaluation which complements what I was able to observe during the children's spontaneous activities during history taking. My mental status evaluation usually includes appropriate verbal and non-verbal tasks such as ball playing, puzzles, blocks, drawing, writing/reading, counting, naming and pointing to pictures, telling a story, and answering questions. The key in evaluating children's comprehension is to avoid giving nonverbal cues like gestures or looking.

Neurologists need to consider for their clinical assessment the characteristics of the child's language listed in Table 4.1. They must pay attention to both the output level (*what the child says and the gestures produced*) and the input level (*how well the child comprehends*), keeping in mind that assessment of comprehension is of necessity inferential because failure to respond may indicate not just lack of comprehension but also negativism or lack of attention or drive to communicate. Especially important is to evaluate the *communicative use of speech (pragmatics)* as it is universally involved in autism, as opposed to hearing loss, DLD or mental retardation uncomplicated by autism.

CLINICAL CLASSIFICATION OF THE LANGUAGE OF VERBAL AND NONVERBAL CHILDREN ON THE AUTISM SPECTRUM

A clinically useful way for neurologists to analyze language clinically is to apply the input–processing–output model to (a) the phonology and grammar levels (intelligibility of words and correctness of multiword utterances) and (b) the semantic level (meaningfulness of what the child is saying), paying particular attention throughout to the adequacy of pragmatics (Table 4.2). Using this approach in the clinic, the late Doris A Allen and I, like many other investigators, divided the developmental language disorders of young children into three broad categories: (1) input (+ processing + output, i.e. mixed receptive–expressive) disorders that affect phonologic decoding and consequently all subsequent language operations; (2) output disorders that affect the programming of a verbal output, in particular phonology; and (3) higher order processing disorders that do not affect phonology and are therefore characterized by intelligibility commensurate with the child's age. We divided each of these major types of disorders into two subtypes on the basis of their severity and other salient characteristics (Table 4.2).

Using this clinical classification scheme, we studied the language disorders of consecutively evaluated children with inadequate development of language, regardless of the severity of their communication skills, which means that we included even minimally verbal or nonverbal children, excluding only those with significant hearing losses or severe mental retardation. We subtyped clinically two cohorts that consisted mainly of preschool children with either an ASD or a DLD (Table 4.3) (Tuchman et al. 1991, Allen and Rapin 1992).

Three main differences between children with autism and those with DLD emerged: (1) deficient pragmatics, especially nonverbal pragmatics, characterizes autism, even its

TABLE 4.2
Allen and Rapin clinically defined developmental language subtypes

1. **Input disorders** – mixed receptive/expressive disorders affecting phonology and, consequently, grammar and semantics
   a. *Verbal auditory agnosia ("deafness in the brain")* – inability to decode phonology via the acoustic channel – precludes all subsequent language operations. Language development extremely delayed or absent. Very severe, rare disorder with an often poor prognosis for the development of oral language
      • Comprehension of connected speech: little or none, but may be able to process language presented to the visual channel
      • Expression:
         —*Phonology, grammar, semantics:* all are profoundly impaired. Child nonverbal or minimally verbal with severely impaired phonologic production (few poorly articulated labored single words). May be associated with oromotor deficit (dysarthria). If child otherwise unimpaired, may be able to acquire a visual language (signed or written)
         —*Pragmatics:* very impaired in children on the autism spectrum. Nonautistic children use gestures, may use Sign, pictures, written words
   b. *Mixed phonologic-syntactic disorder* – less severe, much more frequent subtype, with a better prognosis, although reading acquisition often affected
      • Comprehension of connected speech: limited, equal to or somewhat better than expression
      • Expression: dysfluent, often labored
         —*Phonology:* poorly articulated speech
         —*Grammar:* utterances short and with simplified grammar, e.g. missing articles and other function words and word inflexions
         —*Semantics:* impoverished vocabulary and discourse
         —*Pragmatics:* very impaired in children on the autism spectrum. Nonautistic children use gestures, may use Sign, pictures, written words

2. **Output disorders** – expressive language development delayed, phonologic production impaired, comprehension and processing unimpaired
   a. *Dysfluent (verbal dyspraxia)* – the most severe but relatively infrequent expressive disorder, often associated with, but not caused by, dysarthria (oromotor deficit for non-speech sounds and mouth movements, and in some cases generalized dyspaxia). Prognosis for the acquisition of fluent intelligible speech is guarded, therefore the provision of assisted communication (e.g. Sign, pictures, a communication book, an electronic device) must be considered to give the child a means of expression and to limit frustration
      • Comprehension: almost unimpaired
      • Expression:
         —*Phonology* extremely impaired, especially if associated with a severe dysarthria (which is not causative but contributory!). Verbal output may be limited to vowel sounds or to a few consonant sounds in the face of intact or almost intact comprehension at all levels of language
         —*Grammar:* nonexistent in children limited to single sounds or words
         —*Semantics:* cannot be evaluated but comprehension suggests that potentially intact?
         —*Pragmatics:* presumably unaffected judging from gestures and efforts to communicate nonverbally

(continued over...)

TABLE 4.2
(cont'd)

---

b. *Fluent (or more fluent) – speech programming deficit* – relatively frequent disorder
  - Comprehension: almost unimpaired
  - Expression:
    —*Phonology:* many speech sound omissions/distortions. May produce a more or less unintelligible jargon
    —*Grammar:* unimpaired or impaired by difficulty in programming coherent discourse
    —*Semantics:* unimpaired, but may have word retrieval difficulty
    —*Pragmatics:* unimpaired

3. **Higher order processing disorders** – phonology and syntax almost unimpaired – language development delayed or not delayed
   a. *Lexical–syntactic disorder* – language development delayed. This is a relatively frequent disorder
     - Comprehension: adequate at the word level, impaired for connected speech
     - Expression: fluency variable
       —*Phonology:* early on, frequently jargon; later OK
       —*Grammar:* early on, immature; later OK
       —*Semantics:* early on, severe word finding problems – pseudo-stuttering, lexicon impoverished. Impaired programing of discourse. Elicited speech worse than spontaneous speech
       —*Pragmatics:* impairment is indicative of an autism spectrum disorder
   b. *Semantic–pragmatic disorder* – expressive language development usually not delayed. This disorder is particularly frequent in, but not limited to, children on the autism spectrum who are not, or not severely, mentally retarded, notably those with Asperger syndrome
     - Comprehension: unimpaired at the word or simple sentence level, impaired for discourse, especially for open-ended question forms. Typically comprehension is paradoxically worse than expression
     - Expression: fluency unimpaired, chatty, may be verbose
       —*Phonology:* unimpaired
       —*Grammar:* unimpaired
       —*Semantics:* average or (extremely) large lexicon, often atypical in content. Repetitive or poorly constrained discourse, giving the impression of loose associations (not psychosis!)
       —*Pragmatics:* impaired conversational skill, although nonverbal pragmatics mostly spared in children who are not on the autism spectrum

---

NOTE 1. Pragmatics:
- *Nonverbal pragmatics* universally impaired in the autism spectrum disorders (ASDs), preserved or at most mildly impaired in "specific" (uncomplicated) developmental language disorders (DLDs)
- *Verbal pragmatics* depend largely on the severity of the language disorder, notably comprehension, in both DLDs and ASDs

NOTE 2. Abnormal features suggesting an ASD rather than a DLD:
- *Striking pragmatic impairment*, both nonverbal and verbal, lack of awareness of the power of language, lack of the drive to communicate, speaking to speak rather than to communicate
- *Atypical prosody:* e.g. high pitched, singsong, rising intonation in assertions, robotic rhythm
- *Echolalia:* immediate or delayed (formulaic language, scripted speech), perseveration
- *Esoteric word choices*
- *Comprehension paradoxically more impaired than expression*
- *Purely expressive disorders:* not characteristic of children with an ASD!

TABLE 4.3
Distribution of Allen and Rapin clinical developmental language subtypes in young autistic and dysphasic children

Study	Diagnosis	Language disorder subtypes (% of group)			
		Mixed receptive/expressive		Expressive[1]	Higher order processing[2]
		VAA	Phonologic–syntactic		
Tuchman et al. (1991)	Autistic (N=197)	9	59	0	32
	DLD (N=215)	5	53	33	9
Allen and Rapin (1992)	Autistic (N=229)	63		0	37
	DLD (N=170)	50		35	15

Abbreviations: DLD = developmental language disorder; VAA = verbal auditory agnosia.
[1]Expressive: verbal dyspraxia / speech programming deficit.
[2]Higher order processing: lexical–syntactic / semantic–pragmatic disorder.

least severe variants (including cases now labeled Asperger syndrome); (2) purely expressive disorders do not occur in young children with autism because their comprehension is invariably impaired, with the possible exception of an occasional intelligent child in whom expression is so much worse than comprehension as to perhaps fulfill criteria for verbal dyspraxia; and (3) there is a major difference in the prevalence of language subtypes in autism and DLD, with the semantic–pragmatic disorder being more prevalent in autism than in DLD. The suggestion that verbal auditory agnosia (VAA) or word deafness was also more prevalent in autism was supported in another study (Klein et al. 2000). I stress here that there is a range of severity within the subtypes. The Allen and Rapin clinical subtypes must not be taken as independently validated. They are offered as guidelines suitable for child neurologists and other physicians attempting to characterize the communication deficits of young children with autism or DLDs. Attempts to subtype language disorders in DLD and ASD with standardized language and neuropsychologic tests have generated a number of subtypes but no universally accepted classification scheme.

This clinical view of ASD children as comprising several subtypes of language disorders which map onto some of those of children with DLD represented a major departure from virtually every other study of language in autism over the past quarter century, most of which focused on relatively intelligent verbal – and for the most part older – children, or which compared the language of verbal children with ASD to that of children with DLD or mental retardation (e.g. Baltaxe and Simmons 1975; Bartak et al. 1977; Swisher and Demetras 1985; Tager-Flusberg 1989, 2003; Beitchman and Inglis 1991; Lord and Paul 1997; Wilkinson 1998; Tager-Flusberg and Joseph 2003; Tager-Flusberg et al. 2005). Most studies excluded nonverbal children, assuming that the severity of their autism or associated mental retardation accounted for their lack of speech.

These formal studies emphasized the discrepancy between having higher lexical scores than scores on tests of comprehension of discourse, yet deficient understanding of inferences, metaphors and jokes. Most of the studies attributed these language deficits to cognitive limitations such as concreteness and to impaired theory of mind (see Chapter 3), that is to poor insight into what a conversational partner might be thinking. The classical impression of language in autism was that language is often delayed but that phonologic deficit, if present at all, clears rapidly. These descriptions correspond closely to the higher order language processing deficits of Allen and Rapin, in particular to the semantic–pragmatic disorder subtype for the fully fluent children, and the lexical–syntactic subtype for those with early delay followed by unusually rapid progress in phonology, syntax and vocabulary.

Recent identification of linkage to chromosome 7q31-33 of individuals with autism who have non-autistic family members who spoke or read late – but not of individuals without family members with these deficits (Bradford et al. 2001, Wassink et al. 2001) – provides empirical evidence for the existence of more than one language disorder sub-type in autism. The *FOXP2* gene at the SPCH1 locus on 7q21 is implicated in a family with a severe mixed language disorder inherited as a dominant trait (Lai et al. 2003). Even if linked to some individuals with autism and thus one of many genes relevant to autism, it is not a major autism gene (McCoy et al. 2002, Li et al. 2005).

Study of a school-age group of 82 children who, at preschool, fulfilled criteria for DSM-III-R autistic disorder (Rapin 1996) also supports more than a single subtype of language disorder in autism. Cluster analysis using scores on a standardized test of phono-logic production and one of comprehension of discourse suggested an optimal three-cluster solution (personal data, unpublished). Cluster 1 includes children in whom both production and comprehension of short sentences remain impaired. Children in cluster 2 have low-normal phonology, but comprehension is impaired in the majority. All of those in cluster 3 have unimpaired phonology, and comprehension is adequate or excel-lent in half of them who, by these crude criteria, would no longer be considered language impaired. This latter conclusion may not be valid, however, because the two measures used provide no information on the more complex aspects of language such as lexical retrieval, formulation of discourse, or pragmatic skills, aspects captured in naturalistic clinical evaluation of communication. The clusters are roughly consonant with the clin-ically defined global receptive–expressive disorder (cluster 1), mixed receptive–expressive or lexical–syntactic subtype (cluster 2), and the semantic–pragmatic disorder (cluster 3). Note, however, that the Allen–Rapin subtypes were developed for preschool, not school-age children, and that the cluster study is limited because the children had not been subtyped clinically at preschool; consequently it provides no information on developmental change in language-subtype membership for individual children, or on changes with maturation in the characteristics of the subtypes.

NEUROLOGIC CORRELATES OF LANGUAGE ABNORMALITIES IN AUTISM

Recent technologic advances have made it possible to study the anatomic and physiologic basis of language processing in autism (see Chapters 8 and 10). For example, recent studies of Herbert and collaborators (Herbert et al. 2002, 2005; De Fosse et al. 2004) indicate that reversed asymmetry of language-associated temporo-parietal and frontal areas characterizes both children with autism and those with DLD, which supports the idea that the language disorders of those with autism have overlaps with those of children with DLDs. Functional magnetic resonance imaging (fMRI) studies suggest that acoustic language, as opposed to other sounds, fails to activate temporal auditory association cortex in autistic children (Boddaert and Zilbovicius 2002), that a language task activates right frontal language areas in autism compared to left frontal areas in controls (Takeuchi et al. 2004), and that activation of Wernicke's and Broca's areas is less well synchronized during sentence comprehension in autism than controls (Just et al. 2004).

Detailed audiometric testing and electrophysiology show that auditory processing deficits in children with autism do not involve relays of the subcortical auditory pathway, including the brainstem, unless the child has a hearing loss (Jure et al. 1991, Klin 1993, Gravel et al. 2006). Auditory non-language and language stimuli produce a number of changes in the stimulus-related spectral content of the background electroencephalogram (EEG) and event-related potentials (ERPs) in normally developing children. Steinschneider and Dunn (2002) review some of these changes and others in children with language disorders and in the few studies in children with autism. Several ERP studies confirm atypical hemispheric lateralization of language suggested by MRI morphometry and fMRI studies. In 4- to 8-year-old children with mental retardation and autism, the N1c component of auditory ERPs over temporal auditory association cortex bilaterally was delayed by some 20 ms; it was of lower amplitude than in normal and non-autistic mentally retarded children and its amplitude did not increase with stimulus intensity, as expected, on the left (Bruneau et al. 1999). The mismatch negativity elicited by automatic discrimination of a stimulus change like an infrequent deviant sound was elicited both in 12-year-old mentally retarded boys with autism (Ferri et al. 2003) and in high functioning children with autism, regardless of whether the stimulus was a simple or complex tone or a vowel (Ceponiene et al. 2003). The nature of the stimulus did affect involuntary orienting, indexed by the later P3a component, in that it was normal to both simple and complex tonal changes but not to vowel changes. In the retarded boys the amplitude of both the mismatch negativity and P3a was increased, conceivably as a correlate of heightened sensitivity to sound. In a semantic classification task (animals vs non-animals), there was no amplitude difference to rare non-animal words (targets) than to animals in high functioning children with autism who were as accurate as, albeit slower than, controls (Dunn et al. 1999). This finding is consistent with decreased influence of semantic context on their language (Dunn et al. 1996).

LANGUAGE REGRESSION

The other complaint besides delayed or lack of speech development that often brings young children to the neurologist is parents' awareness that their child's early language skills regressed or disappeared, at a mean age of 18–24 months, usually gradually but occasionally abruptly (Kurita 1985, Shinnar et al. 2001, Sy et al. 2003). When language regression is insidious and occurs before language is fully established, regression of communication may pass unnoticed for many months or until it is obvious that the child is not speaking at all. In some cases parents minimize the importance of language regression because it follows a nonspecific illness, an immunization, or a psychic trauma like the absence of the mother or the birth of a younger sibling. The parents' assumption is that the regression is but a temporary emotional reaction, or an inadequately informed physician may reassure them that it is but an insignificant developmental variation. It is only when regression is abrupt in a child who spoke more than a handful of words or occurs in the context of a seizure or following a significant illness that it will bring the child promptly to a neurologist with the question of whether the regression is the harbinger of an infection or degenerative disease of the brain, a mass lesion, or represents acquired epileptic aphasia (Landau–Kleffner syndrome [LKS], discussed in Chapter 11). Unless asked about regression of behavior and other skills as well as language (Goldberg et al. 2003), parents may not mention it. Consequently they need to be asked specifically about lack of attempts to communicate nonverbally with gestures, failure to respond when called by name, ignoring of other children and persons in the environment, impoverished and repetitive play, rigidity, temper tantrums, and stereotypies such as hand flapping, running around in circles, and gazing at their wiggling fingers or the spinning wheels of a car.

When asked specifically, about a third of all parents of children on the autism spectrum will report that their children underwent a regression of communication *and* other skills. It is important to stress that, whereas regression occurs in some children whose early development gave no cause for concern, careful questioning often elicits evidence for pre-existing, but much milder, autistic features (Werner and Dawson 2005). Prospective studies and earlier video recordings in small groups of children have shown beyond question that autistic/language regression is real (Lord et al. 2004, Luyster et al. 2005, Werner and Dawson 2005). An attractive but thus far unvalidated hypothesis is that regression might result from a "second hit" in a genetically vulnerable child, that is, that an emotional stress or what would be in most children a trivial intercurrent infection or immune mechanism might precipitate the regression (McVicar and Shinnar 2004). Extensive epidemiologic evidence does not support live measles-mumps-rubella vaccine as a likely culprit (Madsen et al. 2002, Fombonne and Cook 2003). Whether regression carries with it a worse prognosis than autism without regression remains controversial (Harper and Williams 1975, Rogers and DiLalla 1990, Kurita 1996, Kobayashi and Murata 1998, Lainhart et al. 2002). Equally controversial is whether autism with and without regression represent two biologically distinct disorders.

Degenerative diseases of the brain and mass lesions are exceedingly rare causes of early language regression with autistic features. Consequently, in the absence of suspicious symptoms in the family or past medical history, or of findings on the neurologic examination, the yield of imaging tests such as MRI for evidence of a structural brain lesion like a neoplasm or other medically treatable condition is very low. The same is true of extensive metabolic or immunologic tests to screen for lysosomal, peroxisomal, mitochondrial and other diagnosable genetic or immune disorders. Because the risk is so low, I strongly recommend these expensive tests *not* be performed routinely (as opposed to the extensive evaluations that need to be carried out with parents' consent in the context of some *formal research studies* designed to further our understanding of the biology of autism). EEG investigation is recommended if there is a history or suspicion of clinical seizures. The more difficult and controversial subject is whether to do an EEG in a child with language regression without clinical seizures. A recent study (McVicar et al. 2005) compared the overnight EEG results of children with isolated language regression to those of children with language and autistic regression. This study found that children with isolated language regression were more likely to have epileptiform discharges than those with both language regression and a more global autistic regression. An interesting and important finding in this study was that the electrical status epilepticus during slow wave sleep (ESES) EEG pattern was almost exclusively (10 of 11 children) found in those with isolated language regression. The present recommendation of the American Academy of Neurology guidelines for autism is to obtain an EEG only if there is a suspicion of subclinical epilepsy in a child with autism and a significant history of regression in language and social communication (Filipek et al. 2000). This recommendation is based in part on weak evidence that medication is indicated unless there is clinical evidence of epilepsy or an ESES pattern is found in the EEG, which do require medication. What to do with a few spikes in the EEG in the absence of clinical seizures remains controversial (Deonna and Roulet-Perez 2005). Simultaneous EEG and video monitoring of the child is cost-effective when it is unclear whether unusual behaviors or staring spells represent seizures or not.

PROGNOSIS

Quantitative tests of language are crucial for formal prognostic studies and individual educational plans. These tests are designed to assess comprehension and production of the language levels listed in Table 4.1, which are the same ones clinicians need to be cognizant of in their clinical evaluations. Although clinical evaluation does not yield quantitative data, it is superior to most formal tests in its sensitivity to the conversational, communicative use of language because attention is automatically paid to nonverbal as well as the verbal pragmatics. Neurologists, like other consumers of quantitative reports, need to be aware that verbal IQ subtests are not language tests, although they do provide a "quick and dirty" comparison with nonverbal cognitive abilities. Neither are questionnaires to parents such as the Autistic Diagnostic Inventory–Revised (ADI-R) (Lord et al. 1994), which enquires specifically about language regression, or the Communication subscale of the Vineland Adaptive Behavior Scales (Sparrow et al. 1984), which provides insight into language use. Valid testing requires "hands-on" assessment of children, not just easier-to-obtain questionnaires to parents or caretakers. Child neurologists need to have observed formal language and neuropsychological testing so that they are aware of the general content of tests and of their limitations.

Speech pathology textbooks exist in many languages that list formal tests for evaluating the distinct levels of language in children of various ages. Likely to be included are some translations of tests developed and extensively validated in another language, which have not necessarily been restandardized to take into account significant cultural differences among languages. Many formal language tests have been standardized on relatively small samples of normally speaking children for use in those with developmental language disorders, and are borrowed for children with autism whose scores may be lowered by other problems such as impaired imitation, lack of motivation or low IQ. Quantitative tests are invaluable, but clinicians need to be aware that they have limitations and that the scores they provide need to be interpreted in light of their own clinical assessment of the individual child.

Prognosis for language is unreliable in the individual toddler. As one would expect, children in whom language develops by school-age have a better prognosis than those who remain nonverbal (Nordin and Gillberg 1998). Language generally improves with age, but improvement depends on the type of language dysfunction, the severity of the cognitive deficits, and the age at which appropriate intervention was made available (Ballaban-Gil et al. 1996, Goldstein 2002, Howlin 2003). The severity of the comprehension deficit interacts with cognitive level to influence prognosis, even in verbal individuals (Tyler et al. 1997; Howlin et al. 2000, 2004; Mawhood et al. 2000). Comprehension may improve in some intelligent children with higher order processing deficits to the point where even metaphors and jokes are understood, but subtle prosodic and more-or-less overt pragmatic deficits tend to persist, and even minor comprehension deficits are likely to jeopardize social and vocational outcomes. Progress in children with mixed receptive/expressive deficits is variable and, as one would expect, poorest in children with VAA who may remain essentially nonverbal and severely cognitively impaired (Klein et al. 2000). As in children with DLD, inadequate phonological skills are often the harbingers of inadequate reading. The importance of early intervention tailored to the child's particular deficits cannot be overemphasized (National Research Council 2001). This recommendation is based on clinical experience and on pre/post studies of change with a variety of interventions, although controlled studies comparing various interventions in well matched samples have yet to be carried out.

INTERVENTION

This chapter will not go in any depth into therapeutic options for children with autism; readers are referred to Chapter 17 for a consideration of recommended interventions. The role of neurologists is to make sure that appropriate referrals for both evaluation and management have been provided and that the interventions offered by specialized teachers and other therapists are focused on each child's particular needs. Inadequate ability to communicate has such serious consequences in everyday life that psychiatric referral may be needed so that these can be addressed more effectively. The major goal of language intervention is to stress to parents and professionals a developmental communication approach and not just the teaching of words out of the context of communicative intent. The concept that communication through any channel is power is something that children with autism need to *learn* early on. Neurologists are often called upon to reassure parents that presenting language by eye as well as by ear will hasten, not delay, the acquisition of oral language, and that the focus of intervention must not be on articulation but on language use in the context of play and everyday activities. Physicians can remind parents that speaking of what is happening in the here and now is helpful because it provides a less fleeting visual referent than the spoken word. Another point that regularly needs emphasis is that comprehension may lag far behind expression in fluent children with sophisticated vocabularies and that making sure that messages have been understood may decrease preschoolers' frustration and tantrums.

Regarding medications, neurologists need to remind themselves and others, in particular parents, that there is no specific medication to help children acquire language. Reports of language improvement in children given fluoxetine (DeLong et al. 1998), or in those with a history or regression treated with steroids, anticonvulsants (Deonna and Roulet-Perez 2005) or immunomodulating treatments, or in children with autistic regression who do not have a structural lesion on MRI or intractable epilepsy treated with neurosurgical approaches such as subpial transection (Nass et al. 1999, Taylor et al. 1999) are still anecdotal and require replication. Neurologists need to tell parents that they do not endorse non-traditional alternative treatments and condemn the use of those for which rigorous well controlled studies have demonstrated lack of efficacy, treatments that are often exploitative. There is of course no point in arguing with parents who make the ultimate decision about what they think is best for their child, but it is the neurologists' and other professionals' duty to try to gain parents' confidence and provide them with scientifically based and updated information as they follow the children.

REFERENCES

Allen DA, Rapin I (1992) Autistic children are also dysphasic. In: Naruse H, Ornitz E, eds. *Neurobiology of Infantile Autism.* Amsterdam: Excerpta Medica, pp. 73–80.

APA (2000) *Diagnostic and Statistical Manual of Mental Disorders, 4th edn, text revision: DSM-IV-TR.* Washington, DC: American Psychiatric Association.

Ballaban-Gil K, Rapin I, Tuchman RF, Shinnar S (1996) Longitudinal examination of the behavioral, language, and social changes in a population of adolescents and young adults with autistic disorder. *Pediatr Neurol* 15: 217–23.

Baltaxe CAM, Simmons JQI (1975) Language in childhood psychosis: A review. *J Speech Hear Disord* 40: 439–58.

Bartak L, Rutter M, Cox A (1977) A comparative study of infantile autism and specific developmental receptive language disorders. III. Discriminant function analysis. *J Autism Child Schizophr* 7: 383-396.

Beitchman JH, Inglis A (1991) The continuum of linguistic dysfunction from pervasive developmental disorders to dyslexia. *Psychiatr Clin N Am* 14: 95–111.

Boddaert N, Zilbovicius M (2002) Functional neuroimaging and childhood autism. *Pediatr Radiol* 32: 1–7.

Bradford Y, Haines J, Hutcheson H, Gardiner M, Braun T, Sheffield V, Cassavant T, Huang W, Wang K, Vieland V, Folstein S, Santangelo S, Piven J (2001) Incorporating language phenotypes strengthens evidence of linkage to autism. *Am J Med Genet* 105: 539–47. Erratum in: *Am J Med Genet* 105: 805.

Bruneau N, Roux S, Adrien JL, Barthelemy C (1999) Auditory associative cortex dysfunction in children with autism: evidence from late auditory evoked potentials (N1 wave-T complex). *Clin Neurophysiol* 110: 1927–34.

Ceponiene R, Lepisto T, Shestakova A, Vanhala R, Alku P, Naatanen R, Yaguchi K (2003) Speech-sound-selective auditory impairment in children with autism: they can perceive but do not attend. *Proc Natl Acad Sci USA* 100: 5567–72.

Condouris K, Meyer E, Tager-Flusberg H (2003) The relationship between standardized measures of language and measures of spontaneous speech in children with autism. *Am J Speech Lang Pathol* 12: 349–58.

De Fosse L, Hodge SM, Makris N, Kennedy DN, Caviness VS, McGrath L, Steele S, Ziegler DA, Herbert MR, Frazier JA, Tager-Flusberg H, Harris GJ (2004) Language-association cortex asymmetry in autism and specific language impairment. *Ann Neurol* 56: 757–66.

DeLong GR, Teague LA, McSwain Kamran M (1998) Effects of fluoxetine treatment on language in young children with autism. *Dev Med Child Neurol* 40: 551–62.

Deonna T, Roulet-Perez E (2005) *Cognitive and Behavioral Disorders of Epileptic Origin in Children. Clinics in Developmental Medicine No. 168.* London: Mac Keith Press.

Dunn M, Gomes H, Sebastian M (1996) Prototypicality of responses in autistic language disordered and normal children in a verbal fluency task. *Child Neuropsychol* 2: 99-108.

Dunn M, Vaughan HG, Kreutzer J, Kurtzberg D (1999) Electrophysiologic correlates of semantic classification in autistic and normal children. *Dev Neuropsychol* 16: 75–99.

Ferri R, Elia M, Agarwal N, Lanuzza B, Musumeci SA, Pennisi G (2003) The mismatch negativity and the P3a components of the auditory event-related potentials in autistic low-functioning subjects. *Clin Neurophysiol* 114: 1671–80.

Filipek PA, Accardo PJ, Ashwal S, Baranek GT, Cook EH, Dawson G, Gordon B, Gravel JS, Johnson CP, Kallen RJ, Levy SE, Minshew NJ, Ozonoff S, Prizant BM, Rapin I, Rogers SJ, Stone WL, Teplin SW, Tuchman RF, Volkmar FR (2000) Practice parameter: screening and diagnosis of autism: report of the Quality Standards Subcommittee of the American Academy of Neurology and the Child Neurology Society. *Neurology* 55: 468–79.

Fombonne E, Cook EH (2003) MMR and autistic enterocolitis: consistent epidemiological failure to find an association. *Mol Psychiatry* 8: 133–4.

Goldberg WA, Osann K, Filipek PA, Laulhere T, Jarvis K, Modahl C, Flodman P, Spence MA (2003) Language and other regression: assessment and timing. *J Autism Dev Disord* 33: 607–16.

Goldstein H (2002) Communication intervention for children with autism: a review of treatment efficacy. *J Autism Dev Disord* 32: 373–96.

Gravel JS, Dunn M, Lee WW, Ellis MA (2006) Peripheral audition of children on the autistic spectrum. *Ear Hear* 27: 299–312.

Harper J, Williams S (1975) Age and type of onset as critical variables in early infantile autism. *J Autism Child Schizophr* 5: 25–36.

Herbert MR, Harris GJ, Adrien KT, Ziegler DA, Makris N, Kennedy DN, Lange NT, Chabris CF, Bakardjiev A, Hodgson J, Takeoka M, Tager-Flusberg H, Caviness VS (2002) Abnormal asymmetry in language association cortex in autism. *Ann Neurol* 52: 588–96.

Herbert MR, Ziegler DA, Deutsch CK, O'Brien LM, Kennedy DN, Filipek PA, Bakardjiev AI, Hodgson J, Takeoka M, Makris N, Caviness VS (2005) Brain asymmetries in autism and developmental language disorder: a nested whole-brain analysis. *Brain* 128: 213–26.

Howlin P (2003) Outcome in high-functioning adults with autism with and without early language delays: implications for the differentiation beween autism and Asperger syndrome. *J Autism Dev Disord* 33: 3–13.

Howlin P, Mawhood L, Rutter M (2000) Autism and developmental receptive language disorder— a follow-up comparison in early adult life. II: Social, behavioural, and psychiatric outcomes. *J Child Psychol Psychiatry* 41: 561–78.

Howlin P, Goode S, Hutton J, Rutter M (2004) Adult outcome for children with autism. *J Child Psychol Psychiatry* 45: 212–29.

Jure R, Rapin I, Tuchman RF (1991) Hearing-impaired autistic children. *Dev Med Child Neurol* 33: 1062–72.

Just MA, Cherkassky VL, Keller TA, Minshew NJ (2004) Cortical activation and synchronization during sentence comprehension in high-functioning autism: evidence of underconnectivity. *Brain* 127: 1811–21.

Klein SK, Tuchman RF, Rapin I (2000) The influence of premorbid language skills and behavior on language recovery in children with verbal auditory agnosia. *J Child Neurol* 15: 36–43.

Klin A (1993) Auditory brain stem responses in autism: Brain stem dysfunction or peripheral hearing loss? *J Autism Dev Disord* 23: 15–35.

Kobayashi R, Murata T (1998) Setback phenomenon in autism and long-term prognosis. *Acta Psychiatr Scand* 98: 296–303.

Kurita H (1985) Infantile autism with speech loss before the age of thirty months. *J Am Acad Child Adolesc Psychiatry* 24: 191–6.

Kurita H (1996) Specificity and developmental consequences of speech loss in children with pervasive developmental disorders. *Psychiatry Clin Neurosci* 50: 181–4.

Lai CS, Gerrelli D, Monaco AP, Fisher SE, Copp AJ (2003) FOXP2 expression during brain development coincides with adult sites of pathology in a severe speech and language disorder. *Brain* 126: 2455–62.

Lainhart JE, Ozonoff S, Coon H, Krasny L, Dinh E, Nice J, McMahon W (2002) Autism, regression, and the broader autism phenotype. *Am J Med Genet* 113: 231–7.

Li H, Yamagata Y, Mori M, Momoi MY (2005) Absence of causative mutations and presence of autism-related allele in FOXP2 in Japanese autistic patients. *Brain Dev* 27: 207–10.

Lord C, Paul R (1997) Language and communication in autism. In: Cohen DJ, Volkmar F R, eds. *Handbook of Autism and Pervasive Developmental Disorders, 2nd edn.* New York: John Wiley, pp. 195-225.

Lord C, Rutter M, Le Couteur A (1994) Autism Diagnostic Interview–Revised: A revised version of a diagnostic interview for caregivers of individuals with possible pervasive developmental disorders. *J Autism Dev Disord* 24: 659–85.

Lord C, Shulman C, DiLavore P (2004) Regression and word loss in autistic spectrum disorders. *J Child Psychol Psychiatry* 45: 936–55.

Luyster R, Richler J, Risi S, Hsu WL, Dawson G, Bernier R, Dunn M, Hepburn S, Hyman SL, McMahon WM, Goudie-Nice J, Minshew N, Rogers S, Sigman M, Spence MA, Goldberg WA, Tager-Flusberg H, Volkmar FR, Lord C (2005) Early regression in social communication in autism spectrum disorders: a CPEA Study. *Dev Neuropsychol* 27: 311–36.

Madsen KM, Hviid A, Vestergaard M, Schendel D, Wohlfahrt J, Thorsen P, Olsen J, Melbye M (2002) A population-based study of measles, mumps, and rubella vaccination and autism. *N Engl J Med* 347: 1477–82.

Mawhood L, Howlin P, Rutter M (2000) Autism and developmental receptive language disorder— a comparative follow-up in early adult life. I: Cognitive and language outcomes. *J Child Psychol Psychiatry* 41: 547–59.

McCoy PA, Shao Y, Wolpert CM, Donnelly SL, Ashley-Koch A, Abel HL, Ravan SA, Abramson RK, Wright HH, DeLong GR, Cuccaro ML, Gilbert JR, Pericak-Vance MA (2002) No association between the WNT2 gene and autistic disorder. *Am J Med Genet* 114: 106–9.

McVicar KA, Shinnar S (2004) Landau–Kleffner syndrome, electrical status epilepticus in sleep, and language regression in children. *Ment Retard Dev Disabil Res Rev* 10: 144–9.

McVicar KA, Ballaban-Gil K, Rapin I, Moshé SL, Shinnar S (2005) Epileptiform EEG abnormalities in children with language regression. *Neurology* 65: 129–31.

Nass R, Gross A, Wisoff J, Devinsky O (1999) Outcome of multiple subpial transections for autistic epileptiform regression. *Pediatr Neurol* 21: 464–70.

National Research Council (2001) *Educating Children with Autism.* Washington DC: National Academy Press.

Nordin V, Gillberg C (1998) The long-term course of autistic disorders: update on follow-up studies. *Acta Psychiatr Scand* 97: 99–108.

Rapin I (1996) Neurological examination. In: Rapin I, ed. *Preschool Children with Inadequate Communication: Developmental Language Disorder, Autism, Low IQ. Clinics in Developmental Medicine No. 139.* London: Mac Keith Press, pp. 98–122.

Rogers SJ, DiLalla DL (1990) Age of symptom onset in young children with pervasive developmental disorders. *J Am Acad Child Adolesc Psychiatry* 6: 863–72.

Shinnar S, Rapin I, Arnold S, Tuchman RF, Shulman L, Ballaban-Gil K, Maw M, Deuel RK, Volkmar FR (2001) Language regression in childhood. *Pediatr Neurol* 24: 185–91.

Sparrow SS, Balla DA, Cicchetti DV (1984) *Vineland Adaptive Behavior Scales: A Revision of the Vineland Social Maturity Scale by Edgar Doll.* Circle Pines, MN: American Guidance Service.

Steinschneider M, Dunn M (2002) Electrophysiology in developmental neuropsychology. In: Segalowitz S, Rapin I, eds. *Handbook of Neuropsychology, vol. 8. Child Neuropsychology, 2nd edn.* Amsterdam: Elsevier Science, pp. 91–146.

Swisher L, Demetras MJ (1985) The expressive language characteristics of autistic children compared with mentally retarded or specific language-impaired children. In: Schopler E, Mesibov G, eds. *Communication Problems in Autism.* New York: Plenum Press, pp. 147–62.

Sy W, Djukic A, Shinnar S, Dharmani C, Rapin I (2003) Clinical characteristics of language regression in children. *Dev Med Child Neurol* 45: 508–14.

Tager-Flusberg H (1989) A psycholinguistic perspective on language development in the autistic child. In: Dawson G, ed. *Autism: Nature, Diagnosis, and Treatment.* New York: Guilford Press, pp. 92–109.

Tager-Flusberg H (2003) Language impairments in children with complex neurodevelopmental disorders: The case of autism. In: Levy Y, Schaeffer J, eds. *Language Competence Across Populations: Toward a Definition of Specific Language Impairment.* Mahwah, NJ: Lawrence Erlbaum, pp. 297–321.

Tager-Flusberg H, Joseph RM (2003) Identifying neurocognitive phenotypes in autism. *Philos Trans R Soc Lond B Biol Sci* 358: 303–14.

Tager-Flusberg H, Paul R, Lord C (2005) Language and communication in autism. In: Volkmar FR, Paul R, Klin A, Cohen D, eds. *Handbook of Autism and Pervasive Developmental Disorders, 3rd edn.* Hoboken, NJ: John Wiley, pp. 335–64.

Takeuchi M, Harada M, Matsuzaki K, Nishitani H, Mori K (2004) Difference of signal change by a language task on autistic patients using functional MRI. *J Med Invest* 51: 59–62.

Taylor DC, Neville BG, Cross JH (1999) Autistic spectrum disorders in childhood epilepsy surgery candidates. *Eur Child Adolesc Psychiatry* 8: 189–92.

Tuchman RF, Rapin I, Shinnar S (1991) Autistic and dysphasic children. I: Clinical characteristics. *Pediatrics* 88: 1211–8.

Tyler LK, Karmiloff-Smith A, Voice JK, Stevens T, Grant J, Udwin O, Davies M, Howlin P (1997) Do individuals with Williams syndrome have bizarre semantics? Evidence for lexical organization using an on-line task. *Cortex* 33: 515–27.

Wassink TH, Piven J, Vieland VJ, Huang J, Swiderski RE, Pietila J, Braun T, Beck G, Folstein SE, Haines JL, Sheffield VC (2001) Evidence supporting WNT2 as an autism susceptibility gene. *Am J Med Genet* 105: 406–13.

Werner E, Dawson G (2005) Validation of the phenomenon of autistic regression using home videotapes. *Arch Gen Psychiatry* 62: 889–95.

Wilkinson P (1998) Profiles of language and communication skills in autism. *Ment Retard Dev Disabil Res Rev* 4: 73–9.

5

STEREOTYPIES AND REPETITIVE BEHAVIORS: CLINICAL ASSESSMENT AND BRAIN BASIS

Jonathan W Mink and David E Mandelbaum

Diagnostic criteria for autism include the presence of "restricted, repetitive and stereo-typed patterns of behavior, interest and activities" (APA 1994). This criterion covers a broad range of behaviors including repetitive movements, more complex compulsive behaviors, excessive preoccupation with cognitive themes, and resisting change in routines. These behaviors typically emerge in early childhood and can persist into adult-hood. While they are part of the diagnostic criteria for autism, none of these behaviors is seen exclusively in autism; they may also occur in individuals with sensory deficits and non-autistic developmental disabilities, or in otherwise normal children. This chapter will review research on stereotyped repetitive behaviors in autism, discuss possible underlying neurobiological mechanisms, and review current knowledge of treatment options.

DEFINITION AND PHENOMENOLOGY

Much has been written about repetitive behaviors in autism. They are often lumped together, but some studies have focused on specific types. Because these behaviors are phenomenologically and may be biologically different, it is reasonable to try to place them into discrete categories. One scheme is contained in the Repetitive Behavior Scale (Bodfish et al. 2000). The categories include stereotypy, self-injury, compulsions, rituals, sameness, and restriction. In addition, individuals with autism may have other repetitive movements including tics and akathisia (Bodfish et al. 2000). Furthermore, individuals with autism are frequently treated with medications that might lead to drug-induced or tardive dyskinesia (Campbell et al. 1990). For studies of repetitive behaviors in autism, it is important to be clear what behaviors are being studied and whether the behaviors are primary or due to medication.

Stereotypies are rhythmic, patterned, repetitive, purposeless, involuntary movements. Examples of stereotypies include body rocking, head nodding, walking in circles, hand flapping or clapping, finger wiggling, and facial grimacing. Some stereotyped movements may occur in the setting of object manipulations, including spinning or twirling items, but manipulation of objects is not required for stereotypies to occur. Stereotypies are rhythmic and continual, and tend to change little over time. By contrast, tics are non-

TABLE 5.1
Comparison of tics and stereotypies*

	Tics	Stereotypies
Age of onset	6–7 years	<2 years
Pattern	Variable, wax and wane	Fixed, identical, patterned, predictable
Movements	Blink, grimace, twist, shrug	Arms/hands (flap, wave), body rocking, pacing
Rhythm	Rapid, sudden, random	Rhythmic
Duration	Intermittent, brief, abrupt	Intermittent, continuous, prolonged
Premonitory urge	Yes	No
Precipitant	Excitement, stress	Excitement, stress, also when engrossed
Suppression	Brief (inner tension)	With distraction, rare conscious effort
Family history	Frequently positive	May be positive
Treatment	Clonidine, neuroleptics	Less responsive

*Modified from Mahone et al. (2004).

rhythmic and discrete, typically change in location and type over time, and wax and wane in frequency and severity (Table 5.1). Akathisia is an internal sensation of restlessness that leads to repetitive movements, such as pacing. However, the movements in response to akathisia are typically not stereotyped and patterned. Thus, while pacing is a common behavior associated with akathisia, the pacing is more variable than with pacing stereotypies. Stereotypies appear purposeless, unlike compulsions and rituals. Other terms have been used to describe stereotypies, including "rhythmic habit patterns", "gratification phenomena", "self-stimulation" and "motor rhythmias".

Self-injurious behaviors are stereotyped, repetitive actions that have the potential to cause injury to oneself. The injury can be minimal or severe. Examples of self-injurious behaviors include hitting oneself with a hand or object, hitting a body part against an object (e.g. head banging), biting, scratching, pulling hair, skin picking, or inserting a finger into an eye or ear. These behaviors are different from stereotypies, but may overlap with compulsions.

Compulsions are repetitive complex behaviors that appear purposeful and are performed according to a rule or until "just right". Examples include ordering or arranging objects, washing, checking, counting, hoarding, completing (e.g. need to have all doors closed or all windows open), and repetition of routine behaviors (e.g. walking through a doorway). Individuals with sufficient cognitive and language capability will be able to say "why" they perform a compulsion. Compulsions may be difficult to differentiate from complex tics in individuals who have both (Leckman and Cohen 1999).

Tics are discrete stereotyped repetitive movements that change over time. They can be simple or complex. Simple tics are rapid, brief, involuntary, non-rhythmic movements. Tics can be motor, such as eye blinking or shoulder shrugging, or vocal, such as throat clearing, sniffing or utterances. Specific tics tend to wax and wane and change over time, in contrast to the persistence of specific movements with stereotypies (Table 5.1). As just noted, complex tics, involving more purposeful appearing movements or a coordinated series of movements may be difficult to distinguish from compulsions. Gilles de la Tourette syndrome (TS) is a disorder characterized by the early onset (2–15 years of age) of chronic motor and vocal tics. The motor and vocal tics of TS may be simple or complex, and may change from simple to complex over different periods of time.

Rituals are the performance of activities of daily living in a repetitive, rigidly identical manner. These can include the ways meals are presented or eaten, bedtime routines, dressing, travel routes, play activities, self-care, or communication (e.g. repeated questioning). Rituals differ from compulsions in that they revolve around routine daily activities, but they also overlap with compulsions in their need to be "just right" and frequent following of "rules".

Sameness is the resistance to change in routine or physical surroundings. Examples include always using the same door, becoming upset in new settings, repetitively viewing part of a movie, listening to the same song over and over, and insisting on having the same schedule every day. There is some overlap between sameness and rituals, but the hallmark of sameness is the resistance to change.

Behavioral *restriction*, or behavioral rigidity, refers to a limited range of behaviors or interests. Examples include apparent attachment to a certain object, fascination with a subject or activity (cars, computer games), and fascination with moving objects or parts. Because restriction leads to a narrow behavioral repertoire, it often manifests as stereotyped repetition of certain behaviors.

Despite the similarities across many of the categories defined above, each category has distinguishing features. In careful studies in adults of rating instruments based on operational definitions, Bodfish and colleagues have shown that stereotypies can be separated categorically from compulsions and self-injury (Bodfish et al. 1995) and from akathisia and dyskinesia (Bodfish et al. 1997). Using such tools, different types of repetitive behaviors can be separated and rated. Specific definition and separate evaluation of repetitive behaviors may have important therapeutic implications.

NATURAL HISTORY OF STEREOTYPIES

Unfortunately, there are few data on the natural history of stereotypies. It is known that stereotypies are present in the majority of autistic children. In two studies of stereotypies in autistic children 100% of the subjects had stereotypies (Campbell et al. 1990, Shay et al. 1993). However, stereotyped, repetitive, rhythmic movements are common and indeed characteristic of infants and toddlers (Thelen 1979, 1981). Particular types of stereotypy develop in correlation with motor development. In the majority of children, these movements decrease and ultimately cease. It has been proposed that rhythmical stereotypies are manifestations of the immature brain, reflecting incomplete cortical control in the maturing motor system (Thelen 1979). Because of the presence of stereotypies during normal development, it is difficult to determine when movements that will ultimately persist as stereotypies begin. In fact, typical infantile stereotypies may develop later in children with autism or developmental disabilities than in normal children (Symons et al. 2005), making it even more difficult to determine the age of onset of stereotypies associated with autism. In a population of non-autistic, non-retarded children, the age of onset of stereotypies was before 3 years of age in 90% (Mahone et al. 2004). As children get older, stereotypies may diminish but they can persist into adulthood in both autistic (Bodfish et al. 2000) and non-autistic children (Mahone et al. 2004).

NEUROBIOLOGY OF STEREOTYPIES

The neurobiological mechanisms underlying stereotypies are not known. However, there are reasons to think that they arise from the basal ganglia or from cortical/basal ganglia/ thalamo-cortical circuits. The majority of involuntary movement disorders arise from the basal ganglia (Mink 2003), and some basal ganglia disorders cause stereotypies (Jankovic 1994). Other disorders characterized by repetitive behaviors or thoughts have been shown to involve basal ganglia and related cortical circuits (Baxter et al. 1988, Baxter 2003). Most animal models of stereotypies have resulted from the administration of medications such as amphetamine and cocaine that augment dopamine in the basal ganglia and frontal lobes. In rodents, it has long been know that administration of direct dopamine agonists into the striatum can induce repetitive stereotyped behaviors (Ernst and Smelik 1966). Furthermore, intrastriatal application of dopamine antagonists blocks amphetamine-induced stereotypies (Bedingfield et al. 1997). Finally, amphetamine-induced stereotypy correlates with immediate early gene expression in the striatum (Canales and Graybiel 2000). These data strongly implicate the basal ganglia and dopamine in drug-induced stereotypies, but other sites may also be important in maintaining these behaviors (Bedingfield et al. 1997).

The rodent models of drug-induced stereotypy have been useful, but questions have been raised as to the relevance of drug-induced stereotypies for understanding naturally occurring human stereotypies in autistic or non-autistic individuals. A recent study in deer mice, a species that has a high rate of spontaneously occurring stereotypies, has shown clear differences between dopamine agonist-induced stereotypies and the spontaneous stereotypies in terms of type of movements and their response to dopamine antagonists (Presti et al. 2004). Thus, while some normally occurring stereotyped sequential behaviors, such as grooming, involve the basal ganglia (Aldridge and Berridge 1998, Baxter 2003) and dopamine mechanisms (Berridge et al. 2005), there may be differences in neural mechanisms underlying different types of stereotypies or other repetitive behaviors. There may also be an important role for serotonin in the maintenance of stereotyped repetitive behaviors. This idea is based in large part on the well-known benefit from selective serotonin reuptake inhibitors (SSRIs) on obsessive–compulsive symptoms. Although the role of dopamine in basal ganglia function is often emphasized, there is also an important input to the basal ganglia and related frontal cortex regions from brainstem serotonergic neurons (Lavoie and Parent 1990). Successful treatment of obsessive–compulsive symptoms with a combination of an SSRI and a dopamine-blocking agent suggests there may be important interactions between the serotonin and dopamine systems in the production and maintenance of stereotypies (McDougle et al. 1994).

Although there have been many human neuroimaging studies in autism (Courchesne et al. 2004), there have been very few studies of stereotypies in autistic or non-autistic individuals. No specific functional imaging studies of stereotypies have been performed. Two small volumetric MRI studies of stereotypies have been published recently. A study of six non-autistic boys with stereotypies reported a trend toward reduced frontal sub-cortical white matter and caudate volumes compared to age-matched controls (Kates et al. 2005). In a study of 17 adults with autism, the volume of the right caudate nucleus was larger than in age-matched controls (Hollander et al. 2005a). In an analysis of data from the autistic adult subjects, the right caudate nucleus volume was positively correlated with the Repetitive and Stereotyped Behaviors domain of the Autistic Diagnostic Inter-view–Revised (Hollander et al. 2005a). Although these two studies involved different types of subjects with stereotypies and reached different conclusions, they both point to a relationship between basal ganglia/cortical circuits and stereotypies.

STEREOTYPIES IN INDIVIDUALS WITHOUT DEVELOPMENTAL DISABILITIES

It has been estimated that stereotypies occur in up to 7% of non-disabled children (Baumeister and Forehand 1973). The term "physiologic stereotypies" has been suggested when they occur in otherwise normal children (Tan et al. 1997, Mahone et al. 2004). Typical movements include repeated, recurrent raising and lowering of the arms, flapping, waving, wrist rotation, and finger wiggling. They are often accompanied by facial move-ments or grimacing. Physiologic stereotypies may be present in any setting, but are most common when the child is excited, mentally engaged, stressed, or bored. They may increase with fatigue. A hallmark of stereotypies is that they usually cease when the child is distracted or engaged in a new activity. Most children appear to be unaware of the stereotypies. When a child is asked during the movement, "Why are you doing that?", the most common response is, "Doing what?"

The clinical characteristics of physiologic stereotypies have been described by Tan et al. (1997) and Mahone et al. (2004). The typical age of onset for childhood stereotypies is less than 2 years. They are more common in boys (almost 2:1). Unlike tics, stereotyp-ies tend not to change in anatomic location or complexity over time. Stereotypies are not preceded by an urge or thought, as is common with tics or compulsions. Physiologic stereotypies last for multiple years in most children. In some children they disappear over time, but in other cases they persist into adulthood. There may be an increased incidence of ADHD or learning disabilities in children with stereotypies.

STEREOTYPES IN SENSORY DISORDERS

Stereotypies occur frequently in children with blindness (Eichel 1978, Fazzi et al. 1999).

In a study of 26 blind children, the more common stereotypies were body-rocking, repetitive handling of objects, finger movements, eye pressing and poking, and jumping (Fazzi et al. 1999). Eye pressing and poking appear to be most specifically associated with blindness, while the other types of stereotypies are similar to those seen in children without visual impairment. Eye pressing or poking was most common in children with peripheral causes of blindness, suggesting that it provided visual sensation through the intact optic nerve. Interestingly, stereotypies were less common in blind children with other disabilities (9/16) than in blind children without other disabilities (10/10). It was proposed that physical limitations or severe brain dysfunction prevented the expression of stereotypies (Fazzi et al. 1999). It was also suggested that anxieties surrounding the sensory deficit are the underlying cause of the stereotypies; however, "the capacity of these children to relate well to objects and to establish a link with the world around them does not exclude the possibility that they will manifest [stereotypies]" (Fazzi et al. 1999). The observation that most stereotypies seen in blind children are similar to those seen in non-blind children supports the impression that the stereotypies do not arise specifically from "anxieties" associated with blindness.

Stereotypies may also be common in children with hearing impairment (Bachara and Phelan 1980). In a study of 320 deaf and hard of hearing students between the ages of 5 and 16 years, rhythmic body rocking was common and was more common in the younger children.[1]

STEREOTYPIES IN OTHER DEVELOPMENTAL DISABILITIES

Stereotypies are well described in individuals with non-autistic developmental disabilities and especially in association with mental retardation (Bartak and Rutter 1976, Bodfish et al. 2000). Most qualitative reports have suggested that stereotypies in autistic and non-autistic mentally retarded individuals are similar phenomenologically (Bartak and Rutter 1976, Campbell et al. 1990). Bodfish et al. (2000) evaluated prospectively repetitive behaviors in 32 autistic and 34 non-autistic adults with mental retardation. The groups were matched for age, gender and IQ. The great majority of the subjects were "severely" or "profoundly" retarded. Both groups had a high incidence of repetitive behaviors including stereotypies, self-injurious behaviors and compulsions, with a somewhat lower incidence of akathisia, dyskinesia or tics. While the autistic group overall had a higher incidence of repetitive behaviors, it was only compulsions that were significantly higher in the autistic individuals (Bodfish et al. 2000). The autistic subjects had more different types of stereotypies and compulsions than the non-autistic group, and there were types

---

[1] These observations have not been replicated, to the knowledge of one of the editors (IR) whose clinical impression after many years of examining hearing impaired children is at odds with this report unless the deaf child is also autistic. Whether some or all the deaf children with stereotypies in the report also had vestibular impairments is not known, but the editor is not aware of studies correlating vestibular impairment with stereotypies.

of stereotypies that appeared to distinguish the two groups. Finally, the severity of stereotypies and compulsions was greater in the autistic group. All of the autistic subjects in that
study had some type of stereotypy; stereotypies were the most common type of repetitive
behavior (Bodfish et al. 2000).

In a large multicenter study, preschool age (4–7 years) children were categorized into
four groups: non-autistic children with developmental language disorders but normal IQ
(DLD), non-autistic children with low nonverbal IQ (<80), and autistic children with
normal or low nonverbal IQ (<80) (Rapin 1996). Neurologists reported stereotypies in
2% of DLD children, 13% of non-autistic children with low IQ, 41% of autistic children
with normal IQ, and 65% of autistic children with low IQ. Thus, stereotypies were more
common in the preschool children with low IQ than in those with normal IQ, and more
common in the autistic than in the non-autistic preschool children. In a follow-up
assessment of these children at school age (ages 7–9 years), neurologists reported stereotypies in 1.5% of DLD children, 13% of non-autistic children with low IQ, 20% of
autistic children with normal IQ, and 72% of autistic children with low IQ (Mandelbaum et al. 2006). Although these studies involved children rather than adults and were
based only on the neurologists' observations, the results are consistent with the systematic
study reported by Bodfish et al. (2000).

Contrary to the hypothesis that stereotypies are pathognomic of autism (Brasic
1999), it seems clear that stereotypies are not unique to autism (Mitchell and Etches
1977, Eichel 1978, Bachara and Phelan 1980, Campbell et al. 1990, Jankovic 1994, Tan
et al. 1997, Bodfish et al. 2000, Mahone et al. 2004). No study to date has found diag-
nostically specific types of stereotypies in autistic individuals. Thus, the mere presence of
stereotypies, of any type, is not a reliable predictor of autism, even though they are suggestive in older non-retarded children with a developmental disorder; and, of course,
neither does the absence of stereotypy in a child with autism negate the diagnosis. These
considerations are important to keep in mind when approaching the diagnostic evaluation
of a child with stereotypies.

STEREOTYPIES – MOVEMENT DISORDER OR SELF-STIMULATION?

Most human behaviors appear purposeful to the casual observer, even if not under
conscious control. However, habits, mannerisms and associated movements are without
clear purpose or function. It can be quite helpful when approaching the evaluation of a
child with unusual movements or behaviors to ask him or her, "Why do you do that?";
the answer can often distinguish tics, compulsions, stereotypies, habits, and mannerisms
(Schlaggar and Mink 2003). In children with autism or other types of communication
impairment such information is often unobtainable, however. There is a long history
of speculation as to why individuals with autism engage in stereotypies or other types of
repetitive behaviors. The sensory self-stimulation hypothesis proposes that movements are
"operant responses" whose reinforcers are the interoceptive and exteroceptive perceptual
consequences of the movements (Lovaas et al. 1987). The high rate of occurrence of

stereotypies in individuals with sensory deficits is used as indirect support of this hypothesis. Accordingly, in those individuals, the function of the stereotypy is thought to be to provide additional sensory stimulation to replace the missing sensations and/or to augment the preserved sensory modalities. An implication of this hypothesis is that a specific sensory modality can be identified through which reinforcement is received and can then be the target for behavioral intervention (Tang et al. 2003). It has also been proposed that the stereotypies may elicit social responses of other people that lead to positive or negative reinforcement of the behavior (Tang et al. 2003). These hypotheses have popular support, but are difficult to test rigorously. They both arise from the underlying assumption that stereotypies are conditioned behaviors that are reinforced by either internal or external responses to the behaviors (Gritti et al. 2003), but there is little objective evidence to support that assumption.

An alternative hypothesis is that stereotypies and other repetitive behaviors are manifestations of an immature or underdeveloped nervous system (Thelen 1979, 1981; Werry et al. 1983; Symons et al. 2005). In this view, stereotyped repetitive movements are a motor output that may be influenced by sensory inputs, but do not function primarily to produce sensory inputs. In this view, stereotypies are akin to other hyperkinetic movement disorders in which the movements are involuntary and arise from abnormal neuronal discharge patterns (Mink 2003). These patterns reflect underlying pathophysiology and not underlying psychopathology. In non-autistic, non-retarded children, it is quite common for the child to be unaware that they are doing the stereotypy unless it is pointed out to them (Mahone et al. 2004). As stated earlier, a common answer to the question "Why are you doing that?" is "Doing what?" Stereotypies typically cease when the child is distracted or redirected. This apparent unawareness of stereotypies is similar to what has been observed for chorea in Huntington disease and dopa-induced dyskinesia in Parkinson disease (Snowden et al. 1998). A careful investigation in patients with Huntington disease was able to reject any psychodynamic contribution to the reduced self-awareness of involuntary movements (Snowden et al. 1998). Similarly, many patients with tic disorders are unaware of some or all of their tics, if they are mild (Pappert et al. 2003). These findings suggest that low awareness of certain kinds of involuntary movements is common and supports the idea that involuntary movements are not done in order to cause sensory stimulation.

TREATMENT OF REPETITIVE BEHAVIORS IN AUTISM

When approaching the treatment of repetitive behaviors in any child, whether or not autistic, the first question should be whether to treat. If the behaviors are not causing discomfort, injury, or social impairment, then it may be preferable not to treat them. If they are causing difficulty, then treatment may be indicated. Treatment options include pharmacological (Lindsay and Aman 2003) and behavioral approaches (Turner 1999).

Many pharmacologic treatments have been reported in single cases or small series. However, most are small open label studies and subject to the usual problems of such studies, i.e. placebo effect and observer bias. Furthermore, most studies in autism have not distinguished among different types of repetitive behaviors. There have been few double-blind placebo-controlled trials with specific measures of repetitive behaviors in individuals with autism. Medications that have been shown to reduce repetitive behaviors in adults with autism include risperidone (McDougle et al. 1998) and fluvoxamine (McDougle et al. 1996). Clomipramine (Gordon et al. 1993), risperidone (McCracken et al. 2002), and fluoxetine (Hollander et al. 2005b) have been shown to reduce repetitive behaviors in children and adolescents with autism.

CONCLUSIONS

Stereotyped repetitive behaviors are common, but not unique, in autism. They occur in many forms that can be categorized as stereotypies, self-injury, compulsions, rituals, sameness, and restriction. The distinctions between categories are supported by studies showing independence of variables on rating scales (Bodfish et al. 2000). It is possible, but not proven, that these distinctions reflect different underlying mechanisms or differential responses to treatments. The neural basis of stereotypies is not known, but is likely to involve basal ganglia and frontal cortical circuits. Whether stereotypies are purposeless or "self-stimulating" is controversial, but it seems in non-autistic individuals with stereotypies that the movements are not done for any specific "purpose". Several pharmacological treatments have been shown to be effective for treatment of repetitive behaviors in autism. The understanding of mechanisms underlying repetitive behaviors and knowledge of treatment options is limited. Substantially more research is needed to determine the impact of these behaviors on the autistic individual and whether treatment is beneficial beyond reducing the behaviors.

REFERENCES

Aldridge J, Berridge K (1998) Coding of serial order by neostriatal neurons: a "natural action" approach to movement sequences. *J Neurosci* 18: 2777–87.

APA (1994) *Diagnostic and Statistical Manual of Mental Disorders, 4th edn (DSM-IV).* Washington, DC: American Psychiatric Association.

Bachara GH, Phelan WJ (1980) Rhythmic movement in deaf children. *Percept Mot Skills* 50: 933–4.

Bartak L, Rutter M (1976) Differences between mentally retarded and normally intelligent autistic children. *J Autism Child Schizophr* 6: 109–20.

Baumeister AA, Forehand R (1973) Stereotyped acts. In: Ellis NR, ed. *International Review of Research in Mental Retardation, vol. 6.* New York: Academic Press, pp. 55–96.

Baxter LR (2003) Basal ganglia systems in ritualistic social displays: reptiles and humans; function and illness. *Physiol Behav* 79: 451–60.

Baxter LR, Schwartz JM, Mazziotta JC, Phelps ME, Pahl JJ, Guze BH, Fairbanks L (1988) Cerebral glucose metabolic rates in non-depressed patients with obsessive–compulsive disorder. *Am J Psychiatry* 145: 518–23.

Bedingfield JB, Calder LD, Thai DK, Karler R (1997) The role of the striatum in the mouse in behavioral sensitization to amphetamine. *Pharmacol Biochem Behav* 74: 833–9.

Berridge KC, Aldridge J, Houchard K, Zhuang X (2005) Sequential super-stereotypy of an instinctual fixed action pattern in hyperdopaminergic mutant mice: a model of obsessive compulsive disorder and Tourette's. *BMC Biol* 3: 4.

Bodfish JW, Crawford TW, Powell SB, Parker DE, Golden RN, Lewis MH (1995) Compulsions in adults with mental retardation: Prevalence, phenomenology, and comorbidity with stereotypy and self-injury. *Am J Ment Retard* 100: 183–92.

Bodfish JW, Newell KM, Sprague RL, Harper VN, Lewis MH (1997) Akathisia in adults with mental retardation: Development of the Akathisia Ratings of Movement Scale (ARMS). *Am J Ment Retard* 101: 413–23.

Bodfish JW, Symons FJ, Parker DE, Lewis MH (2000) Varieties of repetitive behavior in autism: Comparisons to mental retardation. *J Autism Develop Disord* 30: 237–43.

Brasic JR (1999) Movements in autistic disorder. *Med Hypotheses* 53: 48–9.

Campbell M, Locasio J, Choroco MC, Spencer EK, Malone RP, Kafantris V, Overall JE (1990) Sterotypies and tardive dyskinesia: Abnormal movements in autistic children. *Psychopharm Bull* 26: 260–6.

Canales JJ, Graybiel AM (2000) A measure of striatal function predicts motor stereotypy. *Nat Neurosci* 3: 377–83.

Courchesne E, Redcay E, Kennedy DP (2004) The autistic brain: birth through adulthood. *Curr Opin Neurol* 17: 489–96.

Eichel VJ (1978) Mannerism of the blind: A review of the literature. *Impair Blind* 72: 125–30.

Ernst AM, Smelik PG (1966) Site of action of dopamine and apomorphine on compulsive gnawing behavior in rats. *Experientia* 22: 837–8.

Fazzi E, Lanners J, Danova S, Ferrari-Ginevra O, Gheza C, Luparia A, Balottin U, Lanzi G (1999) Stereotyped behaviours in blind children. *Brain Dev* 21: 522–8.

Gordon CT, State RC, Nelson JE, Hamburger SD, Rapoport JL (1993) A double-blind comparison of clomipramine, desipramine, and placebo in the treatment of autistic disorder. *Arch Gen Psychiatry* 50: 441–7.

Gritti A, Bove D, Di Sarno AM, D'Addio AA, Chiapparo S, Bove RM (2003) Stereotyped movements in a group of autistic children. *Funct Neurol* 18: 89–94.

Hollander E, Anagnostou E, Chaplin W, Esposito K, Haznedar MM, Licalzi E, Wasserman S, Soorya L, Buchsbaum M (2005a) Striatal volume on magnetic resonance imaging and repetitive behaviors in autism. *Biol Psychiatr* 58: 226–32.

Hollander E, Phillips A, Chaplin W, Zagursky K, Novotny S, Wasserman S, Iyengar R (2005b) A placebo controlled crossover trial of liquid fluoxetine on repetitive behaviors in childhood and adolescent autism. *Neuropsychopharmacol* 30: 582–9.

Jankovic J (1994) Stereotypies. In: Marsden CD, Fahn S, eds. *Movement Disorders, vol. 3.* Oxford: Butterworth-Heinemann, pp. 501-517.

Kates WR, Lanham DC, Singer HS (2005) Frontal white matter reductions in healthy males with complex stereotypies. *Pediatr Neurol* 32: 109–12.

Lavoie B, Parent A (1990) Immunohistochemical study of the serotoninergic innervation of the basal ganglia in the squirrel monkey. *J Comp Neurol* 299: 1–16.

Leckman J, Cohen D (1999) *Tourette's Syndrome—Tics, Obsessions, Compulsions: Developmental Psychopathology and Clinical Care.* New York: John Wiley.

Lindsay RL, Aman MG (2003) Pharmacologic therapies aid treatment for autism. *Pediatr Ann* 32: 671–6.

Lovaas I, Newsom C, Hickman C (1987) Self-stimulatory behavior and perceptual reinforcement. *J Appl Behav Anal* 20: 45–68.

Mahone EM, Bridges D, Prahme C, Singer HS (2004) Repetitive arm and hand movements (complex motor stereotypies) in children. *J Pediatr* 145: 391–5.

Mandelbaum DE, Stevens M, Rosenberg E, Wiznitzer M, Steinschneider M, Filipek P, Rapin I (2006) Comparison of sensory/motor performance in school-age children with autism, developmental language disorder, or low IQ. *Dev Med Child Neurol* 48: 33–9.

McCracken JT, McGough J, Shah B, Cronin P, Hong D, Aman MG, Arnold LE, Lindsay R, Nash P, Hollway J, McDougle CJ, Posey D, Swiezy N, Kohn A, Scahill L, Martin A, Koenig K, Volkmar F, Carroll D, Lancor A, Tierney E, Ghuman J, Gonzalez NM, Grados M, Vitiello B, Ritz L, Davies M, Robinson J, McMahon D (2002) Risperidone in children with autism and serious behavioral problems. *N Engl J Med* 347: 314–21.

McDougle CJ, Goodman WK, Leckman JF, Lee NC, Heninger GR, Price LH (1994) Haloperidol addition in fluvoxamine-refractory obsessive-compulsive disorder. A double-blind, placebo-controlled study in patients with and without tics. *Arch Gen Psychiatry* 51: 302–8.

McDougle CJ, Naylor ST, Cohen DJ, Volkmar FR, Heninger GR, Price LH (1996) A double-blind, placebo-controlled study of fluvoxamine in adults with autistic disorder. *Arch Gen Psychiatry* 53: 1001–8.

McDougle CJ, Holmes JP, Carlson DC, Pelton GH, Cohen DJ, Price LH (1998) A double-blind, placebo-controlled study of risperidone in adults with autistic disorder and other pervasive developmental disorders. *Arch Gen Psychiatry* 55: 633–41.

Mink J (2003) The basal ganglia and involuntary movements: Impaired inhibition of competing motor patterns. *Arch Neurol* 60: 1365–8.

Mitchell R, Etches P (1977) Rhythmic habit patterns (stereotypies). *Dev Med Child Neurol* 19: 545–50.

Pappert EJ, Goetz CG, Louis ED, Blasucci L, Leurgans S (2003) Objective assessments of longitudinal outcome in Gilles de la Tourette's syndrome. *Neurology* 61: 936–40.

Presti MF, Gibney BC, Lewis MH (2004) Effects of intrastriatal administration of selective dopaminergic ligands on spontaneous stereotypy in mice. *Physiol Behav* 80: 433–9.

Rapin I, ed. (1996) *Preschool Children with Inadequate Communication: Developmental Language Disorder, Autism, Low IQ. Clinics in Developmental Medicine No. 139.* London: Mac Keith Press.

Schlaggar BL, Mink JW (2003) Movement disorders in children. *Pediatr Rev* 24: 39–51.

Shay J, Sanchez L, Cueva J, Armenteros J, Overall JE, Campbell M (1993) Neuroleptic-related dyskinesia and stereotypies in autistic children. *Psychopharm Bull* 29: 359–63.

Snowden JS, Craufurd D, Griffiths HL, Neary D (1998) Awareness of involuntary movements in Huntington disease. *Arch Neurol* 55: 801–5.

Symons FJ, Sperry LA, Dropik PL, Bodfish JW (2005) The early development of stereotypy and self-injury: a review of research methods. *J Intellect Disabil Res* 49: 144–58.

Tan A, Salgado M, Fahn S (1997) The characterization and outcome of stereotypical movements in nonautistic children. *Mov Disord* 12: 47–52.

Tang JC, Patterson TG, Kennedy CH (2003) Identifying specific sensory modalities maintaining the stereotypy of students with multiple profound disabilities. *Res Dev Disabil* 24: 433–51.

Thelen E (1979) Rhythmical stereotypies in normal human infants. *Animal Behav* 27: 699–715.

Thelen E (1981) Rhythmical behavior in infancy: an ethological perspective. *Develop Psychol* 17: 237–57.

Turner M (1999) Repetitive behaviour in autism: a review of psychological research. *J Child Psychol Psychiatry* 40: 839–49.

Werry JS, Carlielle J, Fitzpatrick J (1983) Rhythmic motor activities (stereotypies) in children under five: etiology and prevalence. *J Am Acad Child Psychiatry* 22: 329–36.

6
NEUROBIOLOGY OF AUTISM

Michael V Johnston and Mary E Blue

Although the neurobiology of autism is not well understood, information from neuro-pathology, brain imaging, genetics and developmental neuroscience is providing some insights into the steps in brain development that may be abnormal.

Several neurologic features and behaviors observed in children with autism appear to reflect disorders in developmental programs for neurons and synapses in the immature brain (Rapin 2002). Impaired social and language development suggests disordered circuitry in specific limbic and neocortical areas of cerebral cortex, while altered reactivity to sensorimotor stimuli, stereotyped behaviors (see Chapter 5) and, as discussed in Chapters 14 and 15, other motor abnormalities suggest impairments in brainstem, cerebellar, thalamic and basal ganglia connections (Bailey et al. 1998, Sparks et al. 2002, Bauman and Kemper 2005). In addition, immunological abnormalities have been found in autism; these are discussed in Chapter 6.

Seizures and abnormal EEG patterns, discussed in Chapters 10 and 11, as well as abnormal sleep patterns and electrographic sleep architecture, discussed in Chapter 12, point to possible abnormalities in thalamocortical and other neuronal circuits (Tuchman and Rapin 2002, Limoges et al. 2005). Neuropathology studies have reported neuronal abnormalities in cerebral cortex, including reduced neuronal size and cell packing density in the hippocampus, entorhinal and cingulate cortex (Bauman and Kemper 2005). Casanova et al. (2002) reported abnormalities in the organization of cerebral cortex in autism, with an increase in the number of "minicolumns", the vertical, multi-neuronal structures that form the basic information processing unit. They also found that the size of individual minicolumns is reduced in post-mortem tissue from individuals with autism.

Brain imaging has also demonstrated abnormalities in cerebral cortex. Levitt et al. (2003) used three dimensional magnetic resonance imaging (MRI) mapping to show that the localization of major cortical sulci was shifted in a group of children and adolescents with autism compared to age-matched controls. Herbert et al. (2005) showed that the normal left to right asymmetry in cortical language association areas was reversed in children with developmental language disorders and autism, suggesting problems in growth trajectories and cortical connectivity. Pathological and imaging changes reported in the brainstem and cerebellum may also be related to motor and learning abnormalities in autism (Courchesne 2002, Bauman and Kemper 2005).

ABNORMAL BRAIN GROWTH PATTERN IN AUTISM

Another clue to developmental processes that may be targeted in autism is the observation that early brain growth is accelerated in many children with the disorder (Wallace and Treffert 2004). More than 60 years ago, Kanner (1943) mentioned in his original description of children with autism that they had large heads, and macrocephaly has been one of the most consistent physical characteristics of children with the disorder (Bailey et al. 1993, Stevenson et al. 1997). Enhanced brain growth appears to be most prominent during the time window from a few months after birth to 2–5 years of age (Courchesne et al. 2001, 2003; Carper et al. 2002). This period of overgrowth is bracketed by the neonatal period, in which average head circumference in children with autism spectrum disorders (ASDs) has been reported to be smaller than average, and the period during adolescence and adulthood when it has been reported to be in the normal range (Aylward et al. 2002). Brain imaging indicates that both gray matter and white matter in the brain and cerebellum contribute to the enhanced growth (De Fosse et al. 2004, Herbert et al. 2005). One study suggested that earlier onset and longer duration of accelerated brain growth is associated with more severe clinical signs of autism (Courchesne et al. 2003). The onset of this overgrowth in early infancy suggests that it reflects the impact of underlying developmental disorders or prenatal events, rather than reactions to environmental events in the postnatal period (Courchesne et al. 2003). Accelerated brain growth in ASDs spans the interval when overall brain growth is most rapid in normal infants and when synapses are proliferating at a rapid rate (Fig. 6.1; Johnston et al. 2001). At around 2 years of age, synaptic density in cerebral cortex reaches a peak that is almost twice as high as in the neonate, and after that time synapses are pruned to a level during adolescence and adulthood that is similar to neonates (Huttenlocher 1990). The changes in synaptic counts during development in post-mortem brain tissue correspond to measurements of regional cerebral glucose metabolism using positron emission tomography (PET) in children of different ages (Chugani et al. 1987). Synaptic counts in brains from children with autism have not been reported, but the timing of accelerated growth in autism during this developmental window suggests that enhanced proliferation of synapses and/or reduced pruning during this period may be responsible for macrocephaly in autism. Enhanced myelination could also contribute to this process, although myelination lags behind synaptogenesis, and continues for many years after synaptogenesis is complete (Johnston et al. 2001). The two processes might also be connected since synapse formation and neuronal activity are coordinated processes, and activity in synapses can activate myelination. The hypothesis that *the dynamics of synapse formation and pruning are disrupted in the early postnatal period in children with autism* is an attractive one based on recent information about early brain overgrowth in autism.

NEUROTRANSMITTERS AND BRAIN DEVELOPMENT IN AUTISM

The clinical and pathologic evidence implicating abnormal growth and development of synapses and neuronal circuits in autism has stimulated interest in possible abnormalities

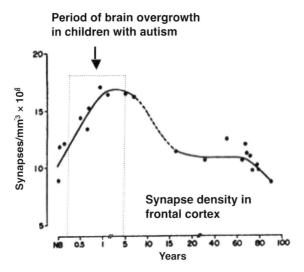

Fig. 6.1. Period of brain overgrowth seen in children with autism shown in the box, and superimposed on a curve of synaptic density in post-mortem cerebral cortex from children of various ages. (Adapted from Huttenlocher 1979.)

in synaptic neurotransmitters. The vast majority of synapses between neurons transmit information using chemicals such as the amino acids glutamate and gamma-aminobutyric acid (GABA), acetylcholine, serotonin, dopamine, norepinephrine and others, including enkephalins and endorphins. Interest in neurotransmitters in autism has come from several directions including clinical responses to drugs that act on neurotransmitter systems and autism- related gene mutations that impact them (Cook et al. 1990, Purcell et al. 2001, DeLong et al. 2002, Chugani 2004). In this section the neurotransmitters serotonin, glutamate and GABA are discussed because they have been implicated in genetic studies, and they play major roles in brain development and function (Johnston and Coyle 1981, McDonald and Johnston 1990). Other sections of the book also deal with neurotransmitters including the catecholamines, dopamine and norepinephrine.

Neurotransmitters play different roles in the fetus and infant compared to the adult, and have roles that extend beyond information transfer to serve as morphogens that influence neuronal structure (Lauder 1990). From fetal life until late childhood, the brain is continuously "under construction" and this development takes place from back to front, with the brainstem maturing before more anterior cortical structures. This allows essential functions such as breathing, feeding and reflex activities to function at birth, while the massive cerebral cortex in humans can continue to expand over a prolonged period. Certain neuronal groups, including those that utilize dopamine, norepinephrine and serotonin as neurotransmitters, originate in the brainstem but send axons upward to the forebrain. In keeping with their brainstem origin, these neuronal groups mature early and

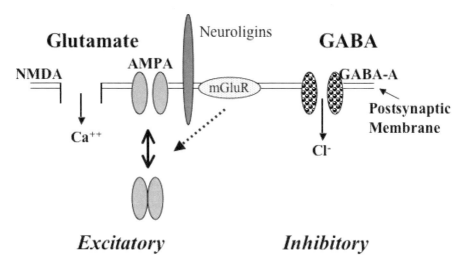

Fig. 6.2. Diagram of excitatory and inhibitory receptors in postsynaptic membrane. Excitatory NMDA, AMPA and metabotropic glutamate receptors (mGluR) are activated by glutamate, and GABA activates inhibitory receptors. NMDA receptor activity increases trafficking of AMPA receptors into the synaptic membrane, while activation of metabotropic receptors favors internalization of AMPA receptors. An increase in AMPA receptors in the synapse potentiates excitatory transmission, while internalization of receptors reduces it. Neuroligins connect pre- and postsynaptic membranes in synapses and anchor receptors and scaffolding molecules. Abnormalities in AMPA receptors, neuroligins and GABA receptors have been associated with autism.

innervation is denser in forebrain areas in the fetus and neonate than in older children and adults (Johnston and Coyle 1981). For example, serotonin neurons appear at 5 weeks gestation in the midbrain raphe in the human brain, and axons expressing serotonin transporters have extended into cerebral cortex by the first trimester (Yew and Chan 1999). Activation of the brainstem neurons in these systems results in the release of neurotransmitters in widespread areas of the cortex and diencephalon where they influence the development of other neurons.

At somewhat later times in fetal development, fibers containing acetylcholine grow out of the nucleus basalis in the basal forebrain into the cerebral cortex where they influence cortical development and activity-dependent plasticity (Nishimura et al. 2002). In contrast to the catecholamine, serotonin and acetylcholine projections that project from the brainstem to the forebrain, neurons that use glutamate or GABA are much more ubiquitous and widely distributed throughout the brain. Glutamate is the major excitatory neurotransmitter of the brain, while GABA is the major inhibitory neurotransmitter; together they control the excitability of most neurons (Fig. 6.2). Unlike biogenic amines such as dopamine and serotonin, which are released regionally and modulate action of other transmitters, glutamate and GABA transmit information by controlling fast activity at discrete synapses in neuronal circuits (McDonald and Johnston 1990). Multiple receptor subtypes for glutamate and GABA allow them to mediate a variety of synaptic responses and play a role in learning, memory and other forms of plasticity (Fig. 6.2).

SEROTONIN AND AUTISM

Serotonin has drawn interest from investigators with several perspectives on autism (Chugani 2004). It was reported almost 40 years ago that a significant proportion of children with autism have elevated levels of serotonin in blood and platelets (Shain and Freedman 1961), and polymorphisms in the 5-HTTLPR serotonin transporter promoter may represent a marker for familial autism (Yirmiya et al. 2001). In some children, free levels of serotonin in blood are not elevated, suggesting that the transporter disorder raises blood levels by elevating transmitter in platelets. Mutations in maternal genotypes for monoamine oxidase-A, an enzyme that metabolizes serotonin, have also been associated with susceptibility to autism in their offspring (Jones et al. 2004). Serotonin levels in spinal fluid from children with autism have been inconsistent. Several studies also suggest changes in blood levels of the serotonin precursor amino acid tryptophan (D'Eufemia et al. 1995). A susceptibility mutation for autism has been reported in the tryptophan 2,3-dioxygenase gene that is a rate limiting enzyme in the metabolism of tryptophan by the kynurenine pathway (Nabi et al. 2004). Serotonin reuptake inhibitors are commonly used to treat stereotyped movements and anxiety in children with autism, and tryptophan depletion leads to worsening symptoms of autism (McDougle et al. 1996). In some patients, a good clinical response has been linked to a family history of major affective disorder (DeLong 1999, Delong et al. 2002).

Some evidence suggests that development of the serotonin innervation in cerebral cortex may be deficient in children with autism. Chugani et al. (1999) measured serotonin synthesis capacity using [^{11}C]-methyl-L-tryptophan and PET in children with and without autism and found that children who did not have autism had a synthesis capacity that was twice as high as adult levels until after age 5 years. Girls declined at an earlier age than boys. In contrast, the serotonin synthesis capacity in children with autism was considerably reduced in younger children, increasing gradually between ages 2 years and 15 years to values that were 1.5 times adult levels. There was no sex difference in the autism group. The results suggest that innervation of cerebral cortex by serotonin-containing axons is delayed, and that a deficit in serotonin during a critical period in cortical development could contribute to neuronal abnormalities in autism.

MODEL OF DEVELOPMENTAL SEROTONIN DEPLETION

A mouse model of neonatal serotonin depletion has been developed to examine the effects of diminished serotonin on developing cerebral cortex and behavior (Berger-Sweeney et al. 1998, Hohmann et al. 2000). In newborn rats, as in humans, cortical levels of serotonin are higher in early postnatal development than at subsequent ages (Hohmann et al. 1988). To deplete serotonin at this time, Hohmann et al. injected the serotonin

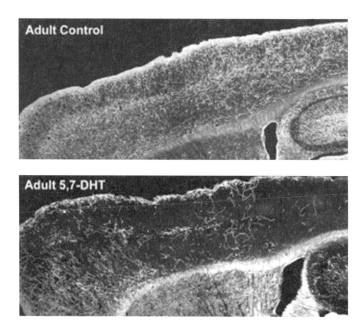

Fig. 6.3. Dark field photomicrographs show serotonin immunostaining in adult (7–9 months old) control versus 5,7-dihydroxytryptamine (5,7-DHT)-lesioned mice. Although the lesion was performed on the day of birth, the cortex of lesioned adult mice has very few serotonergic axons. The greatest degree of serotonin axon sprouting is present in frontal areas of adult cortex.

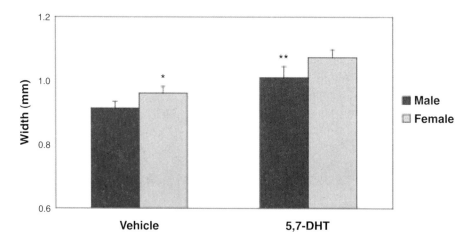

Fig. 6.4. Measurements of the width of entire cortex in the barrel field area show significant increases in cortical width in the neonatally 5,7-DHT-lesioned mice (**$p=0.003$). In addition, the cortex of females was thicker than that in males (*$p=0.05$). Vehicle = sterile saline. (Adapted from Hohmann et al. 2000.)

neurotoxin 5,7-dihydroxytryptamine (5,7-DHT) through a fine cannula into the medial forebrain bundles on both sides of neonatal mice (Berger-Sweeney et al. 1998, Hohmann et al. 2000). This treatment reduced serotonin in cerebral cortex by 86% at 2 weeks of age; regenerative sprouting was limited with frontal areas showing the most extensive regrowth of serotonergic axons (Fig. 6.3). Histological studies of the brains from lesioned mice that were 3–5 months old showed increases in cortical thickness in several regions compared to controls (Hohmann et al. 2000; Fig. 6.4). The effect tended to be greater in female than in male animals. This treatment also reduced levels of norepinephrine due to the proximity of fibers in this system to the lesion site, but separate experiments using a selective toxin for this neurotransmitter system did not show an increase in cortical thickness. These findings for serotonin depletion also contrast with those in which the cholinergic nucleus basalis projection to cerebral cortex is destroyed in the neonatal period (Hohmann et al. 1988). The effect of these lesions is to reduce cortical thickness (Hohmann et al. 2000). Mice with neonatal serotonin lesions displayed retention deficits on passive avoidance and changes in sensorimotor, emotional and cognitive abilities in an open field object recognition task that could be relevant to autism (Hohmann et al. 2000).

The results from the mouse model indicate that serotonin depletion early in the neonatal period causes enhanced cortical thickness, suggesting a parallel with enhanced brain growth in infants with autism. The mechanism for the growth-promoting effect of neonatal serotonin depletion is unclear. These morphologic effects may be relayed through serotonin receptors, which influence the formation of developing dendrites and synapses (Kondoh et al. 2004). While cortical thickness is increased, serotonin depletion has also been shown to delay the maturation of several cortical layers and decrease the size of the mouse cortical barrel field, which receives patterned sensory input from whiskers (Casanova et al. 2002). The barrel field provides a spatial map for processing sensory information, and barrels are specialized examples of the cortical columns found throughout other areas of cortex (Blue et al. 1991, Micheva and Beaulieu 1997). Serotonin fibers have been reported to be necessary for cortical column development (Janusonis et al. 2004). The mouse barrels may be homologues of the minicolumns reported to be abnormal in post-mortem tissue from patients with autism, suggesting that serotonin could be involved in this pathology.

POSSIBLE EFFECTS OF INCREASED PERIPHERAL SEROTONIN

The actual prevalence of low serotonin in the brains of children with autism is unknown, and the mechanism for this abnormality when it occurs is also unclear. However, one hypothesis suggests that reduced brain serotonin could be caused by negative feedback on central serotonin neurons secondary to high levels of serotonin in blood (Whitaker-Azmitia 2005). Administration of the serotonin agonist 5-methoxytryptamine (5-MT) to pregnant rats starting at gestational day 12 until birth and then to pups up to postnatal day 20 leads to behavioral abnormalities. These include reduced vocalizations when pups are removed from their dams, hyper-responsiveness to sound, and seizures and motor stereotypies, which have been compared to autistic behaviors in humans. Animals treated in this way show neuronal abnormalities, including loss of immunoreactivity for oxytocin in neurons in the paraventricular nucleus of the hypothalamus and an increase in calcitonin gene-related peptide (CGRP) in the amygdala. Oxytocin knockout mice have deficits in olfactory-based social recognition and infant ultrasonic vocalizations, suggesting an autism-like behavioral phenotype (Whitaker-Azmitia 2005). Elevations in CGRP, possibly due to loss of serotonin inhibition in the hypothalamus, could be associated with increased fear conditioning. Treatment with 5-MT has also been reported to alter levels of reelin, a glycoprotein produced by Cajal Retzius cells, which is involved in cortical column development (Janusonis et al. 2004). Fatemi et al. (2001) reported that abnormal levels of reelin have been found in human autism brain tissue. These studies suggest that increased peripheral serotonin during development could paradoxically disrupt central neuronal circuits through feedback inhibition and provide a model of autism.

ABNORMALITIES IN GLUTAMATE NEUROTRANSMISSION

Several lines of evidence point to abnormalities in glutamate neurotransmission in autism. Glutamate is intimately involved in control of neuronal excitability, and the increased incidence of seizures in autism suggests a possible connection with abnormal glutamate activity (Tuchman and Rapin 2002). Glutamate is also involved in activity-dependent neuronal plasticity, and defects in plasticity could be involved in the neuropathology as well as the cognitive and behavioral impairments seen in children with autism (McDonald and Johnston 1990). There is considerable interaction between neurons that use serotonin and glutamate in the developing brain. For example, immature thalamocortical axons express serotonin transporters during the neonatal period and transiently "borrow" glutamate as their transmitter (Xu et al. 2004). Additional evidence for abnormal glutamate neurotransmission comes from a study of gene expression using DNA microarray technology in post-mortem cerebellum from patients with autism (Purcell et al. 2001). This study found significant elevations in messenger RNA for the excitatory amino acid transporters 1 and 2, glutamate receptor 1 (GluR1) subunit of the α-amino-3-hydroxy-5-methylisoazole-4-propionic acid (AMPA) receptor and glutamate receptor binding proteins. Western blotting confirmed that the density of AMPA receptors as well as glutamate transporter proteins was also elevated, although autoradiographic studies showed that AMPA receptor binding was reduced. Changes in trafficking of AMPA receptors at excitatory synapses are thought to be important for long term potentiation, an increase in synaptic strength that is a cellular correlate of learning and memory (Fig. 6.2; Malenka 2003). Serajee et al. (2003) also reported the possible association of mutations in the metabotropic glutamate receptor 8 gene in autism. A case of autism with a deletion on 4q leading to hemizygosity for AMPA receptor subunits has also been reported (Ramanathan et al. 2004). Additional evidence linking autism to changes in glutamate synapses comes from reports on individuals with mutations in genes for the cell adhesion molecules neuroligin 3 and 4 (Jamain et al. 2003, Laumonnier et al. 2004). These proteins control the development of both excitatory and inhibitory GABAergic synapses by bridging their pre- and postsynaptic membranes (Chi et al. 2005).

GLUTAMATE ABNORMALITIES AND SYNAPSE DEVELOPMENT IN AUTISM

These changes in molecules associated with excitatory synapses provide additional support for the hypothesis that development and modulation of synapses is disrupted in autism. Construction of excitatory synapses occurs in a stepwise fashion beginning with presynaptic release of glutamate followed by postsynaptic differentiation and accumulation of scaffolding proteins such as the postsynaptic density 95 (PSD-95) protein (Fig. 6.2; Cohen-Cory 2002). The neuroligins, along with beta-neurexin, another cell adhesion molecule, align the presynaptic terminal with the postsynaptic membrane containing glutamate receptors and the PSD-95 protein, which serves as their anchor (Fig. 6.1; Song et al. 1999). *N*-methyl-D-aspartate (NMDA) type glutamate receptors, which are linked to calcium channels, are the first to accumulate in the postsynaptic membrane, followed by AMPA receptors, which are linked to sodium–potassium channels. Increased activation of NMDA receptors leads to reductions in their number along with redistribution of AMPA receptors from intracellular pools to synaptic sites. The morphological maturation of dendritic spines is correlated with the acquisition of functional AMPA receptors, and activity at both NMDA and AMPA receptors modulates axonal and dendritic arbor complexity (Cohen-Cory 2002). This suggests that alterations in AMPA receptors seen in post-mortem brain from individuals with autism could reflect changes in synaptic development. Mutations in neuroligin molecules could have a similar effect. In vitro studies in hippocampal neurons indicate that downregulating neuroligin-1 results in loss of excitatory and inhibitory synapses, with preferential loss of inhibitory synapses, shifting the balance towards excitation (Chi et al. 2005, Hussain and Sheng 2005). Disruption of the functional balance of excitatory and inhibitory synapses could impair synaptic plasticity and alter the dynamics of synapse production and pruning.

ALTERED GLUTAMATE NEUROTRANSMISSION IN FRAGILE-X SYNDROME

A mouse model of fragile X (fra-X) syndrome is also relevant to understanding possible links between abnormalities in brain growth, glutamate neurotransmission and synaptic development in autism (Comery et al. 1997). Fra-X, which may be associated in some individuals with behaviors consistent with the autism phenotype, is also associated with macrocephaly and pathological abnormalities in dendritic spines. Long, thin, immature looking dendritic spines are also seen in post-mortem tissue from individuals with fra-X and in transgenic fra-X gene (*Fmr 1*) knockout mice, that are deficient in fra-X mental retardation protein (FMRP) (Comery et al. 1997). Neurophysiologic assessment of these mice showed that long term depression (LTD) in response to stimulation of type 1 metabotropic glutamate receptors (mGluR) is enhanced in the hippocampus of these mice (Huber et al. 2002, Bear et al. 2004). The effect is mediated by a change in trafficking of AMPA receptors between the cytoplasm and postsynaptic membrane so that AMPA receptors remain internalized, reducing synaptic excitability (Fig. 6.2; Malenka 2003). This change in activity-dependent synaptic plasticity may be related to alterations in dendritic spine morphology, since shortening of spines during maturation is mediated by AMPA receptor activity. The model of fra-X provides additional evidence for an association between abnormal glutamate neurotransmission and neuronal changes in autism.

GABAERGIC INHIBITORY NEUROTRANSMISSION

Genetic linkage studies have implicated genes that code for inhibitory GABA-A receptors in autism. The region on chromosome 15q11-q13 that includes the disease loci for imprinted genes that cause Prader–Willi and Angelman syndromes also includes multiple subunits for GABA-A neurotransmitter receptors (Nurmi et al. 2001). Several studies have found duplications in this region in children with ASDs, and autistic features are part of the Angelman syndrome phenotype. Martin et al. (2000) found suggestive evidence for linkage disequilibrium for a marker near the beta3-subunit of the GABA-A receptor in this region in patients with autism, and Nurmi et al. (2001) found evidence of linkage disequilibrium in a region that contained the *UBE3A* Angelman syndrome gene and multiple GABA-A receptor subunit genes. Casanova et al. (2003) suggested that abnormalities in cortical minicolumns noted in autism involve specific defects in GABAergic inhibitory fibers. Defects in GABA receptor genes might contribute to seizures and abnormal EEG activity in patients with autism and Angelman syndrome. GABA receptor genes regulate membrane excitability at the synapse along with glutamate receptor subtypes, and influence long-term potentiation and cortical plasticity in rodent models (Micheva and Beaulieu 1997). Genetically based disorders in GABA mediated inhibitory neurotransmission during brain development could contribute to the structural and behavioral problems seen in autism.

ABNORMAL SYNAPSE DEVELOPMENT IN AUTISM

In summary, our understanding of the disorders of brain development that contribute to autism is still in its infancy. However, several lines of evidence support the hypothesis that abnormalities in synapses and neuronal circuits are of major importance in autism. Brain overgrowth is one of the most prominent neurologic features of autism, and this occurs during an early postnatal window when synapses are expanding at a rapid rate in infants and toddlers. One of the earliest theories for autism involves abnormalities in metabolism of serotonin, and it is possible to link changes in this neurotransmitter to overgrowth of cerebral cortex and changes in behavior in animal models. Abnormalities in glutamate neurotransmission in autism are suggested by surveys of gene expression using microarrays in autopsy tissue, genetic linkage studies, and results from a mouse model of fra-X. Glutamate is quite important in cortical development and plasticity, and there are interactions between glutamate and serotonin in development of thalamocortical circuits. In addition, changes in inhibitory GABA receptors have also been implicated by genetic studies of the region on chromosome 15 that causes Angelman syndrome. These observations suggest many questions for future exploration.

ACKNOWLEDGMENT

The authors are supported by MRDDRC grant HD-24061 and STAART grant MH066417 from NIH.

REFERENCES

Aylward EH, Minshew NJ, Field K, Sparks BF, Singh N (2002) Effects of age on brain volume and head circumference in autism. *Neurology* 59: 175–83.

Bailey A, Luthert P, Bolton P, Le Couteur A, Rutter M, Harding B (1993) Autism and megalencephaly. *Lancet* 341: 1225–6.

Bailey A, Luthert P, Dean A, Harding B, Janota I, Montgomery M, Rutter M, Lantos P (1998) A clinicopathological study of autism. *Brain* 121: 889–905.

Bauman ML, Kemper TL (2005) Neuroanatomic observations of the brain in autism: a review and future directions. *Int J Dev Neurosci* 23: 183–7.

Bear MF, Huber KM, Warren ST (2004) The mGluR theory of fragile X mental retardation. *Trends Neurosci* 27: 370–7.

Blue ME, Erzurumlu RS, Jhaveri S (1991) A comparison of pattern formation by thalamocortical and serotonergic afferents in the rat barrel field cortex. *Cereb Cortex* 1: 380–9.

Berger-Sweeney J, Libbey M, Arters J, Junagadhwalla M, Hohmann CF (1998) Neonatal monoaminergic depletion in mice (*Mus musculus*) improves performance of a novel odor discrimination task. *Behav Neurosci* 112: 1318–26.

Carper RA, Moses P, Tigue ZD, Courchesne E (2002) Cerebral lobes in autism: early hyperplasia and abnormal age effects. *NeuroImage* 16: 1038–51.

Casanova MF, Buxhoeveden DP, Switala AE, Roy E (2002) Minicolumnar pathology in autism. *Neurology* 58: 428–32.

Casanova MR, Buxhoeveden DP, Gomez J (2003) Disruption in the inhibitory architecture of the cell minicolumn: implications for autism. *Neuroscientist* 9: 496–507.

Chi B, Engelman H, Scheiffele P (2005) Control of excitatory and inhibitory synapse formation by neuroligins. *Science* 307: 1324–8.

Chugani DC (2004) Serotonin in autism and pediatric epilepsy. *Ment Retard Dev Disabil Res Rev* 10: 112–6.

Chugani HT, Phelps ME, Mazziotta JC (1987) Positron emission tomography study of human brain functional development. *Ann Neurol* 22: 487–97.

Chugani DC, Muzik O, Behen M, Rothermel R, Janisse JJ, Lee J, Chugani HT (1999) Developmental changes in brain serotonin synthesis capacity in autistic and nonautistic children. *Ann Neurol* 45: 287–95.

Cohen-Cory S (2002) The developing synapse: construction and modulation of synaptic structures and circuits. *Science* 298: 770–6.

Comery TA, Harris JB, Willems PJ, Oostra BA, Irwin SA, Weiler IJ, Greenough WT (1997) Abnormal dendritic spines in fragile X knockout mice: maturation and pruning deficits. *Proc Natl Acad Sci USA* 94: 5401–4.

Cook EH, Leventhal BL, Heller W, Metz J, Wainwright M, Freedman DX (1990) Autistic children and their first degree relatives: relationships between serotonin and norepinephrine levels and intelligence. *J Neuropychiatr Clin Neuroci* 2: 268–74.

Courchesne E (2002) Abnormal early brain development in autism. *Mol Psychiatry* 7: S21–3.

Courchesne E, Karns BS, Davis BS, Ziccardi R, Carper RA, Tigue ZD, Chisum HJ, Moses P, Pierce K, Lord C, Lincoln AJ, Pizzo S, Schreibman L, Haas RH, Akshoomoff NA, Courchesne RY (2001) Unusual brain growth patterns in early life in patients with autistic disorder: an MRI study. *Neurology* 57: 245–54.

Courchesne E, Carper R, Akshoomoff N (2003) Evidence of brain overgrowth in the first year of life in autism. *JAMA* 290: 337–40.

D'Eufemia P, Finocchiaro R, Celli M, Viozzi L, Monteleone D, Giardini O (1995) Low serum tryptophan to large neutral amino acids ratio in idiopathic infantile autism. *Biomed Pharmacother* 49: 288-292.

De Fosse L, Hodge SM, Makris N, Kennedy DN, Caviness VS, McGrath L, Steele S, Ziegler DA, Herbert MR, Frazier JA, Tager-Flusberg H, Harris GJ (2004) Language-association cortex asymmetry in autism and specific language impairment. *Ann Neurol* 56: 757–66.

DeLong GR (1999) Autism: new data suggest a new hypothesis. *Neurology* 52: 911–6.

DeLong GR, Ritch CR, Burch S (2002) Fluoxetine response in children with autistic spectrum disorders: correlation with familial major affective disorder and intellectual achievement. *Dev Med Child Neurol* 44: 652–9.

Fatemi SH, Stary JM, Halt AR, Realmuto GR (2001) Dysregulation of Reelin and Bcl-2 proteins in autistic cerebellum. *J Autism Dev Disorders* 31: 529–35.

Herbert MR, Ziegler DA, Deutsch CK, O'Brien LM, Kennedy DN, Filipek PA, Bakardjiev AI, Hodgson J, Takeoka M, Makris N, Caviness VS (2005) Brain asymmetries in autism and developmental language disorder: a nested whole-brain analysis. *Brain* 128: 213–26.

Hohmann CF, Brooks AR, Coyle JT (1988) Neonatal lesions of the basal forebrain cholinergic neurons result in abnormal cortical development. *Dev Brain Res* 43: 253–64.

Hohmann CF, Richardson C, Pitts E, Berger-Sweeney J (2000) Neonatal 5,7-DHT lesions cause sex-specific changes in mouse cortical morphogenesis. *Neural Plast* 7: 213–32.

Huber KM, Gallagher SM, Warren, ST, Bear MF (2002) Altered synaptic plasticity in a mouse model of fragile X mental retardation. *Proc Natl Acad Sci USA* 99: 7746–50.

Huttenlocher PR (1979) Developmental changes and effects of aging. *Brain Res* 163: 195–205.

Huttenlocher PR (1990) Morphometric study of human cerebral cortex development. *Neuropsychologia* 28: 517–27.

Hussain NK, Sheng M (2005) Making synapses: a balancing act. *Science* 307: 1207–8.

Jamain S, Quach H, Betancur C, Rastam M, Colineaux C, Gillberg IC, Soderstrom H, Giros B, Leboyer M, Gillberg C, Bourgeron T; Paris Autism Research International Sibpair Study (2003) Mutations of the X-linked genes encoding neuroligins NLGN3 and NLGN4 are associated with autism. *Nat Genet* 34: 27–9.

Janusonis, S, Gluncic V, Rakic P (2004) Early serotonin projections to Cajal–Retzius cells: relevance for cortical development. *J Neurosci* 24: 1652–9.

Johnston MV, Coyle JT (1981) Development of central neurotransmitter systems. *Ciba Found Symp* 86: 251–70.

Johnston MV, Nishimura A, Harum K, Pekar J, Blue ME (2001) Sculpting the developing brain. *Adv Pediatr* 48: 1–38.

Jones MB, Palmour RM, Zwaigenbaum L, Szatmari P (2004) Modifier effects in autism at the MAO-A and DBH loci. *Am J Med Genet B Neuropsychiatr Genet* 126: 58–65.

Kanner L (1943) Autistic disturbances of affective contact. *Nerv Child* 2: 217–50.

Kondoh M, Shiga T, Okado N (2004) Regulation of dendrite formation of Purkinje cells by serotonin through serotonin 1A and serotonin 2A receptors in culture. *Neurosci Res* 48: 101–9.

Lauder JM (1990) Ontogeny of the serotonergic system in the rat: serotonin as a developmental signal. *Ann NY Acad Sci* 600: 297–313.

Laumonnier F, Bonnet-Brilhault F, Gomot M, Blanc R, David A, Moizard MP, Raynaud M, Ronce N, Lemonnier E, Calvas P, Laudier B, Chelly J, Fryns JP, Ropers HH, Hamel BC, Andres C, Barthelemy C, Moraine C, Briault S (2004) X-linked mental retardation and autism are associated with a mutation in the NLGN4 gene, a member of the neuroligin family. *Am J Hum Genet* 74: 552–7.

Levitt JG, Blanton RE, Smalley S, Thompson PM, Guthrie D, McCracken JT, Sadoun T, Heinichen L, Toga AW (2003) Cortical sulcal maps in autism. *Cereb Cortex* 13: 728–35.

Limoges E, Mottron L, Bolduc C, Berthiaume C, Godbout R (2005) Atypical sleep architecture and the autism phenotype. *Brain* 128: 1049–61.

Malenka RC (2003) Synaptic plasticity and AMPA receptor trafficking. *Ann NY Acad Sci* 1003: 1–11.

Martin ER, Menold MM, Wolpert CM, Bass MP, Donnelly SL, Ravan SA, Zimmerman A, Gilbert JR, Vance JM, Maddox LO, Wright HH, Abramson RK, DeLong GR, Cuccaro ML, Pericak-Vance MA (2000) Analysis of linkage disequilibrium in gamma-aminobutyric acid receptor subunit genes in autistic disorder. *Am J Med Genet* 96: 43–8.

McDonald JW, Johnston MV (1990) Physiological and pathophysiological roles of excitatory amino acids during central nervous system development. *Brain Res Rev* 15: 41–70.

McDougle CJ, Naylor ST, Cohen DJ, Aghajanian GK, Heninger GR, Price LH (1996) Effects of tryptophan depletion in drug-free adults with autistic disorder. *Arch Gen Psychiatry* 53: 993–1000.

Micheva KD, Beaulieu C (1997) Development and plasticity of the inhibitory neocortical circuitry with an emphasis on the rodent barrel field cortex: a review. *Can J Physiol Pharmacol* 75: 470–8.

Nabi R, Serajee FJ, Chugani DC, Zhong H, Huq AH (2004) Association of tryptophan 2,3 dioxygenase gene polymorphism with autism. *Am J Med Genet B Neuropsychiatr Genet* 125: 63–8.

Nishimura A, Hohmann CF, Johnston MV, Blue ME (2002) Neonatal electrolytic lesions of the basal forebrain stunt plasticity in mouse barrel field cortex. *Int J Dev Neurosci* 20: 481–9.

Nurmi EL, Bradford Y, Chen Y, Hall J, Arnone B, Gardiner MB, Hutcheson HB, Gilbert JR, Pericak-Vance MA, Copeland-Yates SA, Michaelis RC, Wassink TH, Santangelo SL, Sheffield VC, Piven J, Folstein SE, Haines JL, Sutcliffe JS (2001) Linkage disequilibrium at the Angelman syndrome gene UBE3A in autism families. *Genomics* 77: 105–13.

Purcell AE, Jeon OH, Zimmerman AW, Blue ME, Pevsner J (2001) Postmortem brain abnormalities of the glutamate neurotransmitter system in autism. *Neurology* 57: 1618–28.

Ramanathan S, Woodroffe A, Flodman PL, Mays LZ, Hanouni M, Modahl CB, Steinberg-Epstein R, Bocian ME, Spence MA, Smith M (2004) A case of autism with an interstitial deletion on 4q leading to hemizygosity for genes encoding glutamine and glycine neurotransmitter receptor sub-units (AMPA 2, GLRA3, GLRB) and neuropeptide receptors NPY1R, NPY5R. *BMC Med Genet* 5: 10.

Rapin I (2002) The autistic-spectrum disorders. *N Engl J Med* 347: 302–4.

Serajee FJ, Zhong H, Nabi R, Huq AHMM (2003) The metabotropic glutamate receptor 8 gene at 7q31: partial duplication and possible association with autism. *J Med Genet* 40: e42.

Shain RJ, Freedman DX (1961) Studies on 5-hydroxyindole metabolism in autistic and other mentally retarded children. *Disabil Rehabil* 58: 315–20.

Song J-Y, Ichtchenko K, Sudhof T, Brose N (1999) Neuroligin 1 is a postsynaptic cell-adhesion molecule of excitatory synapses. *Proc Natl Acad Sci USA* 96: 1100–5.

Sparks BF, Friedman SD, Shaw DW, Aylward EH, Echelard D, Artru AA, Maravilla KR, Giedd JN, Munson J, Dawson G, Dager SR (2002) Brain structural abnormalities in young children with autism spectrum disorder. *Neurology* 59: 184–92.

Stevensen RE, Schroer RJ, Skinner C, Fender D, Simensen RJ (1997) Autism and macrocephaly. *Lancet* 349: 1744–5.

Tuchman R, Rapin I (2002) Epilepsy in autism. *Lancet Neurol* 1: 352–8.

Wallace GL, Treffert DA (2004) Head size and autism. *Lancet* 363: 1003–4.

Whitaker-Azmitia PM (2005) Behavioral and cellular consequences of increasing serotonergic activity during brain development: a role in autism? *Int J Dev Neurosci* 23: 75–83.

Xu Y, Sari Y, Zhou FC (2004) Selective serotonin reuptake inhibitor disrupts organization of thalamocortical somatosensory barrels during development. *Brain Res Dev Brain Res* 150: 151–61.

Yew DT, Chan WY (1999) Early appearance of acetylcholinergic, serotonergic and peptigergic neurons and fibers in developing human central nervous system. *Microsc Res Tech* 45: 389–400.

Yirmiya N, Pilowsky T, Nemanov L, Arbelle S, Feinsilver T, Fried I, Ebstein RP (2001) Evidence for an association with the serotonin transporter promotor region polymorphism and autism. *Am J Med Genet* 105: 381–6.

7

GENETIC ASPECTS OF AUTISM

Maria T Acosta and Phillip L Pearl

Multiple lines of evidence converge to suggest that autism, a complex behaviorally defined clinical syndrome, is one of the most heritable neuropsychiatric conditions. Twin and family studies, known chromosomal abnormalities, genetic linkage and association studies, and in some cases genome analysis, provide evidence that there are multiple interacting genes that may contribute to this disorder. Studying specific behavioral domains such as communication or socialization as isolated endophenotypes in affected individuals and family members may help identify subtle albeit specific gene alterations and further our understanding of the genetic basis of autism.

FAMILY AND TWIN STUDIES

The descriptions by Leo Kanner and Hans Asperger in the 1940s and other early studies did not suggest that genetics played a major role in autism. No obvious or consistent chromosomal anomalies were found, and sibling recurrence rates were erroneously thought to be low. Later twin studies altered this view (Folstein and Rutter 1977a; Newschaffer et al. 2002) by revealing substantive differences in concordance for autism between dizygotic (DZ) versus monozygotic (MZ) twin pairs, with concordance rates in MZ twins reaching 96% in some studies (Ritvo et al. 1985). The increased recurrence rate within sibships (Ritvo et al. 1989, Newschaffer et al. 2002) was underestimated until reproductive stoppage was identified as a factor that reduced recurrence in families having an autistic child (Slager 2001). The long identified strong male preponderance remains unexplained (Ritvo et al. 1985, Steffenburg and Gillberg 1986). The genetic contribution to autism is attributed to the combined effects of multiple contributory loci. This conclusion is based partly on lower concordance for dizygotic (DZ) than monozygotic (MZ) twins and partly on the failure to find very strong evidence for linkage in genome-wide studies. The twin data are compatible with oligogenic inheritance combined with a major epigenetic de novo component (Jiang et al. 2004). Genetic factors may produce social and cognitive deficits included in the broad autism phenotype, and an interaction between these and unknown deleterious factors may provide a "second hit" that ultimately produces a more narrow autism phenotype (Folstein and Rutter 1988, Kates et al. 2004). The broader autism phenotype refers to features of autism spectrum disorder (ASD) that involve social or communicative impairment of less severity than what would be considered diagnostic of autistic disorder (Bolton et al. 1994, Bailey et al. 1995).

Results from family and twin studies, summarized in Table 7.1, indicate a strong tendency for autism to cluster in families. There is a particularly strong risk for ASDs among siblings of more severely affected individuals with autistic disorder, with relative risk estimates in the range of 2–6% as compared with the accepted population prevalence rate for autism of 4–6 per 10,000 (Smalley et al. 1988, Newschaffer et al. 2002). The overall recurrence risk in a family appears to be 7–15%. When kinships were analyzed by specific degrees of relationship, it was shown that the familial aggregation of autism appears confined to sib-pairs. This indicates that a single-gene model is unlikely to

TABLE 7.1
Family and twin population studies in autism

Design	Findings	Comments	Reference
MZ twin study: Clinical and neuroimaging studies (16 MZ pairs)	7 pairs concordant, 9 discordant for autism. Both concordant and discordant twin pairs exhibited concordance in cerebral gray and white matter volume. Only the clinically concordant pairs exhibited concordance in cerebellar grey and white matter volume	Differences in cerebellar volume in discordant MZ twins imply that cerebellar morphometry may be mediated by nongenetic factors	Kates et al. (2004)
MZ and DZ twin study (28 MZ pairs; 20 DZ)	High concordance for a broader phenotype		Le Couteur et al. (1996)
Twin study (28 MZ and 20 DZ same sex twin pairs). Includes 19 from the original study by Folstein and Rutter (1977b)	17 MZ, 0 DZ concordance for autism. Using a broader spectrum of related cognitive and social abnormalities, concordance was 26 MZ and 2 DZ	Broadening the clinical spectrum led to increased concordance rates in twins	Bailey et al. (1995)
Large-scale systematic family study	5.8% of siblings of autistic probands had PDD; 12.4% of siblings had "milder phenotype". Mental retardation was an exclusion criterion	No higher association with epilepsy or increase in head size in probands younger than 16 years	Bolton et al. (1994)

continued ↗

TABLE 7.1
(continued)

Design	Findings	Comments	Reference
Epidemiological survey (Utah)	86 autistic subjects linked to genealogical database. Strong tendency for autism to cluster in families	Familial aggregation confined to sib pairs	Jorde et al. (1990)
Epidemiological survey (Utah)	9.7% of 207 families had more than one autistic child. Autism was 215 times more frequent among siblings of autistic children	Overall recurrence risk 8.6%. If first autistic child is male risk is 7%; if female 14.5%	Ritvo et al. (1989)
Population based same sex twin study (Denmark, Finland, Iceland, Norway and Sweden). All twin pairs younger than 25 years with at least one member with ASD (11 MZ, 10 DZ; total 33 with ASD)	Concordance for autism 10 MZ, 0 DZ	In discordant pairs, autistic twin with higher perinatal stress. Fragile-X in 3/33 ASD cases	Steffenburg et al. (1989)
Twin pairs (UCLA registry for genetic studies in autism) (23 MZ, 17 DZ)	Concordance 21 MZ, 4 DZ		Ritvo et al. (1985)
Twin and autistic registry. One or both twins affected (11 MZ, 10 DZ)	Concordance 4 MZ, 0 DZ. In most MZ pairs, the co-twins showed some cognitive impairment	Higher frequency of perinatal complications in affected twin in discordant pairs. Concordance for developmental delay was 9 MZ and 1 DZ	Folstein and Rutter (1977b)

Abbreviations: MZ = monozygotic; DZ = dizygotic; PDD = pervasive developmental disorder; UCLA = University of California at Los Angeles.

account for most cases of autism (Jorde et al. 1990, 1991).

Broadening the phenotype leads to higher identification rates of mild developmental impairments such as varying degrees of social aloofness, lack of friendships and impaired play in parents and siblings than in control families (Bailey et al. 1998). Studies addressing this type of familial involvement are summarized in Table 7.2. Several reports describe a subset of relatives of individuals with autism who display social and language deficits qualitatively similar to those of the autistic proband but milder in severity. Studies have found that co-twins discordant for a diagnosis of autism may yet have similar cognitive and social deficits (Folstein and Rutter 1977b). As early as 1957, Kanner and Eisenberg reported that many of the fathers of autistic children had unusual personality traits such as rigidity and a lack of interest in social interaction. Overall, traits found more commonly in parents of autistic probands than in parents of controls include social reticence, communication difficulties (pragmatic language), preference for routine, and difficulty with change. Generally these traits do not impair functioning (by clinical standards) but they may be a marker of a genetic liability to autism. Delayed onset of speech and reading difficulty are more common in family members than in control families; in contrast, mental retardation has not been found in siblings of autistic children more often than expected by chance, unless the sibling is also autistic (Folstein and Rutter 1977a,b; Folstein and Rosen-Sheidley 2001; Newschaffer et al. 2002).

TABLE 7.2
Autistic traits in family members

Design	Findings in relatives of probands	Comments	Study
Factors influencing the rate and severity of phenotypic expression among 3095 first- and second-degree relatives of 149 autistic probands. Comparison with 36 Down syndrome families	7.5% of relatives classified as falling within the broader phenotype	For probands with intact speech, the phenotype severity in relatives was related to the ICD-10 score in the proband	Pickles et al. (2000)
Evaluation of personality traits of adult relatives of 99 autistic and 36 Down syndrome probands	Increased expression of anxious, impulsive, aloof, shy, over-sensitive traits. Factor analysis revealed 3 groups of traits, 2 (withdrawn and difficult) reflecting impaired social functioning	Scale used: Modified Personality Assessment Schedule	Murphy et al. (2000)

continued ↗

TABLE 7.2
(continued)

Design	Findings in relatives of probands	Comments	Study
Comparison of social and communication deficits in relatives ascertained through two autistic siblings (25 families) compared with Down syndrome (30 families)	Higher rates of social and communication deficits and stereotyped behaviors in relatives within families with multiple-incidence autism		Piven et al. (1997)
Cognitive performance in first-degree relatives of autistic probands and of Down syndrome probands	Relatives of autistic probands tended to have higher verbal scores than those of Down probands	Siblings affected with the broader phenotype had significantly lower IQ scores and poorer reading and spelling performances than unaffected siblings	Fombonne et al. (1997a)
Pragmatic rating scale evaluation in parents of autistic children	As a group, parents of 28 autistic children exhibited greater numbers of atypical pragmatic behaviors that controls. Pragmatic deficits were conceptually similar to the pragmatic language deficits of autism		Landa et al. (1992)
Evaluation of spontaneous narrative–discourse performance	41 parents of 29 autistic children were evaluated. Narratives of autism parents were less complex and coherent than those of controls		Landa et al. (1991)
Estimation of lifetime risk of psychiatric disorders (81 parents of 42 autistic probands; 34 parents of Down syndrome probands)	Lifetime prevalence rate of anxiety significantly greater in parents of autism probands. Lifetime prevalence rates of depression higher in parents of autism probands but not statistically significant	Semistructured investigator-based version of the Schedule for Affective Disorders and Schizophrenia	Piven et al. (1991)

GENETIC CONDITIONS ASSOCIATED WITH AUTISM

Approximately 10–15% of individuals with autism have an identifiable chromosomal aberration or genetic syndrome. Autism is over-represented as part of the behavioral phenotype of several disorders, including fragile-X syndrome (fra-X), tuberous sclerosis, phenylketonuria (PKU), Rett syndrome, and duplications involving chromosome 15q (Gillberg and Wahlstrom 1985, Mariner et al. 1986, Bailey et al. 2001) Most of the associations in the medical literature have been case reports, but several conditions have been studied more systematically (Folstein and Rosen-Sheidley 2001). Some reports have demonstrated that 3–9% of autism patients have chromosomal abnormalities (Fombonne et al. 1997a, Wassink et al. 2001a). These rates vary further depending on whether individuals with mental retardation or dysmorphism are included (Gillberg and Wahlstrom 1985, Wahlstrom et al. 1989, Rutter et al. 1994).

FRAGILE-X SYNDROME

Early estimates reported a prevalence of fra-X in autism as high as 25%; more recent studies suggest a lower percentage (2–5%) (Hagerman et al. 1986a,b; Mariner et al. 1986; Rogers et al. 2001) Current estimates of the prevalence of autistic disorder in fra-X are approximately 15–25% (Hagerman et al. 1986b, Feinstein and Reiss 1998, Bailey et al. 2001) Between 50% and 90% of individuals with fra-X have been reported to have some manifestations of autism such as poor eye contact, hand flapping, hand biting, perseveration in speech and tactile defensiveness, but did not meet full criteria for autistic disorder, although some may well have met criteria for the wider autistic phenotype (ASD, as defined in Chapter 1) (Hagerman et al. 1986, Kerby and Dawson 1994, Bailey et al. 2001). Mazzocco et al. (1997) found that 3% of females with the fra-X full mutation sequence met diagnostic criteria for autistic disorder. Attempts to correlate behavioral ratings, FMR1 protein (FMRP) expression, and the developmental trajectories of boys with fra-X have not demonstrated a relationship between behavior and FMRP (Bailey et al. 2001). The pathophysiologic role of the *FMR1* mutation and its relationship to the autism phenotype thus remains undefined (Rogers et al. 2001).

TUBEROUS SCLEROSIS

In 1932, Critchley and Earl described autistic behavior in tuberous sclerosis complex (TSC) patients (see Curatolo et al. 2004). The prevalence of autistic behaviors in TSC appears to exceed that of cardiac and renal abnormalities for which routine screening is conducted. A review of medical conditions associated with autism concluded that TSC had the highest association with autism and a defined genetic condition (Rutter et al. 1994). Different studies have reported prevalence rates of autism in TSC that range between 19% and 51% (Hunt and Dennis 1987, Hunt and Shepherd 1993, Gillberg et al. 1994). The overall prevalence of TSC in large unselected samples of patients with autism is estimated to be 1–4%, and higher in autism patients with epilepsy.

The *TSC1* and *TSC2* genes are located on chromosomes 9q34 and 16p13, respectively. Alterations in neurogenesis and neuronal migration are believed to underlie the development of cerebral lesions in TSC. Various hypotheses have been proposed to explain the association between TSC and autism. Abnormal brain organization or lesions caused by TSC gene mutations may alter neural networks responsible for autism. A specific autism susceptibility gene(s) may exist in linkage disequilibrium with the TSC genes.

RETT SYNDROME

Careful clinical descriptions served to distinguish Rett syndrome from classic autism before the *MeCP2* gene mutation was identified. The discovery of the *MeCP2* gene has now led to the identification of a broader phenotype than what had been typically associated with the classic clinical features of Rett syndrome. Two preliminary screening studies suggested that *MeCP2* mutation rates may be as high as 3–5% in female autism populations (Lam et al. 2000, Beyer et al. 2002). Rett syndrome is an X-linked disorder with 99.5% of cases being sporadic. Girls with classic Rett syndrome develop normally until approximately 6–8 months of age when acquired microcephaly and lack or loss of purposeful hand skills become evident, followed by failure of speech development with stereotypic hand movements, abnormal breathing patterns, ataxia, and in some cases epilepsy. Autistic behavior tends to be more prominent in early childhood and to abate with age.

The *MeCP2* gene is implicated in DNA methylation and repression of gene expression. Rett syndrome, therefore, appears to be a result of gene overexpression at some point in development. Heterozygous female mice with the *MeCP2* mutation *Mecp2(308/X)* develop neurological and behavioral symptoms at about 9 months of age, after reaching a certain level of maturity. This leads to the hypothesis that the genetic defect might affect brain functioning at a later phase than prenatal or early postnatal development (Chen et al. 2001, Guy et al. 2001) and is consistent with the finding that the MeCP2 protein is expressed after neurons reach a certain level of maturity (Shahbazian et al. 2002a). Male mice hemizygous for *Mecp2(308/Y)* develop symptoms at 6 weeks and eventually manifest many of the core features of Rett syndrome, including stereotyped forelimb movements, less exploration of novel environments, and social dysfunction (Shahbazian et al. 2002b, Moretti 2005).

OTHER DISORDERS ASSOCIATED WITH ASD

Autism has been associated with a variety of disorders. The earliest report of an association between autism and a mendelian condition was phenylketonuria (PKU), in which autistic symptomatology, yet not IQ, improves with delayed institution of dietary treatment after infancy (Folstein and Rutter 1988). Of a population of 100 Swedish thalidomide embryopathy cases, at least four met full criteria for DSM-III-R autistic disorder and ICD-10 childhood autism (Stromland et al. 1994). Gillberg and Rasmussen (1994) described four patients with Williams syndrome who also met criteria for autism. An epidemiologic survey conducted among 325,347 children born in three French départements between 1976 and 1985 found a prevalence rate of autistic disorder of 5.35/10,000 (16.3/10,000 if other pervasive developmental disorders are included), with no differences related to geographical area or social class. Rates of associated medical conditions were: 4.6% sensory impairments, 2.9% chromosomal abnormalities including fra-X, 2.9% cerebral palsy, 1.7% Down syndrome, 1.1% tuberous sclerosis, 0.6% neurofibromatosis, and 0.6% congenital rubella (Fombonne et al. 1997b).

GENETIC MECHANISMS

Studies have emphasized idiopathic cases unassociated with other symptoms. The most parsimonious model is one in which several genes with possibly mild effects interact with each other to produce the phenotype (Folstein and Rosen-Sheidley 2001). Autism would most likely occur in a child who inherits three or four contributory genes from one or both parents. This inheritance may occur as varying combinations of a larger array of predisposing genes. This model provides an explanation for the variation in severity within sibling pairs, and for variable and milder phenotypes of the broadened spectrum in family members. Alternatively, autism may be caused by confluence of a genetic predisposition to language disorders or social reticence combined with a second hit from an environmental or immunogenetic risk factor (Folstein and Mankoski 2000, Folstein and Rosen-Sheidley 2001). The DNA alterations invoked in "autism susceptibility" may involve variance in single nucleotides known as single nucleotide polymorphisms (SNPs). Further, SNPs are now known to be organized into repeated strands or sequences known as copy number polymorphisms, or CNPs. Variations between individuals at the level of CNPs may be the basis of a genetic predisposition to neuropsychiatric syndromes such as autism (Buckley et al. 2005).

Genome-wide scans are a key research strategy that has been employed in multiplex families, i.e. those with more than one affected family member. *Genetic linkage* involves identifying gene markers that segregate with the disorder. Several genome wide scans have been published by various centers over approximately the last decade. In general, the loci identified have not yet been consistent, with the possible exception of chromosome 7q, for which the linkage has been supported by a meta-analysis (Badner 2002). Other regions of interest with strong peaks or multiple supportive studies include chromosomes 2q, 4, 13q and 17p. The evidence of linkage to the X chromosome remains inconsistent despite male predominance (Ritvo et al. 1985, Steffenburg and Gillberg 1986). Methodological improvements such as larger sample sizes or denser mapping will likely yield more markers. Summary results of genome-wide scans in autism are presented in Table 7.3.

CANDIDATE GENES IMPLICATED IN AUTISM

As shown in Table 7.3, genome-wide linkage analyses of families with autism have yielded positive signals for several chromosomal loci (Gutknecht 2001; Shao et al. 2002a,b; Smalley et al. 2002). In particular, 2q and 7q have had the highest LOD scores and

TABLE 7.3
Genome-wide scans in autism

Affected sibling pairs	Chromosome region	Highest LOD scores[1]	Study
87	7q	MLS 2.53	IMGSAC (1998)[2]
	16p	MLS 1.51	
	4p	MLS 1.51	
75	13q	MMLS 2.2	Barrett (1999)
	7q		
51	6q	MMLS 2.23	Philippe (1999)
147	1p	MMLS 2.15	Risch et al. (1999)
118	5q	MMLS 2.55	Liu (2001)
	Xqter	X-MLS 2.56	
	19p	MMLS 2.53	
	Xqter	X-MLS 2.67	
	16p	MMLS 1.93	
	19q	MMLS 1.70	
38	3q	MLS 4.81	Auranen (2002)
	1q	MLS 2.61	
	7q	MLS 3.6	
152	2q	MMLS 4.80	IMGSAC (2001)[2]
	7q	MMLS 3.20	
	16p	MMLS 2.93	
	17q	MMLS 2.34	
96	3p	MLS 1.51	Shao et al. (2002b)
	7q	MLS 1.66	
	Xq	MLS 2.54	
345	17q	MMLS 2.83	Yonan (2003)
	5p	MMLS 2.54	
	11p	MMLS 2.24	
	4q	MMLS 1.72	
	8q	MMLS 1.60	
17 (Asperger)	1q	MLS 3.58	Ylisaukko-oja (2004)
	3p	MLS 3.32	
	13q	MLS 2.86	

[1]LOD = logarithm of the odds; MLS = maximum LOD score; MMLS = multi-point maximum LOD score.
[2]IMGSAC = International Molecular Genetic Study of Autism Consortium.

frequency of detection in different studies (Licinio and Alvarado 2002, Yu et al. 2002). An independent linkage study identified a region on 7q31 as the locus responsible for the speech–language disorder 1 (*SPCH1*) (Fisher et al. 1998). The possible relationship between SPCH1 and autism is supported by increased rates of language impairment in relatives of autistic individuals (Folstein and Mankoski 2000, Warburton et al. 2000).

Chromosomes 7 and 15 have been extensively studied in autism and involve several candidate genes. Table 7.4 specifies the candidate genes referable to these chromosomes. They are chosen on the basis of their position near linkage signals and their plausibility based on their role in fetal brain development. Several groups have been looking closely at 7q22-31 because this region has been implicated in several genome screens.

TABLE 7.4
Candidate genes in chromosomes 7 and 15

Gene	Name	Localization	Function	References
HOXA1	Homeobox A1	7p15-p14.2	Encodes a transcription factor. Expression is spatially and temporally regulated during embryonic development	Hong et al. (1995), Ingram et al. (2000)
RELN	Reelin	7q22	Regulates migration of cortical pyramidal neurons, interneurons and Purkinje cells during brain development	Hong et al. (2000), IMGSAC (2001)
ST7/RAY1	Suppression of tumorigenicity	7q31.1	Tumor suppressor, frequently found in squamous cell carcinomas of head/neck, colon and prostate	Zenklusen et al. (1995), IMGSAC (2001)
IMMP2L	Inner mitochondrial membrane peptidase 2-like	7q31	Encodes the homolog of the yeast inner mitochondrial membrane peptidase subunit-2	IMGSAC (2001)
WNT2	Wingless-type MMTV integration site family member 2	7q31	Influences the development of numerous organs and the central nervous system	IMGSAC (2001), Wassink et al. (2001b)
FOXP2/ SPCH1	Forkhead box P2/Speech and language disorder 1	7q31	Putative transcription factor containing a polyglutamine tract and a forkhead DNA binding domain. It is mutant in developmental verbal dyspraxia	Hurst et al. (1990), Folstein and Mankoski (2000a), Lai et al. (2000), IMGSAC (2001), Newbury and Monaco (2002), Newbury et al. (2002)

continued ↗

TABLE 7.4
Candidate genes in chromosomes 7 and 15

Gene	Name	Localization	Function	References
UBE3A	Ubiquitin-protein ligase E3A	15q11-q13	Encodes a member of a family of functionally related proteins defined by a conserved C-terminal 350-amino acid "hect" domain. Hect E3 proteins appear to be important in substrate recognition and in ubiquitin transfer. Imprinting of the *UBE3A* gene is restricted to brain	Kishino et al. (1997), Nurmi et al. (2001), Jiang et al. (2004), Samaco et al. (2005)
GABRB3	Gamma-aminobutyric acid A receptor beta-3	15q11.2-q12	GABA is the major inhibitory neurotransmitter in the mammalian brain where it acts at GABA-A receptors, which are ligand-gated chloride channels. Chloride conductance of these channels can be modulated by agents such as benzodiazepines that bind to the GABA-A receptor	Maestrini et al. (1999), Buxbaum et al. (2002), Samaco et al. (2005)
HERC2	Hect domain and RCC1-like domain 2	15q11-q13	Encodes a group of unusually large proteins. All members of this gene family have at least 1 copy of an N-terminal region showing homology to the cell cycle regulator RCC1 (regulator chromosome condensation 1) as well as a C-terminal Hect (homologous to E6-AP C terminus) domain found in a number of E3 ubiquitin protein ligases	Smith et al. (2000), Pujana et al. (2002)

RELN

Associations on chromosome 7 with autism have been found for *RELN*, which encodes for reelin, an extracellular protein guiding neuronal migration during fetal brain development. Reelin plays a pivotal role in the development of the cerebral cortex, cerebellum, hippocampus and brainstem (Fatemi 2001; Fatemi et al. 2001a,b). Recent studies have found an association between autism and a GGC repeat located at 5′ on the *RELN* gene (Persico et al. 2001, Skaar et al. 2005). Data from several groups have shown that changes in *RELN* expression exhibit a broad phenotypic spectrum, including several neuropsychiatric disorders (Fatemi et al. 2001a), neuromuscular disorders, and lissencephaly (Hong et al. 2000a).

RAY1

RAY1 (known as *ST7*, or suppression tumorigenicity 7) has been examined carefully without confirmation of linkage. It has a complicated structure, with several isoforms and several coding and non-coding regions (Vincent et al. 2000). Wassink et al. (2001b) found two sib-pair families among 75 in which both affected siblings had mutations of *WNT2* (wingless-type MMTV integration site family member 2), the gene adjacent to *RAY1*. The *WNT* gene family influences the development of numerous organ systems, including the CNS. *WNT2* is located in the region of 7q31-33 linked to autism and was observed to be adjacent to a chromosomal breakpoint in an individual with autism (Wassink et al. 2001b). Furthermore, a mouse knockout of *Dvl1*, a member of a gene family essential for the function of the *WNT* pathway, exhibits a behavioral phenotype characterized primarily by diminished social interaction (Wassink et al. 2001b).

FOXP2 (FORKHEAD BOX 2; FORMERLY REFERRED TO AS *SPCH1*)

FOXP2 has been associated with a developmental language disorder and is located in region 7q31 (Hurst et al. 1990). A point mutation in FOXP2, which encodes a putative transcription factor, was found in affected members of a family with severe speech and language disorder (Lai et al. 2000). Autism and severe language impairment may share a gene in this region (Folstein and Mankoski 2000).

GABA-A RECEPTOR

Special interest has developed in chromosome 15, particularly given the autism phenotype common to some individuals with Angelman syndrome, involving 15q11-13, and a high incidence of chromosome 15 mutations reported in autism. Markers across this region have been screened for evidence of linkage association. Three of the gamma-aminobutyric acid (GABA)-A receptor subunit genes are localized in this critical region. Several studies reported an association with polymorphisms of a GABA-A receptor subtype, *GABRB3*, and autism (Buxbaum et al. 2002) or other nearby genes (Martin et al. 2000, Menold et al. 2001). Other studies have not replicated these findings (Maestrini et al. 1999, Martin et al. 2000). *UBE3A*, an Angelman syndrome gene, has been associated with autism (Slopien and Rajewski 2000, Nurmi et al. 2001).

SEROTONIN TRANSPORTER

Serotonin (5-hydroxytryptamine, 5-HT) is involved in a range of behaviors and psychological processes, including mood, anxiety, obsessive-compulsive symptoms, aggression, impulsivity, sleep and social interaction. The 5-HT transporter gene on chromosome 17, which contains a variable repeat sequence in the promoter region (referred to as the 5-HT-transporter-linked promoter region, HTTLPR), has been examined in several data sets. An initial study found an association between autism and the short allele of HTTLPR (Cook et al. 1997), although further studies showed contradictory results. Studies have shown both positive (Klauck et al. 1997, Tordjman et al. 2001, Yirmiya et al. 2001) and negative (Maestrini et al. 1999, Persico et al. 2000) results for an association with the long allele.

NEUROLIGINS

At least two loci on the X chromosome implicated a novel group of proteins known as neuroligins. These are fundamental in synapse formation. De novo Xp22.3 deletions have been observed in three autistic females (Thomas et al. 1999), and a second locus at Xq13-21 has shown an allele sharing markers DXS7132 and DXS6789 in affected sib pairs (Auranen 2002, Shao et al. 2002a). The transcript KIAA1260 has been identified within the deleted interval on Xp22.3, corresponding to *NLGN4*, a member of the neuroligin family. (Bolliger et al. 2001) An additional neuroligin gene, *NLGN3* (Philibert et al. 2000) (a homolog of *NLGN4*, located at X13 [55-56] cM) has been associated with sib-pairs in autism genome-wide analyses. These genes encode cell-adhesion molecules present at the postsynaptic side of the synapse (Song et al. 1999, Scheiffele et al. 2000). Neuroligin mutations have also been associated with X-linked mental retardation, and it is hypothesized that a defect in *NLGN3* or *NLGN4* may abolish formation, stabilization or recognition of specific synapses essential for communication processes (Jablonka and Lamb 2002, Laumonnier et al. 2004).

GLUR6

The glutamate receptor *GluR6* gene has also been described in association with autism. Glutamate is the principal excitatory neurotransmitter in the brain and is directly involved in cognitive functions such as memory and learning. Jamain et al. (2002) found that 8% of autistic subjects and 4% of the controls had SNPs of *GluR6*. This change seems to be more maternally transmitted to autistic males (p=0.007) than expected.

EPIGENETICS

At one time, "epigenetics" referred to the developmental processes that linked genotype to phenotype and gene–environment relationships, i.e. nature versus nurture. In the modern era of molecular biology, epigenetics has evolved to mean the temporal and spatial processes that regulate gene expression (Jablonka and Lamb 2002, Jablonka et al. 2002). Common modifications include DNA methylation and histone acetylation. Methylation of cytosine residues located in promoter CpG islands prevents binding of transcription factors and shuts down transcription. These modifications allow regulation of both temporal and tissue-specific gene expression (Ingrosso et al. 2003). Hypermethylation of the trinucleotide repeat region in *FMR1* causes fragile X syndrome (in which 15–25% of affected individuals have autistic disorder and up to 90% may have the broader ASD phenotype). Parent of origin effects (i.e. genomic imprinting) depend on DNA methylation and histone modification of a single parental allele. This underlies the maternal chromosome 15q11-q13 duplication that is associated with Angelman syndrome. Histone acetylation is an epigenetic modification that influences chromatin structure. This process is important in the pathophysiology of Rett syndrome. The Rett syndrome gene, *MeCP2*, encodes a protein that, when functional, promotes chromatin condensation at particular points in the genome. In disorders with complex genetic heterogeneity, such as autism, there could be more subtle variations in genes that may encode proteins or RNA molecules that act as regulators of gene expression and thereby perturb multiple systems (Veenstra-Vanderweele et al. 2004).

In addition, there are lines of evidence for environmental influences on gene expression. Exogenous methylation of DNA has been demonstrated in adult humans. Patients on hemodialysis who have elevated homocysteine show impaired DNA methylation and have a resulting shift in expression of imprinted genes that are inappropriately transcribed. Folic acid supplementation, with reduction of homocysteine levels, favors DNA methylation and corrects the pattern of imprinted gene expression (Ingrosso et al. 2003). A second model involves the agouti mouse, whose coat color varies from yellow to black based on a specific genotype. Litters of genetically identical heterozygous agouti mice show remarkable variations in coat pattern that correspond to variable methylation of the gene promoter. However, females with a yellow coat tend to have offspring that appear yellow and mottled, whereas females with a black coat have 20% black offspring (Rakyan et al. 2001). Supplementation with folic acid and other vitamins early in pregnancy is associated with an increased likelihood of bearing offspring with a yellow coat (Waterland and Jirtle 2003), suggesting that dietary modification can cause transmissible, lifelong alterations in phenotype.

There is also evidence for gene-to-gene regulation. *MECP2* deficiency may affect the level of expression of *UBE3A* and neighboring autism candidate gene *GABRB3*. Defects in *UBE3A* expression have been demonstrated in *MeCP2*-deficient mice and in brain tissue from patients with Rett and Angelman syndromes, using microarray and inmunoblot techniques (Samaco et al. 2005). Thus, *MeCP2* appears to have a role in the regulation of *UBE3A* and *GABRB3* expression in the postnatal mammalian brain.

GENETIC/METABOLIC SCREENING

A practice parameter has been published through the auspices of the Child Neurology Society and American Academy of Neurology (Filipek et al. 2000). Karyotype and DNA analysis for fra-X are recommended in the evaluation of patients with autism in the presence of mental retardation (or if mental retardation cannot be excluded), if there is a family history of fra-X or undiagnosed mental retardation, or if dysmorphic features are present. These studies are unlikely to be positive in the presence of high-functioning autism.

Selective metabolic testing should be initiated by the presence of suggestive clinical and physical findings: lethargy, cyclic vomiting or early seizures; the presence of dysmorphic or coarse facial features; evidence of mental retardation or if mental retardation cannot be ruled out; or if there is a question regarding ascertainment of adequate newborn screening.

Consideration of genetic testing leads to ethical questions. Compelling ethical reasons to pursue genetic testing include: (a) identification of rare, albeit treatable, etiologies that, if not treated, would be deleterious to the individual, e.g. PKU; (b) diagnosis of a disorder that may lead to genetic counseling of family members, vis-a-vis recurrence risk, prenatal diagnosis and prognosis; and (c) identification of a suspected disorder that, if confirmed, would obviate the requirement for further extensive diagnostic tests. In clinical practice, testing for specific genetic–metabolic syndromes should be pursued based on clinical suspicion of a disorder. Genome-wide screening for mutation analysis (discussed below) is distinct from the relatively narrow indications for testing in clinical practice and is applicable to the research setting at this time.

ROLE OF RESEARCH STUDIES FOR PATIENTS AND FAMILIES WITH AUTISM

To date, genetic studies of patients and families with autism have been remarkably instructive in our initial understanding of the etiology of autism. Monozygotic twin studies show a concordance rate as high as 96% for the diagnosis of ASD. Milder forms of social and communication abnormalities are remarkably increased in first-degree relatives.

Gene studies have taken various forms. One strategy has been to focus on individuals with well-defined subtypes who appear homogeneous. This reduces the "noise" of pooling subjects, and is designed to facilitate detection of the putative genetic "signal" (Spence 2001). Other study designs include a wide range of clinical and even subclinical forms of the disorder, involving relatives of affected patients. This has enabled detection of increased rates of speech disorders, specific personality traits (e.g. impulsive, aloof, shy, eccentric) and atypical patterns of social behavior (Piven and Palmer 1999). Whole genome screening has become technologically feasible within the last several years. Large populations of patients will be needed so that studies can detect relatively subtle but important changes in the genome. These changes may exist in the forms of single nucleotide polymorphisms, or changes in the sizes of SNP strands known as CNPs, or copy number polymorphisms. There has been an increased understanding of genetic disorders that involve pretranslational problems of RNA, as opposed to proteins themselves. Now that the technology is available for efficient analysis of the human genome, it will become critical in the very near future to recruit large numbers of patients and families into multicenter studies to elucidate the genetic basis of autism. This will have considerably more impact than routine clinical genetic testing of individuals in the absence of risk factors for an underlying identifiable disorder.

CONCLUSION

A primary etiologic factor for autism is a genetic predisposition. Multiple genes are implicated, and include mutations and polymorphisms that are both de novo and inherited, as well as epigenetic factors. Epigenetics involves interactions between genes themselves as well as between genes and the environment. Further research will be spurred by advances in technology that allow for genome-wide screening for subtle gene alterations, but which will require large numbers of affected individuals. Autism displays genetic heterogeneity, where multiple contributory genes with relatively small impact alone appear to interrelate and lead to a decreased threshold to manifest the clinical phenotype described by Kanner and contemporaries over 60 years ago.

REFERENCES

Auranen M (2002) A genomewide screen for autism-spectrum disorders: evidence for a major susceptibility locus on chromosome 3q25-27. *Am J Hum Genet* 71: 777–90.

Badner JA (2002) Regional meta-analysis of published data supports linkage of autism with markers on chromosome 7. *Mol Psychiatry* 7: 56–66.

Bailey A, Le Couteur A, Gottesman I, Bolton P, Simonoff E, Yuzda E, Rutter M (1995) Autism as a strongly genetic disorder: evidence from a British twin study. *Psychol Med* 25: 63–77.

Bailey A, Palferman S, Heavey L, Le Couteur A (1998) Autism: the phenotype in relatives. *J Autism Dev Disord* 28: 369–92.

Bailey DB, Hatton DD, Skinner M, Mesibov G (2001) Autistic behavior, FMR1 protein, and developmental trajectories in young males with fragile X syndrome. *J Autism Dev Disord* 31: 165–74.

Barrett S (1999) An autosomal genomic screen for autism. Collaborative linkage study of autism. *Am J Med Genet* 88: 609–15.

Beyer KS, Blasi F, Bacchelli E, Klauck SM, Maestrini E, Poustka A (2002) Mutation analysis of the coding sequence of the MECP2 gene in infantile autism. *Hum Genet* 111: 305–9.

Bolliger MF, Frei K, Winterhalter KH, Gloor SM (2001) Identification of a novel neuroligin in humans which binds to PSD-95 and has a widespread expression. *Biochem J* 356: 581–8.

Bolton P, Macdonald H, Pickles A, Rios P, Goode S, Crowson M, Bailey A, Rutter M (1994) A case–control family history study of autism. *J Child Psychol Psychiatry* 35: 877–900.

Buckley PG, Mantripragada KK, Piotrowski A, Diaz de Stahl T, Dumanski JP (2005) Copy-number polymorphisms: mining the tip of an iceberg. *Trends Genet* 21: 315–7.

Buxbaum JD, Silverman JM, Smith CJ, Greenberg DA, Kilifarski M, Reichert J Cook EH, Fang Y, Song CY, Vitale R (2002) Association between a GABRB3 polymorphism and autism. *Mol Psychiatry* 7: 311–6.

Chen RZ, Akbarian S, Tudor M, Jaenisch R (2001) Deficiency of methyl-CpG binding protein-2 in CNS neurons results in a Rett-like phenotype in mice. *Nat Genet* 27: 327–31.

Cook EH, Courchesne R, Lord C, Cox NJ, Yan S, Lincoln A, Haas R, Courchesne E, Leventhal BL (1997) Evidence of linkage between the serotonin transporter and autistic disorder. *Mol Psychiatry* 2: 247–50.

Curatolo P, Porfirio MC, Manzi B, Seri S (2004) Autism in tuberous sclerosis. *Eur J Paediatr Neurol* 8: 327–32.

Fatemi SH (2001) Reelin mutations in mouse and man: from reeler mouse to schizophrenia, mood disorders, autism and lissencephaly. *Mol Psychiatry* 6: 129–33.

Fatemi SH, Kroll JL, Stary JM (2001a) Altered levels of Reelin and its isoforms in schizophrenia and mood disorders. *Neuroreport* 12: 3209–15.

Fatemi SH, Stary JM, Halt AR, Realmuto GR (2001b) Dysregulation of Reelin and Bcl-2 proteins in autistic cerebellum. *J Autism Dev Disord* 31: 529–35.

Feinstein C, Reiss AL (1998) Autism: the point of view from fragile X studies. *J Autism Dev Disord* 28: 393–405.

Filipek PA, Accardo PJ, Ashwal S, Baranek GT, Cook EH, Dawson G, Gordon B, Gravel JS, Johnson CP, Kallen RJ, Levy SE, Minshew NJ, Ozonoff S, Prizant BM, Rapin I, Rogers SJ, Stone WL, Teplin SW, Tuchman RF, Volkmar FR (2000) Practice parameter: screening and diagnosis of autism: report of the Quality Standards Subcommittee of the American Academy of Neurology and the Child Neurology Society. *Neurology* 55: 468–79.

Fisher SE, Vargha-Khadem F, Watkins KE, Monaco AP, Pembrey ME (1998) Localisation of a gene implicated in a severe speech and language disorder. *Nat Genet* 18: 168–70.

Folstein SE, Mankoski RE (2000) Chromosome 7q: where autism meets language disorder? *Am J Hum Genet* 67: 278–81.

Folstein SE, Rosen-Sheidley B (2001) Genetics of autism: complex aetiology for a heterogeneous disorder. *Nat Rev Genet* 2: 943–55.

Folstein S, Rutter M (1977a) Genetic influences and infantile autism. *Nature* 265: 726–8.

Folstein S, Rutter M (1977b) Infantile autism: a genetic study of 21 twin pairs. *J Child Psychol Psychiatry* 18: 297–321.

Folstein SE, Rutter ML (1988) Autism: familial aggregation and genetic implications. *J Autism Dev Disord* 18: 3–30.

Fombonne E, Bolton P, Prior J, Jordan H, Rutter M (1997a) A family study of autism: cognitive patterns and levels in parents and siblings. *J Child Psychol Psychiatry* 38: 667–83.

Fombonne E, Du MC, Cans C, Grandjean H (1997b) Autism and associated medical disorders in a French epidemiological survey. *J Am Acad Child Adolesc Psychiatry* 36: 1561–9.

Gillberg C, Rasmussen P (1994) Brief report: four case histories and a literature review of Williams syndrome and autistic behavior. *J Autism Dev Disord* 24: 381–93.

Gillberg C, Wahlstrom J (1985) Chromosome abnormalities in infantile autism and other childhood psychoses: a population study of 66 cases. *Dev Med Child Neurol* 27: 293–304.

Gillberg IC, Gillberg C, Ahlsen G (1994) Autistic behaviour and attention deficits in tuberous sclerosis: a population-based study. *Dev Med Child Neurol* 36: 50–6.

Gutknecht L (2001) Full-genome scans with autistic disorder: a review. *Behav Genet* 31: 113–23.

Guy J, Hendrich B, Holmes M, Martin JE, Bird A (2001) A mouse Mecp2-null mutation causes neurological symptoms that mimic Rett syndrome. *Nat Genet* 27: 322–6.

Hagerman RJ, Chudley AE, Knoll JH, Jackson AW, Kemper M, Ahmad R (1986a) Autism in fragile X females. *Am J Med Genet* 23: 375–80.

Hagerman RJ, Jackson AW, Levitas A, Rimland B, Braden M (1986b) An analysis of autism in fifty males with the fragile X syndrome. *Am J Med Genet* 23: 359–74.

Hong SE, Shugart YY, Huang DT, Shahwan SA, Grant PE, Hourihane JO, Martin ND, Walsh CA (2000) Autosomal recessive lissencephaly with cerebellar hypoplasia is associated with human RELN mutations. *Nat Genet* 26: 93–6. Erratum in: *Nat Genet* 2001, 27: 225.

Hong YS, Kim SY, Bhattacharya A, Pratt DR, Hong WK, Tainsky MA (1995) Structure and function of the HOX A1 human homeobox gene cDNA. *Gene* 159: 209–14.

Hunt A, Dennis J (1987) Psychiatric disorder among children with tuberous sclerosis. *Dev Med Child Neurol* 29: 190–8.

Hunt A, Shepherd C (1993) A prevalence study of autism in tuberous sclerosis. *J Autism Dev Disord*

23: 323–39.

Hurst JA, Baraitser M, Auger E, Graham F, Norell S (1990) An extended family with a dominantly inherited speech disorder. *Dev Med Child Neurol* 32: 352–5.

IMGSAC (1998) A full genome screen for autism with evidence for linkage to a region on chromosome 7q. International Molecular Genetic Study of Autism Consortium. *Human Mol Genet* 7: 571–8.

IMGSAC (2001) A genomewide screen for autism: strong evidence for linkage to chromosomes 2q, 7q, and 16p. *Am J Hum Genet* 69: 570–81.

Ingram JL, Stodgell CJ, Hyman SL, Figlewicz DA, Weitkamp LR, Rodier PM (2000) Discovery of allelic variants of HOXA1 and HOXB1: genetic susceptibility to autism spectrum disorders. *Teratology* 62: 393–405.

Ingrosso D, Cimmino A, Perna AF, Masella L, De Santo NG, De Bonis ML, Vacca M, D'Esposito M, D'Urso M, Galletti P, Zappia V (2003) Folate treatment and unbalanced methylation and changes of allelic expression induced by hyperhomocysteinaemia in patients with uraemia. *Lancet* 361: 1693–9.

Jablonka E, Lamb MJ (2002) The changing concept of epigenetics. *Ann NY Acad Sci* 981: 82–96.

Jablonka E, Matzke M, Thieffry D, Van Speybroeck L (2002) The genome in context: biologists and philosophers on epigenetics. *Bioessays* 24: 392–4.

Jamain S, Betancur C, Quach H, Philippe A, Fellous M, Giros B, Gillberg C, Leboyer M, Bourgeron T; Paris Autism Research International Sibpair (PARIS) Study (2002) Linkage and association of the glutamate receptor 6 gene with autism. *Mol Psychiatry* 7: 302–10.

Jiang YH, Sahoo T, Michaelis RC, Bercovich D, Bressler J, Kashork CD, Liu Q, Shaffer LG, Schroer RJ, Stockton DW, Spielman RS, Stevenson RE, Beaudet AL (2004) A mixed epigenetic/genetic model for oligogenic inheritance of autism with a limited role for UBE3A. *Am J Med Genet A* 131: 1–10.

Jorde LB, Mason-Brothers A, Waldmann R, Ritvo ER, Freeman BJ, Pingree C, McMahon WM, Petersen B, Jenson WR, Mo A (1990) The UCLA–University of Utah epidemiologic survey of autism: genealogical analysis of familial aggregation. *Am J Med Genet* 36: 85–8.

Jorde LB, Hasstedt SJ, Ritvo ER, Mason-Brothers A, Freeman BJ, Pingree C, McMahon WM, Petersen B, Jenson WR, Mo A (1991) Complex segregation analysis of autism. *Am J Hum Genet* 49: 932–8.

Kanner L, Eisenberg L (1957) Early infantile autism, 1943–1955. *Psychiatr Res Rep Am Psychiatr Assoc* Apr(7): 55–65.

Kates WR, Burnette CP, Eliez S, Strunge LA, Kaplan D, Landa R, Reiss AL, Pearlson GD (2004) Neuroanatomic variation in monozygotic twin pairs discordant for the narrow phenotype for autism. *Am J Psychiatry* 161: 539–46.

Kerby DS, Dawson BL (1994) Autistic features, personality, and adaptive behavior in males with the fragile X syndrome and no autism. *Am J Ment Retard* 98: 455–62.

Kishino T, Lalande M, Wagstaff J (1997) UBE3A/E6-AP mutations cause Angelman syndrome. *Nat Genet* 15: 70–3.

Klauck SM, Poustka F, Benner A, Lesch KP, Poustka A (1997) Serotonin transporter (5-HTT) gene variants associated with autism? *Hum Mol Genet* 6: 2233–8.

Lai CS, Fisher SE, Hurst JA, Levy ER, Hodgson S, Fox M, Jeremiah S, Povey S, Jamison DC, Green ED, Vargha-Khadem F, Monaco AP (2000) The SPCH1 region on human 7q31: genomic characterization of the critical interval and localization of translocations associated with speech and language disorder. *Am J Hum Genet* 67: 357–68.

Lam CW, Yeung WL, Ko CH, Poon PM, Tong SF, Chan KY, Lo IF, Chan LY, Hui J, Wong V, Pang

CP, Lo YM, Fok TF (2000) Spectrum of mutations in the MECP2 gene in patients with infantile autism and Rett syndrome. *J Med Genet* 37: E41.

Landa R, Folstein SE, Isaacs C (1991) Spontaneous narrative-discourse performance of parents of autistic individuals. *J Speech Hear Res* 34: 1339–45.

Landa R, Piven J, Wzorek MM, Gayle JO, Chase GA, Folstein SE (1992) Social language use in parents of autistic individuals. *Psychol Med* 22: 245–54.

Laumonnier F, Bonnet-Brilhault F, Gomot M, Blanc R, David A, Moizard MP, Raynaud M, Ronce N, Lemonnier E, Calvas P, Laudier B, Chelly J, Fryns JP, Ropers HH, Hamel BC, Andres C, Barthelemy C, Moraine C, Briault S (2004) X-linked mental retardation and autism are associated with a mutation in the NLGN4 gene, a member of the neuroligin family. *Am J Hum Genet* 74: 552–7.

Le Couteur A, Bailey A, Goode S, Pickles A, Robertson S, Gottesman I, Rutter M (1996) A broader phenotype of autism: the clinical spectrum in twins. *J Child Psychol Psychiatry* 37: 785–801.

Licinio J, Alvarado I (2002) Progress in the genetics of autism. *Mol Psychiatry* 7: 229 (editorial).

Liu J (2001) A genomewide screen for autism susceptibility loci. *Am J Hum Genet* 69: 327–40.

Maestrini E, Lai C, Marlow A, Matthews N, Wallace S, Bailey A, Cook EH, Weeks DE, Monaco AP (1999) Serotonin transporter (5-HTT) and gamma-aminobutyric acid receptor subunit beta3 (GABRB3) gene polymorphisms are not associated with autism in the IMGSA families. The International Molecular Genetic Study of Autism Consortium. *Am J Med Genet* 88: 492–6.

Mariner R, Jackson AW, Levitas A, Hagerman RJ, Braden M, McBogg PM, Smith AC, Berry R (1986) Autism, mental retardation, and chromosomal abnormalities. *J Autism Dev Disord* 16: 425–40.

Martin ER, Menold MM, Wolpert CM, Bass MP, Donnelly SL, Ravan SA, Zimmerman A, Gilbert JR, Vance JM, Maddox LO, Wright HH, Abramson RK, DeLong GR, Cuccaro ML, Pericak-Vance MA (2000) Analysis of linkage disequilibrium in gamma-aminobutyric acid receptor subunit genes in autistic disorder. *Am J Med Genet* 96: 43–8.

Mazzocco MM, Kates WR, Baumgardner TL, Freund LS, Reiss AL (1997) Autistic behaviors among girls with fragile X syndrome. *J Autism Dev Disord* 27: 415–35.

Menold MM, Shao Y, Wolpert CM, Donnelly SL, Raiford KL, Martin ER, Ravan SA, Abramson RK, Wright HH, Delong GR, Cuccaro ML, Pericak-Vance MA, Gilbert JR (2001) Association analysis of chromosome 15 gabaa receptor subunit genes in autistic disorder. *J Neurogenet* 15: 245–59.

Moretti P (2005) Abnormalities of social interactions and home-cage behavior in a mouse model of Rett syndrome. *Hum Mol Genet* 14: 205–20.

Murphy M, Bolton PF, Pickles A, Fombonne E, Piven J, Rutter M (2000) Personality traits of the relatives of autistic probands. *Psychol Med* 30: 1411–24.

Newbury DF, Monaco AP (2002) Molecular genetics of speech and language disorders. *Curr Opin Pediatr* 14: 696–701.

Newbury DF, Bonora E, Lamb JA, Fisher SE, Lai CS, Baird G, Jannoun L, Slonims V, Stott CM, Merricks MJ, Bolton PF, Bailey AJ, Monaco AP; International Molecular Genetic Study of Autism Consortium (2002). FOXP2 is not a major susceptibility gene for autism or specific language impairment. *Am J Hum Genet* 70: 1318–27.

Newschaffer CJ, Fallin D, Lee NL (2002) Heritable and nonheritable risk factors for autism spectrum disorders. *Epidemiol Rev* 24: 137–53.

Nurmi EL, Bradford Y, Chen Y, Hall J, Arnone B, Gardiner MB, Hutcheson HB, Gilbert JR, Pericak-Vance MA, Copeland-Yates SA, Michaelis RC, Wassink TH, Santangelo SL, Sheffield VC, Piven J, Folstein SE, Haines JL, Sutcliffe JS (2001) Linkage disequilibrium at the

Angelman syndrome gene UBE3A in autism families. *Genomics* 77: 105–13.

Persico AM, Militerni R, Bravaccio C, Schneider C, Melmed R, Conciatori M, Damiani V, Baldi A, Keller F (2000) Lack of association between serotonin transporter gene promoter variants and autistic disorder in two ethnically distinct samples. *Am J Med Genet* 96: 123–7.

Persico AM, D'Agruma L, Maiorano N, Totaro A, Militerni R, Bravaccio C, Wassink TH, Schneider C, Melmed R, Trillo S, Montecchi F, Palermo M, Pascucci T, Puglisi-Allegra S, Reichelt KL, Conciatori M, Marino R, Quattrocchi CC, Baldi A, Zelante L, Gasparini P, Keller F; Collaborative Linkage Study of Autism (2001) Reelin gene alleles and haplotypes as a factor predisposing to autistic disorder. *Mol Psychiatry* 6: 150–9.

Philibert RA, Winfield SL, Sandhu HK, Martin BM, Ginns EI (2000) The structure and expression of the human neuroligin-3 gene. *Gene* 246: 303–10.

Philippe A (1999) Genome-wide scan for autism susceptibility genes. Paris Autism Research International Sibpair Study. *Hum Mol Genet* 8: 805–12.

Pickles A, Starr E, Kazak S, Bolton P, Papanikolaou K, Bailey A, Goodman R, Rutter M (2000) Variable expression of the autism broader phenotype: findings from extended pedigrees. *J Child Psychol Psychiatry* 41: 491–502.

Piven J, Palmer P (1999) Psychiatric disorder and the broad autism phenotype: evidence from a family study of multiple-incidence autism families. *Am J Psychiatry* 156: 557–63.

Piven J, Chase GA, Landa R, Wzorek M, Gayle J, Cloud D, Folstein S (1991) Psychiatric disorders in the parents of autistic individuals. *J Am Acad Child Adolesc Psychiatry* 30: 471–8.

Piven J, Palmer P, Jacobi D, Childress D, Arndt S (1997) Broader autism phenotype: evidence from a family history study of multiple-incidence autism families. *Am J Psychiatry* 154: 185–90.

Pujana MA, Nadal M, Guitart M, Armengol L, Gratacos M, Estivill X (2002) Human chromosome 15q11-q14 regions of rearrangements contain clusters of LCR15 duplicons. *Eur J Hum Genet* 10: 26–35.

Rakyan VK, Preis J, Morgan HD, Whitelaw E (2001) The marks, mechanisms and memory of epigenetic states in mammals. *Biochem J* 356: 1–10.

Risch N, Spiker D, Lotspeich L, Nouri N, Hinds D, Hallmayer J, Kalaydjieva L, McCague P, Dimiceli S, Pitts T, Nguyen L, Yang J, Harper C, Thorpe D, Vermeer S, Young H, Hebert J, Lin A, Ferguson J, Chiotti C, Wiese-Slater S, Rogers T, Salmon B, Nicholas P, Petersen PB, Pingree C, McMahon W, Wong DL, Cavalli-Sforza LL, Kraemer HC, Myers RM (1999) A genomic screen of autism: evidence for a multilocus etiology. *Am J Hum Genet* 65: 493–507.

Ritvo ER, Freeman BJ, Mason-Brothers A, Mo A, Ritvo AM (1985) Concordance for the syndrome of autism in 40 pairs of afflicted twins. *Am J Psychiatry* 142: 74–7.

Ritvo ER, Jorde LB., Mason-Brothers A, Freeman BJ, Pingree C, Jones MB, McMahon WM, Petersen PB, Jenson WR, Mo A (1989) The UCLA-University of Utah epidemiologic survey of autism: recurrence risk estimates and genetic counseling. *Am J Psychiatry* 146: 1032–6.

Rogers SJ, Wehner DE, Hagerman R (2001) The behavioral phenotype in fragile X: symptoms of autism in very young children with fragile X syndrome, idiopathic autism, and other developmental disorders. *J Dev Behav Pediatr* 22: 409–17.

Rutter M, Bailey A, Bolton P, Le Couteur A (1994) Autism and known medical conditions: myth and substance. *J Child Psychol Psychiatry* 35: 311–22.

Samaco RC, Hogart A, LaSalle JM (2005) Epigenetic overlap in autism-spectrum neurodevelopmental disorders: MECP2 deficiency causes reduced expression of UBE3A and GABRB3. *Hum Mol Genet* 14: 483–92.

Scheiffele P, Fan J, Choih J, Fetter R, Serafini T (2000) Neuroligin expressed in nonneuronal cells triggers presynaptic development in contacting axons. *Cell* 101: 657–69.

Shahbazian MD, Antalffy B, Armstrong DL, Zoghbi HY (2002a) Insight into Rett syndrome: MeCP2 levels display tissue- and cell-specific differences and correlate with neuronal maturation. *Hum Mol Genet* 11: 115–24.

Shahbazian M, Young J, Yuva-Paylor L, Spencer C, Antalffy B, Noebels J, Armstrong D, Paylor R, Zoghbi H (2002b) Mice with truncated MeCP2 recapitulate many Rett syndrome features and display hyperacetylation of histone H3. *Neuron* 35: 243–54.

Shao Y, Raiford KL, Wolpert CM, Cope HA, Ravan SA, Ashley-Koch AA, Abramson RK, Wright HH, DeLong RG, Gilbert JR, Cuccaro ML, Pericak-Vance MA (2002a) Phenotypic homogeneity provides increased support for linkage on chromosome 2 in autistic disorder. *Am J Hum Genet* 70: 1058–61.

Shao Y, Wolpert CM, Raiford KL, Menold MM, Donnelly SL, Ravan SA, Bass MP, McClain C, von Wendt L, Vance JM, Abramson RH, Wright HH, Ashley-Koch A, Gilbert JR, DeLong RG, Cuccaro ML, Pericak-Vance MA (2002b). Genomic screen and follow-up analysis for autistic disorder. *Am J Med Genet* 114: 99–105.

Skaar DA, Shao Y, Haines JL, Stenger JE, Jaworski J, Martin ER, DeLong GR, Moore JH, McCauley JL, Sutcliffe JS, Ashley-Koch AE, Cuccaro ML, Folstein SE, Gilbert JR, Pericak-Vance MA (2005) Analysis of the RELN gene as a genetic risk factor for autism. *Mol Psychiatry* 10: 563-571.

Slager SL (2001) Stoppage: an issue for segregation analysis. *Genet Epidemiol* 20: 328–39.

Slopien A, Rajewski A (2000) [Genetic studies in autistic disorders]. *Psychiatr Pol* 34: 435–46 (Polish).

Smalley SL, Asarnow RF, Spence MA (1988) Autism and genetics. A decade of research. *Arch Gen Psychiatry* 45: 953–61.

Smalley SL, Kustanovich V, Minassian SL, Stone JL, Ogdie MN, McGough JJ, McCracken JT, MacPhie IL, Francks C, Fisher SE, Cantor RM, Monaco AP, Nelson SF (2002) Genetic linkage of attention-deficit/hyperactivity disorder on chromosome 16p13, in a region implicated in autism. *Am J Hum Genet* 71: 959–63.

Smith M, Filipek PA, Wu C, Bocian M, Hakim S, Modahl C, Spence MA (2000) Analysis of a 1-megabase deletion in 15q22-q23 in an autistic patient: identification of candidate genes for autism and of homologous DNA segments in 15q22-q23 and 15q11-q13. *Am J Med Genet* 96: 765–70.

Song JY, Ichtchenko K, Sudhof TC, Brose N (1999) Neuroligin 1 is a postsynaptic cell-adhesion molecule of excitatory synapses. *Proc Natl Acad Sci USA* 96: 1100–5.

Spence MA (2001) The genetics of autism. *Curr Opin Pediatr* 13: 561–5.

Steffenburg S, Gillberg C (1986) Autism and autistic-like conditions in Swedish rural and urban areas: a population study. *Br J Psychiatry* 149: 81–7.

Steffenburg S, Gillberg C, Hellgren L, Andersson L, Gillberg I C, Jakobsson G, Bohman M (1989) A twin study of autism in Denmark, Finland, Iceland, Norway and Sweden. *J Child Psychol Psychiatry* 30: 405–16.

Stromland K, Nordin V, Miller M, Akerstrom B, Gillberg C (1994) Autism in thalidomide embryopathy: a population study. *Dev Med Child Neurol* 36: 351–6.

Thomas NS, Sharp AJ, Browne CE, Skuse D, Hardie C, Dennis NR (1999) Xp deletions associated with autism in three females. *Hum Genet* 104: 43–8.

Tordjman S, Gutknecht L, Carlier M, Spitz E, Antoine C, Slama F, Carsalade V, Cohen DJ, Ferrari P, Roubertoux PL, Anderson GM (2001) Role of the serotonin transporter gene in the behavioral expression of autism. *Mol Psychiatry* 6: 434–9.

Veenstra-Vanderweele J, Christian SL, Cook EH (2004) Autism as a paradigmatic complex genetic disorder. *Annu Rev Genomics Hum Genet* 5: 379–405.

Vincent JB, Herbrick JA, Gurling HM, Bolton PF, Roberts W, Scherer SW (2000) Identification of a novel gene on chromosome 7q31 that is interrupted by a translocation breakpoint in an autistic individual. *Am J Hum Genet* 67: 510–4.

Wahlstrom J, Steffenburg S, Hellgren L, Gillberg C (1989) Chromosome findings in twins with early-onset autistic disorder. *Am J Med Genet* 32: 19–21.

Warburton P, Baird G, Chen W, Morris K, Jacobs BW, Hodgson S, Docherty Z (2000) Support for linkage of autism and specific language impairment to 7q3 from two chromosome re-arrangements involving band 7q31. *Am J Med Genet* 96: 228–34.

Wassink TH, Piven J, Patil SR (2001a) Chromosomal abnormalities in a clinic sample of individuals with autistic disorder. Psychiatr Genet 11: 57–63.

Wassink TH, Piven J, Vieland VJ, Huang J, Swiderski RE, Pietila J, Braun T, Beck G, Folstein SE, Haines JL, Sheffield VC (2001b) Evidence supporting WNT2 as an autism susceptibility gene. *Am J Med Genet* 105: 406–13.

Waterland RA, Jirtle RL (2003) Transposable elements: targets for early nutritional effects on epigenetic gene regulation. *Mol Cell Biol* 23: 5293–300.

Yirmiya N, Pilowsky T, Nemanov L, Arbelle S, Feinsilver T, Fried I, Ebstein RP (2001) Evidence for an association with the serotonin transporter promoter region polymorphism and autism. *Am J Med Genet* 105: 381–6.

Ylisaukko-oja T (2004) Genome-wide scan for loci of Asperger syndrome. *Mol Psychiatry* 9: 161–8.

Yonan AL (2003) A genomewide screen of 345 families for autism-susceptibility loci. *Am J Hum Genet* 73: 886–97.

Yu CE, Dawson G, Munson J, D'Souza I, Osterling J, Estes A, Leutenegger AL, Flodman P, Smith M, Raskind WH, Spence MA, McMahon W, Wijsman EM, Schellenberg GD (2002) Presence of large deletions in kindreds with autism. *Am J Hum Genet* 71: 100–15.

Zenklusen JC, Weitzel JN, Ball HG, Conti CJ (1995) Allelic loss at 7q31.1 in human primary ovarian carcinomas suggests the existence of a tumor suppressor gene. *Oncogene* 11: 359–63.

8

NEUROANATOMY AND IMAGING STUDIES

Martha R Herbert and Verne S Caviness, Jr

Autism is a behaviorally defined syndrome manifested by disturbances in language, social reciprocity and behavioral flexibility. It is highly heterogenous in multiple respects, both behaviorally and biologically. The atypical behavioral features that define autism undoubtedly reflect a perturbation of central nervous system functioning. Yet at the current time the nature and neural systems basis of this perturbation remain elusive, although we have accumulated a growing number of hints. The purpose of this review is to offer a delineation of the brain findings in autism from the perspectives of analyses based on imaging and post-mortem studies. This will involve an assessment of the classes of findings that have been discerned, the robustness of the findings, and the consistencies and inconsistencies at each level. We will ask what we can know based on evidence about the brain in autism at this point in time, given the complexities and constraints involved in investigating it.

The fact that the pathophysiology underlying the language, social interaction and behavioral impairments does not in itself shorten life – although it may lead to seizures or accidents that cause untimely death – has profoundly constrained autism neuro-anatomical investigation. Early childhood, during which the disorder is recognized, offers only limited possibilities for anatomical investigation. First, the disorder is not generally diagnosed until after the first two years of life, and yet these initial two years are presumably the ones during which the most dynamic postnatal brain changes occur. Second, children in this age range or even a few years older are both unlikely to die (tightly limiting the availability of post-mortem samples) and unlikely to stay still unsedated (hindering the acquisition of adequate quality brain imaging studies). Thus neuro-anatomical studies have been performed almost entirely on brains of autistic individuals years to even decades after the disorder becomes apparent.

Anatomical findings have nonetheless provided important insights at various stages of autism research. Documentation of neuroanatomical abnormalities in early neuro-pathological studies supported the notion that the syndrome had a biological rather than what might have been imagined to be a purely psychiatric or psychodynamic basis. But the step from showing that brain abnormalities exist to identifying which findings are either sufficient or necessary for autism – and in what ways they may be related – has been much more challenging. Most anatomical findings in autism have been inconsistently replicated, which may be a function of the sensitivity of the anatomic methodology, or of variable subject ascertainment and sample size, or of the intrinsic biological heterogeneity of the disorder. Moreover, methodology interacts with underlying assumptions in influencing not only the questions that are asked or not asked and the places (and ways) investigators have looked or not looked in the brain, but also the way investigators have interpreted their findings.

Several basic themes and tensions emerge in studies of the neuroanatomy of autism. One of them is the question of whether abnormalities are anatomically regional, widely distributed or both. Regionally restricted abnormalities, when found, have most often been in limbic system structures and the cerebellum, and yet delimited abnormalities have also been found in a wide variety of other locations. But at the same time not all neuroanatomical abnormalities have been regionally restricted. Many studies have documented an increase in brain size, as will be reviewed below, which is a finding reflecting more widely distributed brain tissue changes. Neurochemical and neuroimmune changes may also be regionally restricted or more widely distributed. Complicated interpretive questions arise here, in particular regarding the functional significance of the neuroanatomical abnormalities detected. On the one hand, some investigators feel that since the neurobehavioral deficits associated with autism are so specific, they must have some focal or modular anatomical correlate. Thus, such findings as alterations in limbic or cerebellar structures have been taken to imply that the behavioral features of autism may largely if not entirely reflect impaired operation of a limited set of specific neural systems. On the other hand, a different class of models holds that autism's neurobehavioral deficits can emerge as consequences of more widely distributed abnormalities, such as altered connectivity or network properties, and so such findings as brain enlargement have been interpreted as providing a substrate for this class of systemic functional disturbances. Abnormalities that are more widely distributed and that alter systems properties might also provide a more parsimonious explanation not only for the primary defining behavioral features of the disorder but also for the various commonly accompanying features such as epilepsy, anxiety, disordered attention, atypical sensory gating, and sleep and immune system abnormalities.

Yet another interpretive issue relates to the kinds of insights that may be gleaned from anatomic findings to date regarding the nature of the underlying pathogenesis of autism. Thus, neuroanatomic findings have been suggested to reflect the consequences of in utero processes that are static and persistent in postnatal life. However, other aspects of the autistic child's health have raised the possibility that there are dynamic metabolic or immunologically based processes active in postnatal life and that these may be substantially significant for the structure and operation of the brain.

Our intention is to provide a critical review of the contributions of neuroanatomical findings, coming both from neuroanatomy and neuroimaging, to an understanding of the neurobiology of autism. The levels at which we will delineate brain findings will include

(1) widespread findings, (2) altered inter-regional relationships, (3) tissue changes, and (4) regional changes. Having laid out the existing evidence, we will address the extent and limits of our knowledge, and the constraints these limits place upon interpretation and hypothesis formulation.

WIDESPREAD FINDINGS

The first category of brain differences we will discuss will be global or widely distributed brain changes. Most prominent among these is the phenomenon of large brains, but some metabolic alterations also may fall under this category of widespread perturbation.

LARGE BRAINS

The single most replicated finding in autism has been a tendency toward unusually large brains. This has been documented through brain weight, head circumference and imaging measures of brain volume. This is not to say that large brains are a biomarker for autism, as the vast majority of people with large heads and large brain volumes are neither autistic nor even mildly on the autism spectrum. The significance of the finding is rather that the mean head or brain size is on average greater than would be predicted for age, at least for younger individuals. This marked tendency toward brain enlargement poses challenges with respect to plausible models of both pathogenesis and mechanisms underlying autistic behaviors (Herbert 2005).

Head size

Measures of head circumference in autistic individuals have been made in many cohorts of individuals with good diagnostic ascertainment. These studies have shown a substantial upward shift in mean head circumference, with the proportion of subjects with head circumference above the 97th percentile ranging from 10% to 30% (Steg and Rapoport 1975, Walker 1977, Bailey et al. 1993, Davidovitch et al. 1996, Rapin 1996, Woodhouse et al. 1996, Lainhart et al. 1997, Stevenson et al. 1997, Fombonne 1999, Fombonne et al. 1999, Ghaziuddin et al. 1999, Fidler et al. 2000, Miles et al. 2000, Aylward et al. 2002, Gillberg and de Souza 2002, Deutsch and Joseph 2003, Dementieva et al. 2005). Macrocephaly is not specific for individuals with autism: it is also common in their first degree relatives (Fidler et al. 2000), in autism spectrum disorder (Woodhouse et al. 1996), ADHD (Ghaziuddin et al. 1999), and developmental language disorder (Herbert et al. 2003b). Nor is it specific for any one autism phenotypic subgroup (Miles et al. 2000), although individuals with Asperger syndrome were found to have a larger mean head circumference than those with autistic disorder (Gillberg and de Souza 2002).

Brain volume

Large brain volume was reported in an abstract by Filipek et al. (1992) in a sample where high functioning autistic school-age children had larger brain volumes than lower functioning (nonverbal; IQ<80) children, and than controls. Piven et al. (1995) studied 20 autistic males and found larger brains due to enlarged tissue and lateral ventricle volume, and in follow-up showed that the enlargement characterized males but not females, and that it was regionalized to temporal, parietal and occipital, but not frontal lobes (Piven et al. 1996). Courchesne et al. (2001) found enlargement of gray and white matter in cerebrum and cerebellum in 2- to 3-year-olds, while Sparks et al. (2002) found cerebral but not cerebellar enlargement in 3- to 4-year-olds. Brain volume was larger for autistic subjects under 12 years of age than for controls (Aylward et al. 2002). For school-age boys with high-functioning autism, brain enlargement bordered on significance (Herbert et al. 2003a). Lotspeich et al. (2004) compared high functioning and low functioning autism and Asperger syndrome in individuals aged from mid-childhood through adolescence versus controls, and found cerebral gray matter but not white matter enlargement.

Brain weight

Findings from post-mortem specimens, though consistent with those from imaging and head circumference measurements, are confounded by lack of control over diagnostic comorbidities, with many brains coming from individuals with histories of metabolic, seizure or other disorders, and/or of mental retardation. One must also recognize the likelihood of other methodological confounds inherent in the study of brains post-mortem, in particular the inevitable brain swelling associated with the terminal illness and the interval between death and tissue fixation. Neuropathological investigations have not consistently reported total brain weight, but when reported, it tended to be markedly above average, particularly in younger subjects (Courchesne et al. 1999), although this was not always the case (the early sample of Williams et al. (1980) included 4 brains all weighing within 2 SD of the mean for age). Kemper and Bauman (1998) reported that of 19 brains for which weight was available, 8 of the 11 where subjects were aged under 12 years had increased weight compared to controls, while 6 of 8 brains from individuals aged over 18 years weighed less than expected. Of the 6 brains in the Bailey et al. (1998) sample, 4 were frankly above the normal range derived from Dekaban and Sadowsky (1978), while the remaining 2 were near the upper limit of that range. However, of note, while there are localized alterations in cell size or packing density, no widespread tissue-level change has been identified in any neuropathological study to date that establishes a tissue basis at the cellular level for the increased brain weight.

Hypoperfusion and Glucose Metabolism

Another finding that is either widespread or of variable focality is brain hypoperfusion. SPECT (single photon emission computerized tomography) and PET (positron emission tomography) scans have been available for some time, and one of their applications is to assess brain perfusion. Many studies have been performed, and almost without exception their orientation has been confined to attempts to uncover local brain correlates of the autism behavioral phenotype. From that vantage point these studies have been inconclusive, showing a substantial amount of variability. However, if examined through the lens of attempting to characterize abnormal brain function and its pathophysiology, it becomes possible to perceive a substantial thread of consistency among the studies. While Zilbovicius et al. (1992) found no cortical dysfunction, and Herold et al. (1988) found no cerebral differences in blood flow from controls, the preponderance of other SPECT and a few PET studies showed perfusion decreases that in some cases were highly significant (Sherman et al. 1984, George et al. 1992, Chiron et al. 1995, Mountz et al. 1995, Ryu et al. 1999, Hashimoto et al. 2000, Ohnishi et al. 2000, Starkstein et al. 2000, Zilbovicius et al. 2000, Kaya et al. 2002, Wilcox et al. 2002). Not all of the differences were significant, but the trends were virtually entirely in the direction of lower perfusion. Interestingly, none of these investigators discussed the potential mechanisms that might underlie this diminished perfusion, revealing an implicit but untested assumption that these changes are stable and presumably static properties of the brain.

In studies of widespread patterns of glucose metabolism, the direction of abnormality is not as consistent as in the perfusion studies. Rumsey et al. (1985) reported a widespread elevation of glucose metabolism, but Herold et al. (1988) using somewhat different methods found no significant differences. In the patients with PET abnormalities in the study by Schifter et al. (1994), 16 of 195 regions showed hypometabolism while no regions showed hypermetabolism; these hypometabolic areas sometimes had anatomical correlates on MRI. Galuska et al. (2002) in a 99mTc-ECD-SPECT and FDG-PET study report a "perfusion-metabolism mismatch", with decreased bitemporal and bifrontal perfusion and increased frontal metabolism.

ALTERED PROPORTIONS, GROWTH RATES AND PATTERNING

A second category of brain differences is alteration in the proportions or relationships among different brain regions. In volumetrics, brain proportionality is highly conserved across mammalian species (Finlay et al. 2001), with differences being related to varying adaptive demands of ecological niches (Barton and Harvey 2000). Altered brain proportionality in autism is thus a phenomenon that may be associated with altered behavioral repertoires. Altered inter-regional relationships may involve differing growth trajectories over time and may also be detectable cross-sectionally. They may involve volume, metabolism, connectivity, altered asymmetry or other functional features. Identifying altered relationships among brain regions and structures may be relevant since altered proportionality among components of distributed systems can reflect altered systems properties (Mesulam 1990, Andrews et al. 1997).

Atypical developmental trajectories: brain size

Longitudinal studies would be highly valuable for learning about brain development in autism, but at the current time these are only just getting underway. A further problem, mentioned in the introduction, is the impossibility of studying infants and young toddlers with autism other than through hard-to-perform "at-risk" studies, given that diagnosis is made after these first few years. Therefore inferences about developmental trajectory have been made in other ways. In retrospective studies of head circumference in children diagnosed with autism, this brain volume increase appears to occur postnatally. Several studies reported that most autistic individuals with macrocephaly were not that way at birth but experienced head growth subsequently (Mason-Brothers et al. 1990, Lainhart et al. 1997, Stevenson et al. 1997, Hultman et al. 2002, Dementieva et al. 2005), while Courchesne et al. (2003) reported a mean of 30th percentile at birth with 59% experiencing growth of two standard deviations in the first two years after birth.

Brain volume measures in autism have been reported in 0- to 2-year-olds (Hazlett et al. 2005) and in 2- to 4-year-olds (Courchesne et al. 2001). Two-year-olds showed generalized enlargement of gray and white matter cerebral volumes, but not of cerebellar volumes, as well as indirect evidence that the onset of increased growth rate may have occurred late in the first year of life (Hazlett et al. 2005). Among the 2- to 4-year-olds, 90% had brain volumes above average, and up to 37% were frankly macrocephalic (Redcay and Courchesne 2005). Initial large size relative to controls does not, however, persist. In older autistic subjects, smaller brain volume has been found to coexist with larger head circumference, suggesting that the brains in these subjects were larger when the subjects were younger (Aylward et al. 2002), with the implication that volume has been lost over time. While this could conceivably be related to the neuropathological observation of Bauman and Kemper (1994) that cytological findings differed by age, with younger subjects having larger cells while older subjects had smaller cells in portions of the inferior olive and cerebellar nuclei, those cytological findings were regionally restricted and would not be sufficient to explain a more generalized volume increase in younger subjects nor volume loss in older autistic individuals.

Atypical developmental trajectories: brain metabolism
Change across age has also been reported in metabolic measures. Wilcox et al. (2002) noted a change with age in the pattern of hypoperfusion, with an initial effect noted in the prefrontal area and an effect in left temporal and frontal areas noted only in mid- and late childhood and beyond, suggesting that location/perfusion varied with age, and possibly illuminating aspects of language development. Zilbovicius et al. (1995) reported frontal hypoperfusion in 2- to 4-year-old autistic children that resolved by the age of 5–7 years.

Non-uniform regional volume patterns
There are a modest number of studies of altered volumetric scaling and proportion in autistic brains. While some studies have reported proportional as well as absolute volumes as a way of addressing the influence of increased total brain volume, only more recently has it become technically easier for studies to include multiple measures obtained from the same brains. Thus the data on relationship among different findings, including ratios and scaling, are more sparse than the data to be presented further below on regions of interest.

Several investigators have found atypical relationships between the frontal lobe and the cerebellum. Carper and Courchesne (2000) found that larger frontal lobe volume was correlated with reduction of size of cerebellar vermal lobules VI–VII. However, while similar reductions in areas of cerebellar vermal lobules VI–VII were observed by Ciesielski et al (1997), and were found to be related to frontal lobe function (not volume), these reductions did not appear to be specific to autism (although that may not gainsay their functional relevance). Tsatsanis et al. (2003) have reported a loss of correlation in an autistic group compared with controls between thalamic and total brain volume.

In the first whole brain morphometric profile of autism, Herbert et al. (2003a) reported that the brain volume increase is non-uniform, with the volume differences from controls varying by structure. These increases yielded three factors, with white matter alone being disproportionately larger (in regard to both absolute and proportional volume [i.e. adjusted in relation to overall volume increase]; cerebral cortex and hippocampus–amygdala being absolutely no different but relatively smaller; and the remaining structures being proportionally larger, with greater absolute volumes but scaled volumes no different from controls. In this study, white matter made up only about 28% (for controls) to 30% (for the autistic sample) of cerebral volume, but contributed disproportionately to the overall volume increase, accounting for 66% of the volume increase in autistic subjects over controls.

White matter volume increase and its regionalization
Several studies suggest that increased brain volume in young autistic individuals appears to be largely driven by an increase in white matter. In Courchesne and coworkers' (2001) study of 2- to 16-year-olds, white matter enlargement (18% more cerebral and 38% more cerebellar white matter) was found in 2- to 3-year-old autistic children, whereas 12- to 16-year-old autistic children had less white matter than controls. In a comprehensive volumetric profile of high functioning autistic boys, Herbert et al. (2004) reported that white matter was 15% larger in 6- to 12-year-old autistic boys than in age-matched controls, and was also the only structure of the brain that was disproportionately larger in autism. This group performed a further analysis to characterize regional biases in this white matter volume increase, utilizing a method of topographical white matter parcellation based upon the neuroanatomy of white matter tracts (Makris et al. 1999, Meyer et al. 1999). This study showed that the volume increase is confined to the radiate zone, i.e. the subcortical white matter primarily comprised of corona radiata and U-fibers; the deeper white matter, including major sagittal tracts, internal capsule and corpus callosum, showed no volume increase over controls (Herbert et al. 2004). The frontal lobe white matter showed the greatest enlargement over controls (27%), a finding also reported by Carper et al. (2002), with the prefrontal proportion even more strongly affected (36%) (Herbert et al. 2004).

In older autistic individuals voxel-based methods have shown less white matter "concentration" (a different measure than volume: Giuliani et al. 2005) than in age-matched controls (Chung et al. 2004, Waiter et al. 2005). The one diffusion tensor imaging study of autism published to date found multiple clusters of reduced fractional anisotropy (since this measures the non-randomness of water diffusion in the brain, one might cautiously infer that a reduction in this measure implies less coherency in the directionality of white matter) in white matter adjacent to ventromedial prefrontal cortices, in anterior cingulate, in temporoparietal junctions, near the amygdala, in occipitotemporal tracts, and in the corpus callosum (Barnea-Goraly et al. 2004).

Since corpus callosum normally varies to the ⅔ power of brain volume (Jancke et al. 1997), one would expect that in the light of brain and white matter volume increases, corpus callosum should be larger as well; however, this structure has consistently been measured to be no different or smaller in autistic brains than in controls, albeit with different callosal subdivisions emphasized across studies. Two studies found the corpus callosum to be smaller in autism, mostly posteriorly (Egaas et al. 1995, Piven et al. 1997a). Manes et al. (1999) found volume reduction in mentally retarded autistic subjects, mostly in the body of the corpus callosum. Hardan et al. (2000) found volume reduction in the anterior of the corpus. Herbert et al. (2004) found no difference in mid-sagittal area of the corpus callosum, either as a whole or in any subregion, although there was a trend toward relative volume decrease in the anterior callosum, which paradoxically connects the parts of the white matter showing the greatest enlargement in the same brains.

ALTERED INTER-REGIONAL RELATIONSHIPS

Reduced inter-regional covariance

Horwitz et al. (1988), in an early PET study, pioneered an analysis of interrelationships between many regions of the autistic brain. They looked at 861 possible correlations, and found that the regional intercorrelations were reduced. Looking at correlations among ratios of global and regional metabolic rates, they found that 70% of the 861 possible correlations had lower values in the group with autism; moreover, there were significantly fewer robust correlations in the group with autism than in the control group. Of note, point by point statistical comparisons were not sensitive to this pattern, since only 4 of 31 regional cerebral metabolic rates for glucose differed between groups. Following this study, Starkstein et al. (2000) calculated a correlation matrix with 42 correlations and found that the control group had 26 of 42 correlations above this r-value, as compared to only 8 of 42 correlations for the autistic group (χ^2=18.4, df=1, p=0.0001).

While the Horwitz and Starkstein studies were of resting brain activity, two recent functional MRI studies, one of sentence comprehension and one of working memory, both showed a reduced degree of synchronization of the time series of functional activation between the various participating cortical areas (Just et al. 2004, Koshino et al. 2005). In the first paper, Just reported consistently lower functional connectivity in autism as compared with controls, with the level of functional connectivity between pairs ranking from higher to lower in the same order in autism as in controls, but at a lower level. He placed this finding in the framework of "underconnectivity theory", a formulation following upon his co-author Minshew's earlier formulation of autism as a disorder of complex information processing (Minshew et al. 1997), but discussed how the "under-connectivity" functional data and formulation now further integrate functional and neurobiological components of this model (Koshino et al. 2005).

Asymmetry shifts: volumetric and metabolic studies

A few studies have documented asymmetries in the altered metabolic relationships among regions. Chiron et al. (1995) reported reversed left-to-right rCBF (regional cerebral blood flow) indices, while Muller et al. (1999) reported reversed hemispheric dominance to auditory stimulation. Altered asymmetry has also been reported volumetrically. In an early report, Hier et al. (1979) reported that the right parieto-occipital zone was wider on the right than the left. Herbert et al. (2005) in a whole brain survey of asymmetry, noted a lack of asymmetry in high functioning autistic boys when large regions were examined, but found widespread alterations of asymmetry when examining cortical subunits. These brains, previously reported to be larger with increased radiate white matter, showed a substantial increase in rightwardly asymmetric cortex as well as a reversal of the right:left cortical asymmetry ratio, Greater degrees of abnormality in the right hemisphere have also been found in some magnetoencephalogram (MEG) studies (Gage et al. 2003, Flagg et al. 2005).

TISSUE CHANGES

Metabolites

Magnetic resonance spectroscopy (MRS) has been employed in autism to study brain metabolism. However, these studies to date have been scattered and varied in methodology. Using proton MRS, reduced NAA (a metabolite associated with neurons) was found in a number of studies (Chugani et al. 1999b, Friedman et al. 2003), with the former study also finding increased lactate. Levitt et al. (2003) showed altered choline and creatinine metabolism in the left anterior cingulate gyrus, in both caudate nuclei, and in the right occipital cortex. An increased choline/creatine ratio has also been reported (Sokol et al. 2002). An early 31P-MRS study found that as test performance declined in the autistic subjects, levels of the most labile high energy phosphate compound and of membrane building blocks decreased, while levels of membrane breakdown products increased. These results were inferred to imply an energy deficit (Minshew et al. 1993).

Neurotransmitters

Alterations in multiple neurotransmitters and their associated receptors have been documented; these are considered in more detail in Chapters 6 and 15. A particularly striking contribution to this domain was made utilizing the PET ligand 11C-alpha-methyltryptophan (AMT), a serotonin precursor used to measure local serotonin synthesis in the brain. Asymmetries of serotonin synthesis were found in frontal cortex, thalamus, and dentate nucleus of the cerebellum in all 7 boys, but not in the 1 autistic girl studied (Chugani et al. 1997); and a different developmental trajectory of serotonin synthesis was seen in autism, with a gradual increase between 2 and 15 years of age as compared with controls who showed double the adult level of synthesis until age 5 with a subsequent decline toward adult values (Chugani et al. 1999a). In a more recent study some of the same investigators demonstrated that if there was hemispheric asymmetry in AMT uptake, left hemisphere reduction correlated with language impairment while right hemisphere reduction correlated with a higher prevalence of left and mixed handedness (Chandana et al. 2005).

Neuroinflammation
The finding of chronic tissue changes involving activated microglia and inflammatory cytokine profiles in post-mortem autistic brain tissue (Vargas et al. 2005) are reviewed in Chapter 9. Of note, this type of abnormality was found in subjects ranging in age from 5 to 44, and represents a chronic set of immune and metabolic changes of a different class than alterations of size or proportion of gray and white matter components that have usually been considered in autism volumetric investigations. On this account it widens the range of factors that now must be considered in interpreting anatomical findings.

Cytoarchitecture
Casanova et al. (2002) analyzed digitized images of lamina III in Brodman areas 9 (in the superior and middle frontal gyrus), 21 (middle temporal gyrus), and 22 (Tpt – temporal–parietal auditory area). Minicolumns were detected using a computerized column detection routine. Minicolumns were defined as vertical clusters of large neurons delimited by cell-sparse areas on either side. Minicolumn width, peripheral neuropil space and compactness were considered to be significantly reduced in autism as compared with controls. While 4 of the 9 autistic cases had brain weights greater than two standard deviations above the mean (though one of these had edema), these findings did not appear to be correlated to minicolumn width, although assessment was limited as brain weights were available for only one control. These findings of an increased number of narrower columns, if confirmed with additional study in more subjects, have implications for connectivity – related both to interneuron changes with associated diminution of inhibitory function that would alter connectivity properties (Casanova et al. 2003), and to an increase predominantly in short-range connecting fibers (Casanova 2004).

Cytology
Abnormalities of the cerebral cortex have been reported by a number of investigators. Although focal origins for autistic deficits had been posited, a report of abnormal glucose metabolism (Rumsey et al. 1985) suggesting diffuse abnormalities prompted Coleman et al. (1985) to count cells in Brodmann cortical areas 21 (auditory association), 41 (primary auditory) and 44 (Broca's area) for 1 autistic and 2 control brains, with results being

roughly the same on three runs. There was considerable interindividual variability between the control brains, so that while 26 of 42 comparisons showed statistically significant differences among the 3 brains, in 20 of these 26 the two controls differed more from each other than the autistic brain did from either control. However, there was a trend for the glia/neuron ratio to be smaller than the average for the two control brains, although this did not reach statistical significance. While none of the 6 brains studied by Bailey et al. (1998) had abnormal frontal cortex neuronal counts, 4 showed some subtle evidence of cortical dysgenesis, such as slight laminar abnormalities, abnormal pyramidal cell orientation or thickened cortices. In 9 brains studied by Kemper and Bauman (1998), with the exception of a minor orbitofrontal cortical malformation in 1, the non-limbic cortices had no identified pathology.

REGIONAL CHANGES

Because autism is defined by a set of behavioral abnormalities, it has seemed logical to pursue the identification of regional abnormalities that may underlie these defining behaviors. Damasio and Maurer (1978) contributed a set of hypotheses, positing that autism arose from abnormalities in the mesolimbic structures associated with neurotransmitter imbalance that might be a consequence of perinatal viral infection, insult to the periventricular watershed area, or genetically determined neurochemical abnormalities; they also posited basal ganglia circuitry abnormalities based on the presence of gait and movement abnormalities. When studies have been designed to investigate regions of interest based on a priori hypotheses, mesolimbic and also cerebellar structures have thus often been investigated, with abnormalities frequently though not entirely consistently discerned.

LIMBIC SYSTEM

In early neuropathological studies, neurons in the limbic system were found to be small and densely distributed in six subjects (Kemper and Bauman 1998), although except for the first subject for whom cell counts were published, this evaluation was reported qualitatively. The finding appeared to be consistent, though with variability in the degree of involvement of some limbic system components. Raymond et al. (1996) examined the morphology of hippocampal neurons in 2 further subjects using Golgi stain, and reported smaller CA4 cell bodies and less branching of pyramidal neurons in CA4 and CA1 but no difference in perikaryon area and no dysmorphic features. However, Guerin et al. (1996), in their examination of the brain of a single 16-year-old subject who had microcephaly with dilated ventricles and thin corpus callosum, characterized the limbic structures as normal, though the features examined to make this assessment were not detailed. In the study by Bailey et al. (1998) of 6 autistic brains, the examination of hippocampal neuronal density in a subgroup discerned no statistically significant increase in cell density, and while 2 subjects were described as having relatively high hippocampal neuronal density, only 1 of these cases showed this density increase in all CA subfields.

In volumetric neuroimaging studies, measures of amygdala and hippocampus have varied considerably. The amygdala was measured to be both absolutely and relatively smaller in one study, in which the hippocampus was found to be only relatively but not absolutely smaller (Aylward et al. 1999, Herbert et al. 2003a). However, it was measured to be larger in several other studies using a variety of methods (Abell et al. 1999, Howard et al. 2000, Sparks et al. 2002), with the last of these studies reporting a subgroup with proportional enlargement and another subgroup with greater than proportional enlargement. No amygdala volume differences were found by Haznedar et al. (2000). Another limbic system structure, the cingulate gyrus, has been measured less often in neuroanatomical studies; it was smaller anteriorly on the right, as well as metabolically less active, in two studies by the same group (Haznedar et al. 1997). Small structures are particularly vulnerable to methodological problems, with both differences among individual raters doing the analyses in the same laboratory and differences in techniques among laboratories potentially contributing to inconsistent results (Haznedar et al. 2000).

An association between reduced cingulate volume metabolic decrease in the same area has also been observed (Haznedar et al. 1997, 2000). As noted above, Levitt et al. (2003) found reduced choline in the left inferior anterior cingulate. The anterior cingulate has frequently been implicated, as well, in functional MRI investigations (Luna et al. 2002).

Although neuropathological abnormalities in the limbic system have helped motivate neuroimaging investigations of these structures, there may be a disconnect between microanatomical abnormalities and macroanatomically detectable volume change. For example, in the neuropathological studies of Bauman and Kemper (1994) the limbic system was found to have an increased number of small cells that were densely packed, but the volumetric implications of such a combination of findings are not obvious, since trends for cell size, number and organization are not all in the same direction.

CEREBELLUM

One of the earliest findings in autism, commonly but not universally replicated, is reduced numbers of cerebellar Purkinje cells. In an early study of 4 autistic brains by Williams et al. (1980), there was a general reduction in Purkinje cell number in the subject suspected (due to a similarly affected sibling) of having an inherited metabolic disorder, but not in either the 2 subjects with apparently idiopathic autism or the 1 with PKU. Guerin et al. (1996) also reported no Purkinje cell reduction. Ritvo et al. (1986), however, found a reduction of Purkinje cell counts in all 4 autistic subjects in their study that was highly statistically significant, even though there was notable interindividual variability, which they pointed out argued for the importance of using total counts. Fatemi et al. (2002b) noted reduced Purkinje cell size, though not density, in 5 matched subjects. Kemper, Bauman and colleagues published a series of studies noting a variable but symmetrical loss of cerebellar Purkinje and granule cells, and also reported involvement of deep cerebellar nuclei as well as of the inferior olivary nucleus. The presence or absence of these findings did not appear to be consistently related to the presence or absence of a history of seizure activity in the patients. However, a recent study by the same group used calbindin rather than Nissl stain as 2 of 10 brains showed significantly lower Purkinje cell counts with Nissl than with calbindin (Whitney et al. 2004). With calbinden, no significant difference in Purkinje cell count between 6 autistic and 4 control subjects was discerned, possibly suggesting that inadequate Nissl staining (perhaps related to agonal changes or post-mortem handling), might have led to lower Purkinje cell counts in earlier studies.

Cerebellar abnormalities have been found in neuroimaging as well as in neuropathology. Cerebellar area, requiring definition of regional boundaries in one sagittal plane, has been measured more often than volume, which requires summation of multiple measures. An early report of cerebellar vermal lobules VI–VII hypoplasia (Courchesne et al. 1988) was followed by a substantial number of papers reporting measurements of the midline sagittal area of the cerebellum vermal lobules. These have been reviewed and discussed in detail elsewhere (Courchesne et al. 1995, Filipek 1995, Piven and Arndt 1995, Courchesne 1999, Piven et al. 1999). While some of the papers replicated the findings of hypoplasia, others did not. Smaller cerebellar vermal lobules VI–VII were found in several studies (Gaffney et al. 1987, Courchesne et al. 1988, Murakami et al. 1989, Saitoh et al. 1995), while some later studies discerned a subgroup with an area increase (e.g. Courchesne et al. 1994). However, several other studies found no difference in cerebellar vermal lobules (Rumsey and Hamburger 1988; Nowell et al. 1990; Filipek et al. 1992; Garber and Ritvo 1992; Holttum et al. 1992; Kleiman et al. 1992; Piven et al. 1992, 1997; Elia et al. 2000). It was also argued that vermal hypoplasia was found in a number of other neurodevelopmental disorders, and therefore was not specific to autism (Schaefer et al. 1996).

Cerebellar volume increase has been found in all of the studies making this measurement, although to different degrees. Piven et al. (1997b) and Sparks et al. (2002) showed cerebellar increase proportional to increased total brain volume. Herbert et al. (2003a) similarly found that total cerebellar volume was greater in autism than in controls, but not different after adjustment for total brain volume; this finding was in the same set of brains where earlier analysis had found no difference in midline vermal lobule VI–VII areas (Filipek et al. 1992). However, Hardan et al. (2001) found cerebellar volumes to be both relatively and absolutely larger. Using a different method whose measures are not directly comparable to those used in the above studies, Abell et al. (1999) in a voxel-based morphometry study also found increased gray matter bilaterally in the cerebellum. Improvements in posterior fossa resolution have more recently allowed the segmentation of cerebellar gray and white matter; this measure has led to findings suggesting that overall cerebellar volume increase may be due to an increase in cerebellar white matter, as in the only study in which this was measured, cerebellar white matter was as much as 39% larger in 2- to 4-year-olds with autism than in controls (Courchesne et al. 2001). Boddaert et al. (2004) found a mean decrease in the voxel-based morphometry measure discussed above of "white matter concentration" in 21 school-age children with autism, though the relationship between this measure and volume measures needs systematic study.

LANGUAGE AREAS

A reversal of typical leftward asymmetry in frontal-related language cortex was reported in high-functioning autistic boys by Herbert et al. (2002). This finding was replicated in an independent sample of language impaired autistic boys and also in non-autistic boys with specific language impairment, but was not found in either non-language impaired autistic boys or typically developing controls (De Fosse et al. 2004). Rojas et al. (2002) reported a smaller left planum temporale, while Herbert et al. (2002) reported a larger planum temporale in autistic boys. Late development of aberrant language asymmetry was reported by Flagg in a recent MEG study (Flagg et al. 2005).

FUSIFORM GYRUS

Since individuals with autism have been demonstrated through psychological investigations to have impairments in face processing, functional neuroimaging studies endeavored to identify altered neural circuitry associated with this activity. Three studies of face processing in autism demonstrated deviations from the typical pattern of fusiform face area activation (Critchley et al. 2000, Schultz et al. 2000, Pierce et al. 2001); however, the deviations varied among the studies. In the study by Schultz et al., with a task related to face and object discrimination, face processing showed greater activation in autistic subjects than controls of the inferior temporal gyrus, an area associated in both autistic subjects and controls with the processing of objects. However, Hadjikhani et al. (2004) reported that subjects with autism do succeed in activating the fusiform face area with face processing and proposed that face processing deficits in autism are due to more complex anomalies in the distributed network of brain areas involved in social perception and cognition. Dalton et al. (2005) showed that diminished fusiform activation was associated with diminished gaze fixation, which in turn was associated with amygdalar activation.

BRAINSTEM

In those studies that have examined the brainstem, some abnormalities have been found. Bauman and Kemper (Bauman 1991, Kemper and Bauman 1998) reported abnormal size of neurons in the inferior olive that differed by age, with 3 younger subjects showing larger neurons, and 3 older subjects showing smaller, pale neurons; in addition a tendency was reported across these subjects for the neurons to cluster at the periphery of the convolutions. Bailey et al. (1998) found various brainstem abnormalities including olivary abnormalities in 3 of 5 subjects for whom relevant sections were available, accompanied by neuronal ectopia in 2 of these subjects as well as in a third who did not have olivary dysplasia. Also noted in this sample were abnormalities in the medulla, pons, locus ceruleus, stria medullaris and arcuate nuclei in individual subjects but not consistently across the sample. Some perivascular lymphocytic infiltrates and microglial nodules were noted in the 16-year-old subject examined by Guerin et al. (1996). Rodier et al. (1996) sectioned through the lower cranial nerve nuclei of a single subject and reported multiple abnormalities, including markedly reduced neuronal cell counts as well as abnormal presence of myelinated fibers at the level of the facial nucleus. Also noted was an absence of superior olivary cells, and a shortened distance between landmarks in the trapezoid body and the inferior olive, the region from which the facial nucleus was absent. The hypoglossal nucleus did not have reduced cell number but contained an atypical bilateral structure whose fibers on one side could be traced into the medial longitudinal fasciculus. However, a recent abstract from the Bauman and Kemper research group (Thevarkunnel et al. 2004) reported abnormalities in the inferior olivary complex comparable to those described by Bailey et al. (1998) not only in 6 autistic but also in 7 control brains. In contrast to the findings of Rodier et al. (1996), there was no absence of the superior olivary complex in any of these autistic brains, while the facial nucleus was comparably formed between autistic and control groups. Welsh et al. (2005) presented experimental findings related to the potential functional role of inferior olivary abnormalities in leading to brain desynchronization. Whereas these findings may be taken at face value, it is premature to be confident that they have specific relevance to the pathogenetic origins of autism.

ASSOCIATION CORTEX

Evidence that associational cortex shows greater differences from controls than primary or unimodal association cortices has been found in both volumetric and functional studies. Herbert et al. (2005) showed widespread cortical asymmetry shifts that were most different from controls in higher order association cortex, and were nearly the same in both autism and developmental language disorder, suggesting a systematic rather than a random pattern of change. Carper and Courchesne (2005) showed that volume differences from controls were most pronounced and growth trajectory was most different in dorsolateral frontal cortex. Reduced activation in associational or modality independent cortex were also found by Castelli et al. (2002), Luna et al. (2002), and Belmonte and Yurgelun-Todd (2003).

DISCUSSION

Neuropathology and neuroimaging studies in autism clearly have yielded a range of findings, by no means all consistent, related to the brain basis of this behaviorally defined syndrome. Neuropathological studies have resolution at the microscopic level not available to neuroimaging, but they labor under the constraints of fixation artifact, general lack of adequate subject ascertainment, lack of control for or consistency in conditions of death or post-mortem interval, and inclusion in some of the studies of individuals with other identifiable diagnoses, such as Rett syndrome. While neuroimaging studies do not have microscopic resolution, they are in vivo studies and also are more likely to involve an adequate sample size that includes prospectively assessed subjects meeting consistent criteria and free of identifiable artifacts or confounds.

Neuroanatomical findings can be organized in relation to how well they have been replicated. The single most robust neuroanatomical finding in autism is the tendency toward unusually large brain size in young autistic individuals – an upward shift in mean brain size. This result has been found repeatedly by every measure, whether brain volume, brain weight or head circumference. This early brain overgrowth appears to be driven strongly, though not entirely, by an increase in white matter volume. Altered scaling appears to be a neuroanatomical feature that persists, though with changing proportions, over time. Cerebellar, limbic and brainstem changes have been prominently documented, but not uniformly. Perfusion appears to be lower than normal but in a varying distribution among studies. Minicolumn and neuroinflammatory changes are highly suggestive but require further study. An understanding of the relationship between neurotransmitter and neuroanatomical abnormalities is in its infancy. Metabolic changes documented by spectroscopy are suggestive but at this time only preliminary. Functional MRI findings appear to be highly dependent upon experimental conditions.

One of the major challenges in interpreting neuroanatomical data in autism is figuring out which separately documented changes travel together. Autism is likely to be both heterogeneous and dynamic over time at the level of biology, and we do not yet know how to characterize subgroups. On this account, given that findings are generally measured in separate cohorts, often of different ages, it is hard to know whether disparate phenomena represent separate subgroups and/or stages of development, or whether they are pieces of the same picture. As a consequence, our pathoetiological notions of what factors or features are more primary and what are secondary is based almost entirely on inference and speculation.

For example, it has been argued that autism is a disorder of neural information processing that involves impaired coordination among multiple processing components and impairment of complex processing. Placed alongside the phenomenon of large brain and white matter volume, it is tempting to infer that aberrant volume leads to suboptimal connectivity. But we do not know whether the underlying mechanism is consistent with this interpretation, since currently our knowledge of the timing of autism brain overgrowth is greater than our knowledge of its tissue composition. Hopefully this will change soon, as neuroimaging and neuropathological studies targeted at clarifying this question are planned or underway. But until we know this we cannot be sure at what level the phenomenon of large brains is related to that of reduced functional connectivity. There is the further question of why autistic features persist even when brain growth falls behind that of neurotypical controls. Adolescents and adults still by and large meet criteria for autism even though their brains are on average no longer abnormally large compared to typically developed controls, and may even be significantly smaller. So we must admit that we have not documented just what it is about these transiently larger brains that underlies the functional impairments.

Regarding function, from a cognitive neuroscience point of view, we can start with the idea that a certain class of computational disturbance is likely to be a common neural information processing-level substrate of the observed features that define autism. From this starting point, the next question would be whether there are one or multiple biological routes to that type of computational perturbation. For example, proposed or conceivable tissue substrates for disturbed connectivity have included white matter enlargement (structural) (Herbert et al. 2004), pyramidal cell abnormalities (Courchesne and Pierce 2005), altered connectivity secondary to abnormal cortical minicolumns (structural/neurochemical) (Casanova et al. 2003, Casanova 2004, Courchesne and Pierce 2005) increased excitation/inhibition ratios (neurochemical) (Rubenstein and Merzenich 2003), abnormal interneurons (Levitt et al. 2004), and impaired oscillatory function of the inferior olive (structural/electrophysiological) (Welsh et al. 2005). Might these represent distinct subgroups or could some of them be interrelated?

Regarding development, early or prenatal onset of autism has been inferred because of smaller, tightly packed cells in the limbic system, because brainstem changes would be due to changes very early in gestation (Rodier et al. 1996), or because of the high heritability of the disorder. But it is possible that mechanisms other than delayed or curtailed development may account for at least some of these cytological changes. Some neuropathological researchers have held that since the brains lack major dysmorphology, they are unlikely to have suffered significant insult prior to the late gestational or early postnatal period (Ciaranello et al. 1982, Coleman et al. 1985, Raymond et al. 1996) Recent identification of neuroinflammation in autistic brains (Vargas et al. 2005), new knowledge about the role of cytokines and immune receptors in brain development (Boulanger and Shatz 2004), postnatal brain enlargement in animal models of in utero viral infection (Fatemi et al. 2002a), and the identification of environmental factors to which Purkinje cells are vulnerable (Kern 2003) all suggest that we cannot be overconfident in inferences made diachronically backwards into development from synchronic tissue or imaging studies, because many mechanisms may potentially be involved beyond the genetically modulated perturbations of brain development that may most easily come to mind in interpreting volumetric or cytological findings.

Regarding pathoetiology, if neural information processing abnormalities sufficient to cause autism can be the outcome of a heterogeneous set of underlying biological abnormalities, then it is conceivable that cases with prenatal origins can coexist alongside cases of regressive autism that had a normal prenatal course, with various histories and mechanisms still leading to a child who meets full criteria for autism. There is no evidence-based way at this time to exclude this possibility. The picture is further complicated by case reports of patients with certain metabolic diseases and autistic symptoms who, when treated for their metabolic disorders, experience an improvement of some aspects and intensity of their symptom burden (Page 2000). Such recoveries suggest that there may be other routes to autism than altered brain structure, and that perhaps among the various underlying pathophysiologies are some that may not be entirely immutable.

The clinical implications of our inferences and uncertainties include that we cannot be certain that any one etiology or neuroanatomic abnormality underlies the clinical situation in any one patient. The research implications include that we need a more systematic approach both to the biology of this disorder and to sorting out its multifactorial character. From the point of view of research, multimodal imaging studies, where two or more different classes of measures (e.g. perfusion, volumetrics, metabolic studies, EEG/MEG, functional neuroimaging) are assessed in tandem, will allow clarification of the interrelationships among the different classes of findings. Even better would be to additionally collect other biomarker data beyond imaging, including not only genetics but also proteomics, metabolomics, biochemistry, neurochemistry and immune markers – all of which go beyond, or perhaps "beneath", the behavioral realm. With these kind of data at hand the likelihood of discerning subgroups would be greatly increased. Once we can begin to discern subgroups, issues of which features measured to date are necessary or sufficient for autism can be addressed more systematically. Furthermore, given that treatment targets will almost certainly differ among subgroups, such a research program is likely to substantially speed the progress for treatments for significant subgroups of autistic individuals. Identifying targets for effective treatments would be one of the best possible outcomes of our research enterprise.

REFERENCES

Abell F, Krams M, Ashburner J, Passingham R, Friston K, Frackowiak R, Happe F, Frith C, Frith U (1999) The neuroanatomy of autism: a voxel-based whole brain analysis of structural scans. *Neuroreport* 10: 1647–51.

Andrews TJ , Halpern SD, Purves D (1997) Correlated size variations in human visual cortex, lateral geniculate nucleus, and optic tract. *J Neurosci* 17: 2859–68.

Aylward EH, Minshew NJ, Goldstein G, Honeycutt NA, Augustine AM, Yates KO, Barta PE, Pearlson GD (1999) MRI volumes of amygdala and hippocampus in non-mentally retarded autistic adolescents and adults. *Neurology* 53: 2145–50.

Aylward EH, Minshew NJ, Field K, Sparks BF, Singh N (2002) Effects of age on brain volume and head circumference in autism. *Neurology* 59: 175–83.

Bailey A, Luthert P, Bolton P, LeCouteur A, Rutter M (1993) Autism and megalencephaly. *Lancet* 34: 1225–6.

Bailey A, Luthert P, Dean A, Harding B, Janota I, Montgomery M, Rutter M, Lantos P (1998) A clinicopathological study of autism. *Brain* 121: 889–905.

Barnea-Goraly N, Kwon H, Menon V, Eliez S, Lotspeich L, Reiss AL (2004) White matter structure in autism: preliminary evidence from diffusion tensor imaging. *Biol Psychiatry* 55: 323–6.

Barton RA, Harvey PH (2000) Mosaic evolution of brain structure in mammals. *Nature* 405: 1055–8.

Bauman M (1991) Microscopic neuroantomic abnormalities in autism. *Pediatrics* 87: 791–6.

Bauman ML, Kemper TL (1994) Neuroanatomic observations of the brain in autism. In: Bauman ML, Kemper TL, eds. *The Neurobiology of Autism.* Baltimore: Johns Hopkins University Press, pp. 119–45.

Belmonte MK, Yurgelun-Todd DA (2003) Functional anatomy of impaired selective attention and compensatory processing in autism. *Brain Res Cogn Brain Res* 17: 651–64.

Boddaert N, Chabane N, Gervais H, Good CD, Bourgeois M, Plumet MH, Barthelemy C,

Mouren MC, Artiges E, Samson Y, Brunelle F, Frackowiak RS, Zilbovicius M (2004) Superior temporal sulcus anatomical abnormalities in childhood autism: a voxel-based morphometry MRI study. *Neuroimage* 23: 364–9.

Boulanger LM, Shatz CJ (2004) Immune signalling in neural development, synaptic plasticity and disease. *Nat Rev Neurosci* 5: 521–31.

Carper RA, Courchesne E (2000) Inverse correlation between frontal lobe and cerebellum sizes in children with autism. *Brain* 123: 836–44.

Carper RA, Courchesne E (2005) Localized enlargement of the frontal cortex in early autism. *Biol Psychiatry* 57: 126–33.

Carper RA, Moses P, Tigue ZD, Courchesne E (2002) Cerebral lobes in autism: early hyperplasia and abnormal age effects. *Neuroimage* 16: 1038–51.

Casanova MF (2004) White matter volume increase and minicolumns in autism. *Ann Neurol* 56: 453; author reply 454.

Casanova MF, Buxhoeveden DP, Switala AE, Roy E (2002) Minicolumnar pathology in autism. *Neurology* 58: 428–32.

Casanova MF, Buxhoeveden D, Gomez J (2003) Disruption in the inhibitory architecture of the cell minicolumn: implications for autism. *Neuroscientist* 9: 496–507.

Castelli F, Frith C, Happe F, Frith U (2002) Autism, Asperger syndrome and brain mechanisms for the attribution of mental states to animated shapes. *Brain* 125: 1839–49.

Chandana SR, Behen ME, Juhasz C, Muzik O, Rothermel RD, Mangner TJ, Chakraborty PK, Chugani HT, Chugani DC (2005) Significance of abnormalities in developmental trajectory and asymmetry of cortical serotonin synthesis in autism. *Int J Dev Neurosci* 23: 171–82.

Chiron C, Leboyer M, Leon F, Jambaque I, Nuttin C, Syrota A (1995) SPECT of the brain in childhood autism: evidence for a lack of normal hemispheric asymmetry. *Dev Med Child Neurol* 37: 849–60.

Chugani DC, Muzik O, Rothermel R, Behen M, Chakraborty P, Mangner T, da Silva EA, Chugani HT (1997) Altered serotonin synthesis in the dentatothalamocortical pathway in autistic boys. *Ann Neurol* 42: 666–9.

Chugani DC, Muzik O, Behen M, Rothermel R, Janisse JJ, Lee J, Chugani HT (1999a) Developmental changes in brain serotonin synthesis capacity in autistic and nonautistic children. *Ann Neurol* 45: 287–95.

Chugani DC, Sundram BS, Behen M, Lee ML, Moore GJ (1999b) Evidence of altered energy metabolism in autistic children. *Prog Neuropsychopharmacol Biol Psychiatry* 23: 635–41.

Chung MK, Dalton KM, Alexander AL, Davidson RJ (2004) Less white matter concentration in autism: 2D voxel-based morphometry. *Neuroimage* 23: 242–51.

Ciaranello RD, VandenBerg SR, Anders TF (1982) Intrinsic and extrinsic determinants of neuronal development: relation to infantile autism. *J Autism Dev Disord* 12: 115–45.

Ciesielski KT, Harris RJ, Hart BL, Pabst HF (1997) Cerebellar hypoplasia and frontal lobe cognitive deficits in disorders of early childhood. *Neuropsychologia* 35: 643–55.

Coleman P, Romano J, Lapham L, Simon W (1985) Cell counts in cerebral cortex of an autistic patient. *J Autism Dev Disord* 15: 245–55.

Courchesne E (1999) An MRI study of autism: the cerebellum revisited. *Neurology* 52: 1106–7.

Courchesne E, Pierce K (2005) Brain overgrowth in autism during a critical time in development: implications for frontal pyramidal neuron and interneuron development and connectivity. *Int J Dev Neurosci* 23: 153–70.

Courchesne E, Yeung-Courchesne R, Pres GA, Hesselink JR, Jernigan TL (1988) Hypoplasia of cerebellar vermal lobules VI and VII in autism. *N Engl J Med* 318: 1349–54.

Courchesne E, Saitoh O, Yeung-Courchesne R, Press GA, Lincoln AJ, Haas RH, Schreibman L (1994) Abnormality of cerebellar vermian lobules VI and VII in patients with infantile autism: identification of hypoplastic and hyperplastic subgroups with MR imaging. *Am J Roentgenol* 162: 123–30.

Courchesne E, Townsend J, Saitoh O (1995) Reply from the authors to Piven and Arndt. *Neurology* 45: 399–402.

Courchesne E, Muller RA, Saitoh O (1999) Brain weight in autism: normal in the majority of cases, megalencephalic in rare cases. *Neurology* 52: 1057–9.

Courchesne E, Karns CM, Davis HR, Ziccardi R, Carper RA, Tigue ZD, Chisum HJ, Moses P, Pierce K, Lord C, Lincoln AJ, Pizzo S, Schreibman L, Haas RH, Akshoomoff NA, Courchesne RY (2001) Unusual brain growth patterns in early life in patients with autistic disorder: An MRI study. *Neurology* 57: 245–54.

Courchesne E, Carper R, Akshoomoff N (2003) Evidence of brain overgrowth in the first year of life in autism. *JAMA* 290: 337–44.

Critchley HD, Daly EM, Bullmore ET, Williams SC, Van Amelsvoort T, Robertson DM, Rowe A, Phillips M, McAlonan G, Howlin P, Murphy DG (2000) The functional neuroanatomy of social behaviour: changes in cerebral blood flow when people with autistic disorder process facial expressions. *Brain* 123: 2203–12.

Dalton KM, Nacewicz BM, Johnstone T, Schaefer HS, Gernsbacher MA, Goldsmith HH, Alexander AL, Davidson RJ (2005) Gaze fixation and the neural circuitry of face processing in autism. *Nat Neurosci* 8: 519–26.

Damasio A, Maurer R (1978) A neurological model for childhood autism. *Arch Neurol* 35: 777–86.

Davidovitch M, Patterson B, Gartside P (1996) Head circumference measurements in children with autism. *J Child Neurol* 11: 389–93.

De Fosse L, Hodge SM, Makris N, Kennedy DN, Caviness VS, Mcgrath L, Steele S, Ziegler DA, Herbert MR, Frazier JA, Tager-Flusberg H, Harris GJ (2004) Language-association cortex asymmetry in autism and specific language impairment. *Ann Neurology* 56: 757–66.

Dekaban A, Sadowsky D (1978) Changes in brain weight during the span of human life: relation of brain weights to body heights and weights. *Ann Neurol* 4: 345–56.

Dementieva YA, Vance DD, Donnelly SL, Elston LA, Wolpert CM, Ravan SA, DeLong GR, Abramson RK, Wright HH, Cuccaro ML (2005) Accelerated head growth in early development of individuals with autism. *Pediatr Neurol* 32: 102–8.

Deutsch CK, Joseph RM (2003) Brief report: cognitive correlates of enlarged head circumference in children with autism. *J Autism Dev Disord* 33: 209–15.

Egaas B, Courchesne E, Saitoh O (1995) Reduced size of corpus callosum in autism. *Arch Neurol* 52: 794–801.

Elia M, Ferri R, Musumeci SA, Panerai S, Bottitta M, Scuderi C (2000) Clinical correlates of brain morphometric features of subjects with low- functioning autistic disorder. *J Child Neurol* 15: 504–8.

Fatemi SH, Earle J, Kanodia R, Kist D, Emamian ES, Patterson PH, Shi L, Sidwell R (2002a) Prenatal viral infection leads to pyramidal cell atrophy and macrocephaly in adulthood: implications for genesis of autism and schizophrenia. *Cell Mol Neurobiol* 22: 25–33.

Fatemi SH, Halt AR, Realmuto G, Earle J, Kist DA, Thuras P, Merz A (2002b) Purkinje cell size is reduced in cerebellum of patients with autism. *Cell Mol Neurobiol* 22: 171–5.

Fidler DJ, Bailey JN, Smalley SL (2000) Macrocephaly in autism and other pervasive developmental disorders. *Dev Med Child Neurol* 42: 737–40.

Filipek PA (1995) Quantitative magnetic resonance imaging in autism: the cerebellar vermis. *Curr*

Opin Neurol 8: 134–8.

Filipek P, Richelme C, Kennedy D, Rademacher J, Pitcher D, Zidel S, Caviness V (1992) Morphometric analysis of the brain in developmental language disorders and autism. *Ann Neurol* 32: 475 (abstract).

Finlay BL, Darlington RB, Nicastro N (2001) Developmental structure in brain evolution. *Behav Brain Sci* 24: 263–78; discussion 278–308.

Flagg EJ, Oram Cardy JE, Roberts W, Roberts TP (2005) Language lateralization development in children with autism: insights from the late field magnetoencephalogram. *Neurosci Lett* 386: 82–7.

Fombonne E (1999) The epidemiology of autism: a review. *Psychol Med* 29: 769–86.

Fombonne E, Roge B, Claverie J, Courty S, Fremolle J (1999) Microcephaly and macrocephaly in autism. *J Autism Dev Disord* 29: 113–9.

Friedman SD, Shaw DW, Artru AA, Richards TL, Gardner J, Dawson G, Posse S, Dager SR (2003) Regional brain chemical alterations in young children with autism spectrum disorder. *Neurology* 60: 100–7.

Gaffney GR, Tsai LY, Kuperman S, Minchin S (1987) Cerebellar structure in autism. *Am J Dis Child* 141: 1330–2.

Gage NM, Siegel B, Callen M, Roberts TP (2003) Cortical sound processing in children with autism disorder: an MEG investigation. *Neuroreport* 14: 2047–51.

Galuska L, Szakall S, Emri M, Olah R, Varga J, Garai I, Kollar J, Pataki I, Tron L (2002) [PET and SPECT scans in autistic children.] *Orv Hetil* 143: 1302–4 (Hungarian).

Garber HI, Ritvo ER (1992) Magnetic resonance imaging of the posterior fossa in autistic adults. *Am J Psychiatry* 149: 245–7.

George MS, Costa DC, Kouris K, Ring HA, Ell PJ (1992) Cerebral blood flow abnormalities in adults with infantile autism. *J Nerv Ment Dis* 180: 413–7.

Ghaziuddin M, Zaccagnini J, Tsai L, Elardo S (1999) Is megalencephaly specific to autism? *J Intellect Disabil Res* 43: 279–82.

Gillberg C, de Souza L (2002) Head circumference in autism, Asperger syndrome, and ADHD: a comparative study. *Dev Med Child Neurol* 44: 296–300.

Giuliani NR, Calhoun VD, Pearlson GD, Francis A, Buchanan RW (2005) Voxel-based morphometry versus region of interest: a comparison of two methods for analyzing gray matter differences in schizophrenia. *Schizophr Res* 74: 135–47.

Guerin P, Lyon G, Barthelemy C, Sostak E, Chevrollier V, Garreau B, Lelord G (1996) Neuropathological study of a case of autistic syndrome with severe mental retardation. *Dev Med Child Neurol* 38: 203–11.

Hadjikhani N, Joseph RM, Snyder J, Chabris CF, Clark J, Steele S, McGrath L, Vangel M, Aharon I, Feczko E, Harris GJ, Tager-Flusberg H (2004) Activation of the fusiform gyrus when individuals with autism spectrum disorder view faces. *Neuroimage* 22: 1141–50.

Hardan AY, Minshew NJ, Keshavan MS (2000) Corpus callosum size in autism. *Neurology* 55: 1033–6.

Hardan AY, Minshew NJ, Harenski K, Keshavan MS (2001) Posterior fossa magnetic resonance imaging in autism. *J Am Acad Child Adolesc Psychiatry* 40: 666–72.

Hashimoto T, Sasaki M, Fukumizu M, Hanaoka S, Sugai K, Matsuda H (2000) Single-photon emission computed tomography of the brain in autism: effect of the developmental level. *Pediatr Neurol* 23: 416–20.

Hazlett H, Poe M, Gerig G, Smith R, Provenzale J, Ross A, Gilmore J, Piven J (2005) Magnetic resonance imaging and head circumference study of brain size in autism: birth through age 2 years. *Arch Gen Psychiatry* 62: 1366–76.

Haznedar MM, Buchsbaum MS, Metzger M, Solimando A, Spiegel-Cohen J, Hollander E (1997) Anterior cingulate gyrus volume and glucose metabolism in autistic disorder. *Am J Psychiatry* 154: 1047–50.

Haznedar MM, Buchsbaum MS, Wei TC, Hof PR, Cartwright C, Bienstock CA, Hollander E (2000) Limbic circuitry in patients with autism spectrum disorders studied with positron emission tomography and magnetic resonance imaging. *Am J Psychiatry* 157: 1994–2001.

Herbert MR (2005) Large brains in autism: the challenge of pervasive abnormality. *Neuroscientist* 11: 417–40.

Herbert MR, Harris GJ, Adrien KT, Ziegler DA, Makris N, Kennedy DN, Lange NT, Chabris CF, Bakardjiev A, Hodgson J, Takeoka M, Tager-Flusberg H, Caviness VS (2002) Abnormal asymmetry in language association cortex in autism. *Ann Neurol* 52: 588–96.

Herbert MR, Ziegler DA, Deutsch CK, O'Brien LM, Lange N, Bakardjiev A, Hodgson J, Adrien KT, Steele S, Makris N, Kennedy D, Harris GJ, Caviness VS (2003a) Dissociations of cerebral cortex, subcortical and cerebral white matter volumes in autistic boys. *Brain* 126: 1182–92.

Herbert MR, Ziegler DA, Makris N, Bakardjiev A, Hodgson J, Adrien KT, Kennedy DN, Filipek PA, Caviness VS (2003b) Larger brain and white matter volumes in children with developmental language disorder. *Dev Sci* 6: F11–22

Herbert MR, Ziegler DA, Makris N, Filipek PA, Kemper TL, Normandin JJ, Sanders HA, Kennedy DN, Caviness VS (2004) Localization of white matter volume increase in autism and developmental language disorder. *Ann Neurol* 55: 530–40.

Herbert MR, Ziegler DA, Deutsch CK, O'Brien LM, Kennedy DN, Filipek PA, Bakardjiev AI, Hodgson J, Takeoka M, Makris N, Caviness VS (2005) Brain asymmetries in autism and developmental language disorder: a nested whole-brain analysis. *Brain* 128: 213–26.

Herold S, Frackowiak RS, Le Couteur A, Rutter M, Howlin P (1988) Cerebral blood flow and metabolism of oxygen and glucose in young autistic adults. *Psychol Med* 18: 823–31.

Hier DB, LeMay M, Rosenberger PB (1979) Autism and unfavorable left-right asymmetries of the brain. *J Autism Dev Disord* 9: 153–9.

Holttum JR, Minshew NJ, Sanders RS, Phillips NE (1992) Magnetic resonance imaging of the posterior fossa in autism. *Biol Psychiatry* 32: 1091–101.

Horwitz B, Rumsey JM, Grady CL, Rapoport SI (1988) The cerebral metabolic landscape in autism. Intercorrelations of regional glucose utilization. *Arch Neurol* 45: 749–55.

Howard MA, Cowell PE, Boucher J, Broks P, Mayes A, Farrant A, Roberts N (2000) Convergent neuroanatomical and behavioural evidence of an amygdala hypothesis of autism. *Neuroreport* 11: 2931–5.

Hultman CM, Sparen P, Cnattingius S (2002) Perinatal risk factors for infantile autism. *Epidemiology* 13: 417–23.

Jancke L, Staiger JF, Schlaug G, Huang Y, Steinmetz H (1997) The relationship between corpus callosum size and forebrain volume. *Cereb Cortex* 7: 48–56.

Just MA, Cherkassky VL, Keller TA, Minshew NJ (2004) Cortical activation and synchronization during sentence comprehension in high-functioning autism: evidence of underconnectivity. *Brain* 127: 1811–21.

Kaya M, Karasalihoglu S, Ustun F, Gultekin A, Cermik TF, Fazlioglu Y, Ture M, Yigitbasi ON, Berkarda S (2002) The relationship between 99mTc-HMPAO brain SPECT and the scores of real life rating scale in autistic children. *Brain Dev* 24: 77–81.

Kemper TL, Bauman M (1998) Neuropathology of infantile autism. *J Neuropathol Exp Neurol* 57: 645–52.

Kern JK (2003) Purkinje cell vulnerability and autism: a possible etiological connection. *Brain Dev* 25: 377–82.

Kleiman MD, Neff S, Rosman NP (1992) The brain in infantile autism: Are posterior fossa structures abnormal? *Neurology* 42: 753–60.

Koshino H, Carpenter PA, Minshew NJ, Cherkassky VL, Keller TA, Just MA (2005) Functional connectivity in an fMRI working memory task in high-functioning autism. *Neuroimage* 24: 810–21.

Lainhart JE, Piven J, Wzorek M, Landa R, Santangelo SL, Coon H, Folstein SE (1997) Macrocephaly in children and adults with autism. *J Am Acad Child Adolesc Psychiatry* 36: 282–90.

Levitt JG, O'Neill J, Blanton RE, Smalley S, Fadale D, McCracken JT, Guthrie D, Toga AW, Alger JR (2003) Proton magnetic resonance spectroscopic imaging of the brain in childhood autism. *Biol Psychiatry* 54: 1355–66.

Levitt P, Eagleson KL, Powell EM (2004) Regulation of neocortical interneuron development and the implications for neurodevelopmental disorders. *Trends Neurosci* 27: 400–6.

Lotspeich LJ, Kwon H, Schumann CM, Fryer SL, Goodlin-Jones BL, Buonocore MH, Lammers CR, Amaral DG, Reiss AL (2004) Investigation of neuroanatomical differences between autism and Asperger syndrome. *Arch Gen Psychiatry* 61: 291–8.

Luna B, Minshew NJ, Garver KE, Lazar NA, Thulborn KR, Eddy WF, Sweeney JA (2002) Neocortical system abnormalities in autism: an fMRI study of spatial working memory. *Neurology* 59: 834–40.

Makris N, Meyer JW, Bates JF, Yeterian EH, Kennedy DN, Caviness VS (1999) MRI-based topographic parcellation of human cerebral white matter and nuclei II. Rationale and applications with systematics of cerebral connectivity. *Neuroimage* 9: 18–45.

Manes F, Piven J, Vrancic D, Nanclares V, Plebst C, Starkstein SE (1999) An MRI study of the corpus callosum and cerebellum in mentally retarded autistic individuals. *J Neuropsychiatry Clin Neurosci* 11: 470–4.

Mason-Brothers A, Ritvo ER, Pingree C, Petersen PB, Jenson WR, McMahon WM, Freeman BJ, Jorde LB, Spencer MJ, Mo A, et al. (1990) The UCLA–University of Utah epidemiologic survey of autism: prenatal, perinatal, and postnatal factors. *Pediatrics* 86: 514–9.

Mesulam MM (1990) Large-scale neurocognitive networks and distributed processing for attention, language, and memory. *Ann Neurology* 28: 597–613.

Meyer JW, Makris N, Bates JF, Caviness VS, Kennedy DN (1999) MRI-based topographic parcellation of human cerebral white matter. *Neuroimage* 9: 1–17.

Miles JH, Hadden LL, Takahashi TN, Hillman RE (2000) Head circumference is an independent clinical finding associated with autism. *Am J Med Genet* 95: 339–50.

Minshew NJ, Goldstein G, Dombrowski SM, Panchalingam K, Pettegrew JW (1993) A preliminary 31P MRS study of autism: Evidence for undersynthesis and increased degradation of brain membranes. Biol Psychiatry 33: 762–73.

Minshew NJ, Goldstein G, Siegel DJ (1997) Neuropsychologic functioning in autism: profile of a complex informational processing disorder. *J Int Neuropsychol Soc* 3: 303–16.

Mountz JM, Tolbert LC, Lill DW, Katholi CR, Liu HG (1995) Functional deficits in autistic disorder: characterization by technetium-99m-HMPAO and SPECT. J Nucl Med 36: 1156–62.

Muller RA, Behen ME, Rothermel RD, Chugani DC, Muzik O, Mangner TJ, Chugani HT (1999) Brain mapping of language and auditory perception in high-functioning autistic adults: a PET study. *J Autism Dev Disord* 29: 19–31.

Murakami JW, Courchesne E, Press GA, Yeung-Courchesne R, Hesselink JR (1989) Reduced cerebellar hemisphere size and its relationship to vermal hypoplasia in autism. *Arch Neurol* 46: 689–94.

Nowell MA, Hackney DB, Muraki AS, Coleman M (1990) Varied MR appearance of autism: fifty-three pediatric patients having the full autistic syndrome. *Magn Reson Imaging* 8: 811–6.

Ohnishi T, Matsuda H, Hashimoto T, Kunihiro T, Nishikawa M, Uema T, Sasaki M (2000) Abnormal regional cerebral blood flow in childhood autism. *Brain* 123: 1838–44.

Page T (2000) Metabolic approaches to the treatment of autism spectrum disorders. *J Autism Dev Disord* 30: 463–69.

Pierce K, Muller RA, Ambrose J, Allen G, Courchesne E (2001) Face processing occurs outside the fusiform 'face area' in autism: evidence from functional MRI. *Brain* 124: 2059–73.

Piven J, Arndt S (1995) The cerebellum and autism. *Neurology* 45: 398–99.

Piven J, Nehme E, Simon J, Barta P, Pearlson G, Folstein SE (1992) Magnetic resonance imaging in autism: Measurement of the cerebellum, pons, and fourth ventricle. *Biol Psychiatry* 31: 491–504.

Piven J, Arndt S, Bailey J, Havercamp S, Andreasen NC, Palmer P (1995) An MRI study of brain size in autism. *Am J Psychiatry* 152: 1145–9.

Piven J, Arndt S, Bailey J, Andreasen N (1996) Regional brain enlargement in autism: a magnetic resonance imaging study. *J Am Acad Child Adolesc Psychiatry* 35: 530–6.

Piven J, Bailey J, Ranson BJ, Arndt S (1997a) An MRI study of the corpus callosum in autism. *Am J Psychiatry* 154: 1051–6.

Piven J, Saliba K, Bailey J, Arndt S (1997b) An MRI study of autism: the cerebellum revisited. *Neurology* 49: 546–51.

Piven J, Saliba K, Bailey J, Arndt S (1999) An MRI study of autism: the cerebellum revisited – Reply. *Neurology* 52: 1106–7.

Rapin I, ed. (1996) *Preschool Children with Inadequate Communication: Developmental Language Disorder, Autism, Low IQ. Clinics in Developmental Medicine No. 139.* London: Mac Keith Press.

Raymond GV, Bauman ML, Kemper TL (1996) Hippocampus in autism: a Golgi analysis. *Acta Neuropathol* 91: 117–9.

Redcay E, Courchesne E (2005) When is the brain enlarged in autism? A meta-analysis of all brain size reports. *Biol Psychiatry* 58: 1–9.

Ritvo ER, Freeman BJ, Scheibel AB (1986) Lower Purkinje cell counts in the cerebella of four autistic subjects. *Am J Psychiatry* 143: 862–6.

Rodier PM, Ingram JL, Tisdale B, Nelson S, Romano J (1996) Embryological origins for autism: Developmental anomalies of the cranial nerve motor nuclei. *J Comp Neurol* 370: 247–61.

Rojas DC, Bawn SD, Benkers TL, Reite ML, Rogers SJ (2002) Smaller left hemisphere planum temporale in adults with autistic disorder. *Neurosci Lett* 328: 237–40.

Rubenstein JL, Merzenich MM (2003) Model of autism: increased ratio of excitation/inhibition in key neural systems. *Genes Brain Behav* 2: 255–67.

Rumsey JM, Hamburger SD (1988) Neuropsychological findings in high-functioning men with infantile autism residual state. *J Clin Exp Neuropsychol* 10: 201–21.

Rumsey J, Duara R, Grady C, Rapoport JL, Margolin RA, Rapoport SI, Cutler NR (1985) Brain metabolism in autism: Resting cerebral glucose utilization rates as measured with positron emission tomography. *Arch Gen Psychiatry* 42: 448–55.

Ryu YH, Lee JD, Yoon PH, Kim DI, Lee HB, Shin YJ (1999) Perfusion impairments in infantile autism on technetium-99m ethyl cysteinate dimer brain single-photon emission tomography: comparison with findings on magnetic resonance imaging. *Eur J Nucl Med* 26: 253–9.

Saitoh O, Courchesne E, Egaas B, Lincoln AJ, Schreibman L (1995) Cross-sectional area of the posterior hippocampus in autistic patients with cerebellar and corpus callosum abnormalities. *Neurology* 45: 317–24.

Schaefer GB, Thompson JN, Bodensteiner JB, McConnell JM, Kimberling WJ, Gay CT, Dutton WD, Hutchings DC, Gray SB (1996) Hypoplasia of the cerebellar vermis in neurogenetic syndromes. *Ann Neurol* 39: 382–85.

Schifter T, Hoffman JM, Hatten HP, Hanson MW, Coleman RE, DeLong GR (1994) Neuro-imaging in infantile autism. *J Child Neurol* 9: 155–61.

Schultz RT, Gauthier I, Klin A, Fulbright RK, Anderson AW, Volkmar F, Skudlarski P, Lacadic C, Cohen DJ, Gore JC (2000) Abnormal ventral temporal cortical activity during face dis-crimination among individuals with autism and Asperger syndrome. *Arch Gen Psychiatry* 57: 331–40.

Sherman M, Nass R, Shapiro T (1984) Brief report: regional cerebral blood flow in autism. *J Autism Dev Disord* 14: 439–46.

Sokol DK, Dunn DW, Edwards-Brown M, Feinberg J (2002) Hydrogen proton magnetic reso-nance spectroscopy in autism: preliminary evidence of elevated choline/creatine ratio. *J Child Neurol* 17: 245–9.

Sparks BF, Friedman SD, Shaw DW, Aylward EH, Echelard D, Artru AA, Maravilla KR, Giedd JN, Munson J, Dawson G, Dager SR (2002) Brain structural abnormalities in young children with autism spectrum disorder. *Neurology* 59: 184–92.

Starkstein SE, Vazquez S, Vrancic D, Nanclares V, Manes F, Piven J, Plebst C (2000) SPECT findings in mentally retarded autistic individuals. *J Neuropsychiatry Clin Neurosci* 12: 370–5.

Steg J, Rapoport J (1975) Minor physical anomalies in normal, neurotic, learning disabled, and severely disturbed children. *J Autism Child Schizophr* 5: 299–307.

Stevenson RE, Schroer RJ, Skinner C, Fender D, Simensen RJ (1997) Autism and macrocephaly. *Lancet* 349: 1744–5.

Thevarkunnel S, Martchek MA, Kemper TL, Bauman ML, Blatt GJ (2004) A neuroanatomical study of the brainstem nuclei in autism. Program no. 1028.10. Abstract Viewer/Itinerary Planner. Washington, DC: Society for Neurosciences (online: http://sfn.scholarone.com/itin2004).

Tsatsanis KD, Rourke BP, Klin A, Volkmar FR, Cicchetti D, Schultz RT (2003) Reduced thalamic volume in high-functioning individuals with autism. *Biol Psychiatry* 53: 121–9.

Vargas DL, Nascimbene C, Krishnan C, Zimmerman AW, Pardo CA (2005) Neuroglial activation and neuroinflammation in the brain of patients with autism. *Ann Neurol* 57: 67–81.

Waiter GD, Williams JH, Murray AD, Gilchrist A, Perrett DI, Whiten A (2005) Structural white matter deficits in high-functioning individuals with autistic spectrum disorder: a voxel-based investigation. *Neuroimage* 24: 455–61.

Walker H (1977) Incidence of minor physical anomaly in autism. *J Autism Child Schizophr* 7: 165–76.

Welsh JP, Ahn ES, Placantonakis DG (2005) Is autism due to brain desynchronization? *Int J Dev Neurosci* 23: 253–63.

Whitney ER, Kemper TL, Bauman ML, Blatt GJ (2004) Calcium-binding proteins in cerebellar Purkinje cells in the autistic cerebellum. Program no. 116.11. Abstract Viewer/Itinerary Planner. Washington, DC: Society for Neurosciences (online: http://sfn.scholarone.com/itin2004).

Wilcox J, Tsuang MT, Ledger E, Algeo J, Schnurr T (2002) Brain perfusion in autism varies with age. *Neuropsychobiology* 46: 13–6.

Williams RS, Hauser SL, Purpura DP, DeLong GR, Swisher CN (1980) Autism and mental re-tardation: neuropathologic studies performed in four retarded persons with autistic behavior. Arch Neurol 37: 749–53.

Woodhouse W, Bailey A, Rutter M, Bolton P, Baird G, Le Couteur A (1996) Head circumference in autism and other pervasive developmental disorders. *J Child Psychol Psychiatry* 37: 665–71.

Zilbovicius M, Garreau B, Tzourio N, Mazoyer B, Bruck B, Martinot JL, Raynaud C, Samson Y, Syrota A, Lelord G (1992) Regional cerebral blood flow in childhood autism: a SPECT study. *Am J Psychiatry* 149: 924–30.

Zilbovicius M, Garreau B, Samson Y (1995) Delayed maturation of the frontal cortex in childhood autism. *Am J Psychiatry* 158, 248–52.

Zilbovicius M, Boddaert N, Belin P, Poline JB, Remy P, Mangin JF, Thivard L, Barthelemy C, Samson Y (2000) Temporal lobe dysfunction in childhood autism: a PET study. Positron emission tomography. *Am J Psychiatry* 157: 1988–93.

9

NEUROIMMUNOLOGY AND NEUROTRANSMITTERS IN AUTISM

Andrew W Zimmerman, Susan L Connors and Carlos A Pardo-Villamizar

Potential relationships between the immune system and neurotransmitters have been posited in autism as well as other neurological disorders. For example, in Sydenham's chorea antibodies form to the basal ganglia following streptococcal pharyngitis (Church et al. 2003); in Tourette syndrome antineuronal antibodies occur but have uncertain significance (Singer 2005); and in Rett syndrome systemic immune findings may occur in parallel to changes in the central nervous system (CNS) due to a known genetic cause (Fiumara et al. 1999). In autism, both immune factors and neurotransmitters are likely to participate in mechanisms of disease that do not alter the basic shape of the brain but can affect neurophysiology and brain function beginning in fetal life.

In this chapter we will review abnormalities of the immune system, several neurotransmitters and autonomic functions in autism. Recent findings of neuroinflammation in the brain and CSF from patients with autism suggest that innate immune dysfunction in the CNS may contribute to the pathogenesis of the autistic syndromes (Vargas et al. 2005). Prenatal overstimulation of the beta-2 adrenergic receptor, which occurs with stress and the use of tocolytics such as terbutaline, may contribute to the development of autism (Connors et al. 2005). In turn, disordered development of certain neurotransmitter systems may also contribute to neuroinflammation, possibly through abnormal cytokine signaling that is genetically determined.

IMMUNE ABNORMALITIES IN AUTISM

Although the neurobiological basis for the autism spectrum disorders (ASDs) remains poorly understood, several lines of research now support the view that genetic, environmental, neurological and immunological factors contribute to their development (Newschaffer et al. 2002). In particular, reports of differences in systemic immune findings over the past 30 years have led to speculation that autism may represent, *in some patients*, an immune mediated or autoimmune disorder (Licinio et al. 2002; Ashwood and Van de Water 2004). Recent reviews of immune dysfunction in autism have sought to understand these findings in the clinical context of the syndrome (Korvatska et al. 2002, Lipkin and Hornig 2003, Chez et al. 2004, Zimmerman 2005).

Abnormalities of both humoral and cellular immune functions have been described in small studies of children with autism (N = 10–36), and include decreased production of immunoglobulins or B- and T-cell dysfunction (Warren et al. 1986, 1990b). Early studies suggested that prenatal viral infections might damage the immature immune system and induce viral tolerance (Stubbs and Crawford 1977), while later studies showed altered T-cell subsets and activation, consistent with the possibility of an autoimmune pathogenesis (Warren et al. 1990b, Gupta et al. 1998). Odell et al. (2005) confirmed earlier reports of a 4-fold increase in the serum complement (C4B) null allele (i.e. no protein produced) in 85 children with autism, compared to controls. In most of these studies, phenotyping was limited to descriptions of the subjects as "autistic" based on criteria of the *Diagnostic and Statistical Manual* of the American Psychiatric Association. "Abnormal" immune findings occurred in 15–60% of children with autism. For some parameters, unaffected siblings showed intermediate values, and a background of such "abnormalities" was noted in normal controls as well. In all studies, measurements have been reported at single time points and among subjects of different ages. Since these differences in systemic immune findings in autism have not been followed in the same patients over time, it is not clear whether they reflect true immune dysfunction or may represent dysmaturation that changes with age.

Circulating autoantibodies directed against CNS antigens have been described in patients with autism, reacting to myelin basic protein (MBP; Singh et al. 1993, 1998), frontal cortex (Todd et al. 1988, Plioplys et al. 1989), cerebral endothelial cells (Connolly et al. 1999), and neuronal–axon filament protein (NAFP; Singh et al. 1997). Recently, Silva et al. (2004) found consistent serum reactivity to an epitope in human brain tissue by quantitative immunoblotting, which was similar (but not identical) to MBP, in children with autism and not other family members. Sera from autistic children also reacted more frequently to rat caudate nucleus, compared to cerebellum and hippocampus (Singh and Rivas 2004). However, such reactions were not replicated when autism sera were reacted against human brain tissue (Harvey Singer, personal communication 2005).

AUTOIMMUNITY AND AUTISM

The significance of autoantibodies in serum from patients with autism has been difficult to determine. Their presence might imply that autism is an autoimmune disorder. However, several criteria, including the necessity to demonstrate the autoimmune disease after passive transfer of antibodies into animals, would be necessary to establish the role of these autoantibodies as pathogenic effectors (Rose and Bona 1993), and this evidence is still lacking. Even though several antibodies in serum from subjects with autism have been demonstrated to react against human brain tissue, their pathogenicity has not been demonstrated in autism post-mortem brain tissue from individuals with autism.

Of equal interest to serum reactivity in children, however, have been studies in maternal sera. Warren et al. (1990a) demonstrated reactivity of mothers' sera to their autistic children's lymphocytes. Maternal serum has also been shown to cause antibody binding to fetal Purkinje cells when it was injected into pregnant mice (Dalton et al. 2003). Maternal antibodies may therefore be relevant to prenatal brain development (Vincent et al. 2003) by interfering with cell signaling in the developing brain, and possibly thereby disturbing normal patterns of CNS organization.

Autoimmune disorders, such as rheumatoid arthritis, lupus and thyroid disorders, have been found at increased rates in surveys of family members of children with autism, rather than in the children themselves, compared to controls. This was first observed in one family by Money et al. (1971), and subsequently in three clinical surveys (Comi et al. 1999, Sweeten et al. 2003; Cynthia Molloy, personal communication 2005). However, these associations were not found in another study after review of medical records (Micali et al. 2004). A recent study of mothers with autistic children reported an association with psoriasis but not other autoimmune disorders, and a two-fold increased risk of having an autistic child for those mothers with asthma and allergies during the second trimester (Croen et al. 2005). The meaning of these studies for autism is still not clear, but they suggest that maternal immunological effects might be important during gestation. They are also consistent with reported increases in frequencies of HLA-DR4 and related alleles in children with autism and their mothers (Burger and Warren 1998, Torres et al. 2002). HLA-DR4, a class II antigen, has been identified as one of the susceptibility markers for certain autoimmune diseases, such as rheumatoid arthritis, and is strongly associated with others such as hypothyroidism and autoimmune diabetes (Wordsworth et al. 1989, Levin et al. 2004).

INFECTIONS AND AUTISM

Infections have been associated with autism in small numbers of children, and include prenatal rubella (Chess 1977) and cytomegalovirus (Yamashita et al. 2003, Sweeten et al. 2004a), and postnatal herpes encephalitis (DeLong et al. 1981, Gillberg 1991). Given the variety of viruses and their pathogenic effects that can be associated with autism, the location of the pathology and the neural networks affected appear to be more important than the specific types of viruses. For example, reversible symptoms of autism have been reported with bilateral temporal lobe involvement in herpes simplex virus encephalitis (DeLong et al. 1981).

Autism rarely results from known infectious causes, and the immune abnormalities or variants described in autism studies have not been consistent with typical immune deficiency states that would predispose to such infections. Furthermore, there have been no documented increased rates of infection in children with autism (Comi et al. 1999). Although persistence of measles virus in the gastrointestinal tract and peripheral mononuclear cells has been reported in children with autism (Kawashima et al. 2000, Uhlmann et al. 2002), replication and further study of its possible relevance to autism in CSF and brain tissue are needed. Animal models of autism using prenatal infections (Patterson 2002) lend credence to the importance of gestational effects on fetal brain development, as is the association of maternal influenza and the increased risk of schizophrenia (Shi et al. 2003). Autistic behaviors also have been induced experimentally in a rat model using neonatal Borna disease virus (Pletnikov et al. 2002).

NEUROGLIAL ACTIVATION AND NEUROINFLAMMATION IN THE BRAIN

Although most studies in the peripheral immune system have found differences in autism that suggested possible immune involvement, neuroanatomical studies, until recently, have demonstrated few overt signs of immune effects in post-mortem brain tissue (Bailey et al. 1998, Kemper and Bauman 1998). In particular, no signs of previous or current infections have been documented, and only infrequent lymphocyte infiltration has been shown. Further, no astrocytic or microglial (i.e. neuroglial) activation has been noted using standard Nissl and other standard staining procedures.

Neuroglial cells such as astrocytes and microglia, along with perivascular macrophages and endothelial cells, play important roles in neuronal function and homeostasis (Aloisi 2001, Dong and Benveniste 2001, Neumann 2001, Prat et al. 2001). Both microglia and astroglia are fundamentally involved in cortical organization, neuro-axonal guidance and synaptic plasticity (Fields and Stevens-Graham 2002). Neuroglial cells contribute in a number of ways to the regulation of immune responses in the CNS. Astrocytes, for example, play an important role in the detoxification of excess excitatory amino acids (Nedergaard et al. 2002), maintenance of the integrity of the blood–brain barrier (Prat et al. 2001), and production of neurotrophic factors (Bauer et al. 2001). In normal homeostatic conditions, astrocytes facilitate neuronal survival by producing growth factors and mediating uptake/removal of excitotoxic neurotransmitters, such as glutamate, from the synaptic microenvironment (Nedergaard et al. 2002). However, during astroglial activation secondary to injury or in response to neuronal dysfunction, astrocytes can produce several factors that may modulate inflammatory responses; they secrete pro-inflammatory cytokines, chemokines and metalloproteinases that can magnify immune reactions within the CNS (Bauer et al. 2001, Benn et al. 2001, Rosenberg 2002). Similarly, microglial activation is an important factor in the neuroglial responses to injury or dysfunction. Microglia are involved in synaptic stripping, cortical plasticity and immune surveillance (Graeber et al. 1993, Aloisi 2001). Changes in astroglia and microglia can therefore produce marked neuronal and synaptic changes that are likely to contribute to CNS dysfunction observed in autism. Neuronal dysfunction and abnormalities in cortical organization may also be responsible for pathophysiological responses that may lead to neuroglial activation, reactions that may subsequently increase the magnitude of neuronal dysfunction.

Evidence of neuroglial activation, and a role for neuroimmune responses mediated by innate immunity in the neuropathology of autism, has recently been demonstrated by our laboratory (Vargas et al. 2005). Based on neuropathological analysis of post-mortem brain tissues from 11 autistic patients (age range 5–44 years), we have demonstrated the presence of an active and ongoing neuroinflammatory process in the cerebral cortex and white matter, and notably in the cerebellum. Immunocytochemical studies of brain tissues from these 11 autistic patients showed marked activation of microglia and astroglia as compared with controls. The neuroglial activation was particularly prominent in the granular cell layer and white matter of the cerebellum, a brain region well known by imaging studies to be abnormal in autism (Courchesne 1997, Allen et al. 2004). We also noted subsets of Purkinje cells with morphological changes consistent with degeneration.

Additional assessment of immune mediators such as cytokines and chemokines in the CNS tissues revealed increases in subsets of pro-inflammatory and anti-inflammatory mediators. Protein array profiling of cytokines indicated that MCP-1, a chemoattractant protein for monocytes and macrophages, and TGF-β1, a pleotropic anti-inflammatory cytokine mainly derived from activated neuroglia, were the most prevalent cytokines in brain tissues. Other cytokines such as IL-6, known for pro-inflammatory action, were also increased in some regions of the cortex such as the anterior cingulate gyrus.

Our studies also indicated that CSF from patients with autism following developmental regression (N=6), when compared with control subjects (N=9), had a unique pro-inflammatory profile of cytokines, including a marked increase in MCP-1 (12-fold increase), and IFN-γ (232-fold increase), findings that support the view that an active inflammatory process occurs in the brain of some autistic patients. Our findings also indicate that innate neuroimmune reactions are part of the pathological processes involved in autism and that immune responses are likely among the factors that produce CNS dysfunction in autism.

The previously noted evidence obtained from neuropathological studies strongly suggests that *innate* neuroimmune responses rather than *adaptive* immunity are part of the immunopathogenic mechanisms associated with autism. Despite the presence of autoantibodies against neural epitopes and abnormalities in cytokine profiles in the peripheral immune system, the only solid evidence shown in brain from subjects with autism up to the present is the activation of innate immune reactions mediated by neuroglial cells. Current anecdotal reports of clinical improvements after treatments that target mostly the *adaptive* immune system (such as prednisone and IVIG) are not supported by our findings of activation of the *innate* immune system. Further studies should focus on the potential presence of adaptive immune responses in earlier stages of the disorder and even during early phases of brain development.

IMMUNOGENETICS IN AUTISM

Some of the most promising findings linking the immune system to autism come from the study of the HLA genes, as noted above. HLA types are important genetic determinants of immune function within the major histocompatibility complex (MHC), and could reflect important antigenic differences between parents and their affected children. Other genetic loci associated with autoimmune and inflammatory disorders appear to cluster with those for autism (as well as those for Tourette syndrome), and suggest a genetic relationship that may result in immune dysregulation in these disorders (Becker et al. 2003). In the case of HLA genes, the association of specific antigens/alleles with autoimmunity suggests that autistic patients (with increased frequencies of HLA-DR4) may exhibit a similar pattern of association with autoimmune phenomena. However, it should be emphasized that autism does not meet criteria as an autoimmune disorder based on current evidence.

Immunogenetic host factors, such as genes for HLA, for cytokines and chemokines and their receptors, may influence the natural course of autism through their effects on the immune system. Allelic variations, or point mutations (single nucleotide polymorphisms, SNPs), in regulatory regions of cytokine genes, have been demonstrated to affect gene transcription or levels of cytokine expression, and to produce interindividual variation in cytokine production (Meenagh et al. 2002). These variations in cytokine expression may predispose toward, or confer resistance to, immune mediated disorders and may influence the strength and duration of the immune response. This theory has been supported by numerous reports of the association of some cytokine alleles and expression phenotypes with immune mediated or autoimmune disorders (Bidwell et al. 1999, 2001; Haukim et al. 2002). Likewise, similar findings of SNPs have been reported in CNS disorders. For example, a polymorphism of the *MCP-1* gene (A-2518G) is associated with an increased risk of HIV dementia (Gonzalez et al. 2002), early onset of Parkinson's disease (Nishimura et al. 2003), and increased resistance to antipsychotic therapy in schizrenia (Mundo et al. 2005). Diverse effects from a single SNP therefore may be found in different disorders. In the case of autism, such variables may be difficult to tease out due to its inherent clinical heterogeneity.

AUTONOMIC NERVOUS SYSTEM FUNCTION IN AUTISM

Differences in autonomic nervous system function have been noted in patients with autism, both by published research and anecdotal report. These include sleep disorders (discussed in Chapters 12 and 15) in up to 80% of children (Gillberg and Coleman 2000, Thirumalai et al. 2002), and gastrointestinal issues such as chronic constipation or diarrhea (Wakefield et al. 2000). Studies of the peripheral autonomic nervous system in autism have shown abnormal skin conductance responses (Van Engeland 1984), blunted autonomic arousal (heart rate and galvanic skin responses) to social stimuli (Palkovitz and Wiesenfeld 1980, Hirstein et al. 2001), and increased tonic electrodermal activity (Barry and James 1988). In addition, Murphy et al. (2000) found some improvements in patients with autistic behaviors and epilepsy from the use of a vagal nerve stimulator, though it is not clear how much of the improvements in behavior were due to better seizure control, or other factors. In our clinical experience, many parents of autistic patients also have reported abnormal autonomic symptoms in their children, such as urinary retention, cool clammy extremities, and sluggish pupillary responses to light.

Recently, Ming et al. (2005) have used a device called the Neuroscope® to measure cardiovascular tone in autistic children. They have shown low baseline cardiac parasympathetic activity, with evidence of elevated sympathetic tone in children with autism compared to controls, whether or not the patients had symptoms or signs of autonomic dysfunction. The cardiovascular parameters investigated reflect measures of brainstem function. Their findings implicate the sympathetic nervous system and catecholamines in the etiology of autism, and may be the basis for future clinical testing and diagnosis of children with this disorder, though more research is needed to expand the study to larger groups of children and to standardize Neuroscope® testing for normal healthy children in the general population. Because autism is a heterogeneous disorder, further investigations are also needed to correlate subgroups within the autism spectrum to clinical response categories that could be defined by Neuroscope® testing.

NEUROTRANSMITTER INVOLVEMENT IN AUTISM

Although several hypotheses have been proposed in attempts to link abnormalities in the peripheral immune system in autism to causation in the brain, none has been proven (Zimmerman 2005). It is more likely that the abnormal immune activation reported in brain and CSF of autistic subjects (Vargas et al. 2005) and circulating immune system differences develop in parallel, due to interference with one or more mechanisms affecting both systems in early prenatal development. Perturbations of neurotransmitters or their receptor signaling during fetal brain development may lead to a cascade of abnormalities that evolve over time, may affect the immune system within the brain as well as systemically, and would also affect autonomic functions throughout development and later life.

All neurotransmitter systems are important for normal fetal brain development and interact synchronously to produce normal maturation. An abnormality in any of the earliest appearing neurotransmitter systems, such as the catecholamines (Fig. 9.1), would impact the development of the other systems. For example, the beta-2 adrenergic receptor (B2AR), part of the catecholamine system, is expressed on nearly every cell type and is important for normal brain and tissue maturation (Slotkin et al. 1994, Wagner et al. 1995). Overstimulation of this receptor with a tocolytic beta-2 agonist drug, terbutaline, has been linked to concordance for autism spectrum disorders in a study of 37 sets of dizygotic twins, as have certain polymorphisms of the receptor's gene in the same study (Connors et al. 2005).

Support for the hypothesis that prenatal interference with beta-2 adrenergic receptor signaling may contribute to the development of autism can be found in animal studies. Treatment of pregnant rats with terbutaline results in offspring with many neuropathological changes in the brain that are analogous to differences seen in autism, such as decreased numbers of cerebellar Purkinje cells, small cells in the hippocampus, and increased expression of GFAP (Rhodes et al. 2003). Animal studies have also shown that overstimulation of the B2AR with terbutaline during the second and early third trimesters in rats results in postnatal B2AR signaling in brain and peripheral tissues of the offspring (measured by receptor function in membrane preparations) that is similar to that in fetal life (Slotkin et al. 2003). In these animal offspring, receptor signaling *sensitizes*, instead of *desensitizes*, to repeated ligand binding, and produces high cellular levels of second

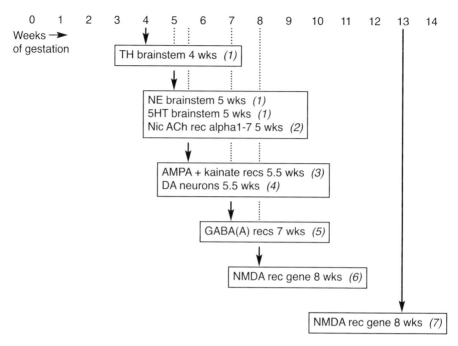

Fig. 9.1. Ontogeny of neurotransmitter systems in the human brain.

The diagram indicates the order of appearance of neurotransmitters during human embryonic brain development. Catecholamines are among the earliest appearing neurotransmitters, based on currently available data. In some studies, the age of the tissue in which the receptors were detected was the earliest examined (3, 5, 6).

Key: TH = tyrosine hydroxylase; NE = norepinephrine; 5HT: serotonin (5-hydroxytryptamine); Nic ACh rec alpha1-7 = nicotinic acetylcholine receptor alpha subunits 1–7; AMPA = α-amino-3-hydroxy-5-methyl-4-isoxazole propionic acid; kainite recs = kainite receptors; DA = dopamine; GABA = gamma-amino-butyric acid; NMDA = N-methyl-D-aspartate; M1/M2 = muscarinic acetylcholine receptors type 1and 2; nic recs = other nicotinic receptor subunits or functional receptors.

References: *(1)* Sundstrom et al. (1993), number (N) of specimens = 29; *(2)* Hellstrom-Lindahl et al. (1998), N=21; *(3)* Bardoul et al. (1998), N=8; *(4)* Verney et al. (2001), N=8; *(5)* Hebebrand et al. (1988), N=24; *(6)* Ritter et al. (2001), N=12; *(7)* Perry et al. (1986), N=15.

messengers such as cyclic AMP (cAMP) and protein kinase A (PKA). If this animal model proves analogous to autism, the resulting increased levels of second messengers that would be expected, as well as cell physiology reminiscent of fetal life, could contribute to the immune activation noted in brain of individuals with autism (discussed below) and to the circulating immune system differences reported in this disorder. For example, decreased natural killer cell activity in autism (Warren et al. 1987) could then theoretically be due to increased cAMP levels (Whalen and Bankhurst 1990); decreased production of interleukin-2 in stimulated immune cells in autism (Gupta et al. 1998) would hypothetically reflect fetal and very early infant physiology (Zola et al. 1998); and increased levels of immunoglobulin G1 in autism (Trajkovski et al. 2004) might be due to increased B2AR signaling, as in fetal life (Podojil and Sanders 2003).

Many of the cytokines reported by Vargas et al. (2005) as elevated in CSF and brain from autistic patients act as growth and differentiation factors during prenatal brain development (Meng et al. 1999, Dame and Juul 2000), and their increased expression may reflect a retained fetal pattern. HLA-DR expression, as well as reflecting microglial (immune) activation, may also be related to fetal life. HLA-DR antigen-positive microglia are present in human brain from the second trimester onward, and are thought to be involved in normal development (Wierzba-Bobrowicz et al. 2000a,b). The expression of HLA-DR molecules is also increased in glioblastoma cells in response to cAMP (Basta et al. 1989), one of the second messengers produced by increased B2AR signaling as occurs during fetal life. Microglia also may be more numerous in autistic brain, due to fetal levels of growth factors, such as basic fibroblast growth factor, whose transcription is increased by B2AR stimulation (Di Pucchio et al. 1996, Riva et al. 1998). There may be "incomplete" immune activation due to delays in the normal progression of cell programming for further inflammatory pathways. The rat model of prenatal B2AR overstimulation (Rhodes et al. 2003) may also be useful to demonstrate pathways by which astroglial activation arises and may persist beyond fetal brain development, because neuroinflammation has been observed in this model (AWZ, unpublished personal observations).

In this example of prenatal B2AR overstimulation, multiple downstream pathways for immune activation that involve other neurotransmitter systems could be triggered over the course of development. This may be especially true for the glutamate pathways; signaling through glutamate receptors is enhanced by the B2AR's second messengers, cAMP and PKA (Raman et al. 1996, Banke et al. 2000). Increased glutamate signaling, involving astrocytes and microglia, could lead to excitotoxicity in vulnerable tissues, and perhaps to developmental regression.

Abnormalities have been reported in every neurotransmitter system investigated in autism to date (see also Chapters 6 and 15). Several are summarized in Table 9.1. The catecholamine system has been implicated in the etiology of autism, in excess, as well as in deficiency in central and peripheral studies. Consideration of all these studies together may suggest dysregulation, which could be true if the system were severely delayed in development.

Other neurotransmitter systems may be involved in autism as well, either directly or indirectly as they interact with the catecholamine system. The earlier in prenatal development that one disordered neurotransmitter system starts to impact the process, the greater the number of signaling pathways, and the more patterns and numbers of receptor expression in other systems that will be affected. The effects would be brain region- and timing-specific, depending on the developmental period in which B2AR overstimulation occurred.

TABLE 9.1

Findings among several neurotransmitter systems reported in autism

System	Source	N	Abnormality	Reference
Catecholamine	CSF	25	Increased dopamine metabolite HVA compared to controls	Gillberg and Svennerholm (1987)
	Urine	156	Increased urinary dopamine metabolites (HVA and 3MT) compared to controls	Martineau et al. (1992)
	DNA multiplex families	37 families	Lower maternal DBH activity in multiplex autism families	Robinson et al. (2001)
	CSF	17	No significant difference between autism and controls in HVA levels	Narayan et al. (1993)
	Platelets, plasma, serum, urine	13	No significant difference between autism and controls in serum tyrosine*, or in urinary excretion of catecholamines	Croonenberghs et al. (2000)
	DNA	25	Missense mutation (L88F) all dopamine receptors, α1- and β-adrenergic receptors	Feng et al. (1998)
	Concordance in DZ twins after prenatal terbutaline	37 twin sets	Increased relative risk for concordance in ASDs in terbutaline exposed twins	Connors et al. (2005)
GABA	Post-mortem autism and control parietal and cerebellar cortices	5	Reduced levels of GAD 65 and 67 in autism compared to controls	Fatemi et al. (2002)
	Postmortem autism and control hippocampi	4	Reduced GABA(A) and BZ receptor binding in autism	Blatt et al. (2001)
	DNA	100	Abnormalities of chromosome 15q, including genes for 3 GABA(A) receptor subunits	Schroer et al. (1998)

continued ↗

TABLE 9.1
(continued)

System	Source	N	Abnormality	Reference
Acetylcholine	Post-mortem cerebral cortex, autism and controls	7	Decreased cortical M1 receptor binding; decreased $\alpha4\beta2$ nicotinic receptor binding cortex compared to controls	Perry et al. (2001)
	Post-mortem cerebellar cortex, autism and controls	8	Decreased cerebellar nicotinic $\alpha4\beta2$ receptors; increased cerebellar nicotinic $\alpha7$ receptors	Lee et al. (2002)
Nitric oxide	Plasma	29	Increased levels of metabolites of nitric oxide	Sweeten et al. (2004b)
	RBC	27	Increased nitric oxide levels in autism	Sogut et al. (2003)

*Tyrosine is a precursor for norepinephrine.
Abbreviations: HVA = homovanillic acid; 3MT = 3-methoxytryamine; DBH = dopamine beta-hydroxylase; ASD = autism spectrum disorder, GABA = gamma-aminobutyric acid; GAD = glutamic acid decarboxylase; BZ = benzodiazepine; M1 = muscarinic receptor type 1; RBC = red blood cell count.

The gamma-amino-butyric acid (GABA)-ergic system seems a likely candidate for involvement in the development of autism since it appears early in embryonic/fetal life, and its main function is one of inhibition, a deficiency of which may explain some clinical features of the disorder, such as epilepsy and anxiety reported in a proportion of autistic individuals. Several studies have reported abnormalities in this system in autism (Table 9.1). It is possible, however, that an earlier process, i.e. dysregulation of the catechol-amines, is responsible for the abnormal development of the GABA system during very early gestation. For example, low levels of the GAD enzymes and GABA(A)/BZ receptors documented in post-mortem brain from individuals with autism could reflect high levels of B2AR second messengers such as cAMP (Salero-Coca et al. 1995) correlating with our B2AR model, or they could result from delayed maturation, since GABA(A) subunit receptor expression tends to be varied, transient and regionally specific during brain development (Poulter et al. 1992). Additionally, in animal studies normal inhibitory functioning of GABA receptors in several areas of the brain has been shown to be dependent on the integrity of adrenergic signaling (Saitow et al. 2000, Ciranna et al. 2004).

Abnormalities have been reported in the cholinergic system in autism. These are summarized in Table 9.1. Although nicotinic receptors are early appearing in brain development (Fig. 9.1), and these findings may correlate with attentional problems and pain perception in autism and may be relevant to future therapeutic interventions, it is also possible that these receptor abnormalities are an effect of the mechanism(s) leading to autism, rather than their cause. For example, cortical muscarinic type 1 acetylcholine receptors increase from postnatal day 7 in rats (equivalent to the late second trimester in humans) until adulthood (Lee et al. 1990). Lower levels than controls would be expected if there were a maturational delay in autism, correlating with our hypothesis of prenatal B2AR overstimulation. The cerebellar increase in $\alpha7$ nicotinic receptor expression reported in autism may also reflect delayed maturation, as in our B2AR model, since these receptors are increased in this brain region at a postnatal period in rats (postnatal days 8–15) that is roughly equivalent to the third trimester in humans (Dominguez del Toro et al. 1997). Finally, $\alpha4$ nicotinic receptor expression is dependent (in the rat) on PKA, a B2AR second messenger (Nakayama et al. 1993).

Several studies have suggested a role for nitric oxide in the development of a number of neuropsychiatric disorders, including autism (Table 9.1). Nitric oxide, generated by nitric oxide synthase (NOS), serves as a neurotransmitter in brain and a signaling molecule in peripheral tissues. It is involved in a number of physiological functions, but is also a marker for oxidative stress, which can impair neuronal function and result in cell death. Metabolites and enzymes associated with oxidative stress have not yet been studied in CSF or brain tissue in autism. Nitric oxide is involved in a great number of pathways in many tissues including the brain and immune system, and, if abnormal, could certainly contribute to clinical symptoms seen in autism, such as regression, resulting from oxidative stress and neuronal dysfunction. Increased levels of nitric oxide metabolites could be expected from our B2AR model since B2A receptor stimulation activates NOS in many tissues, such as human umbilical vein endothelium and human platelets (Ferro et al. 1999, Queen et al. 2000), though not in *adult* rat microglia in vitro (Mori et al. 2002).

SUMMARY

Findings from research on the immune system in autism may have relevance to the development of neurotransmitter systems in the brain, such as we have demonstrated for the beta-2 adrenergic receptor. Disordered development of one important transmitter system may result in a failure of synchronous and orderly maturation of others, in the CNS as well as in other tissues such as the immune system. Single nucleotide polymorphisms in cytokines, chemokines and their receptors may also contribute to neuroimmune activation and downstream effects in an already disordered developing nervous system.

At this time there are no established clinical markers of immune dysfunction that are indicated for routine evaluation of patients with autism spectrum disorders. This may change as current research studies that include large (N>50) groups of well-defined subjects and controls begin to clarify differences in immune parameters, both in the peripheral immune system and CNS, during development. If further research confirms our findings related to neuroinflammation and changes in cytokines in the brain and CSF in autism, we would predict that such measures might become useful clinical markers that are relevant to the pathogenesis of autism and suggest possible avenues for meaningful treatments. However, it remains to be seen whether such changes in the CNS also might have reliably detectable systemic counterparts.

REFERENCES

Allen G, Muller RA, Courchesne E (2004) Cerebellar function in autism: functional magnetic resonance image activation during a simple motor task. *Biol Psychiatry* 56: 269–78.

Aloisi F (2001) Immune function of microglia. *Glia* 36: 165–79.

Ashwood P, Van de Water J (2004) Is autism an autoimmune disease? *Autoimmune Rev* 3: 557–62.

Bailey A, Luthert P, Dean A, Harding B, Janota I, Montgomery M, Rutter M, Lantos P (1998) A clinicopathological study of autism. *Brain* 121: 889–905.

Banke TG, Bowie D, Lee H-K, Huganir RL, Schousboe A, Traynelis SF (2000) Control of GluR1 AMPA receptor function by cAMP-dependent protein kinase. *J Neurosci* 20: 89–102.

Bardoul M, Levallois C, Konig N (1998) Functional AMPA/kainate receptors in human embryonic and foetal central nervous system. *J Chem Neuroanat* 14: 79–85.

Barry RJ, James AL (1988) Coding of stimulus parameters in autistic, retarded, and normal children: evidence for a two-factor theory of autism. *Int J Psychophysiol* 6: 139–49.

Basta PV, Moore TL, Yokota S, Ting JP (1989) A beta-adrenergic agonist modulates DR alpha gene transcription via enhanced cAMP levels in a glioblastoma multiforme line. *J Immunol* 142: 2895–2901.

Bauer J, Rauschka H, Lassmann H (2001) Inflammation in the nervous system: the human perspective. *Glia* 36: 235–43.

Becker KG, Freidlin B, Simon RM (2003) Comparative genomics of autism, Tourette syndrome and autoimmune/inflammatory disorders. Online: www.grc.nia.nih.gov/branches/rrb/dna/pubs/cgoatad.pdf.

Benn T, Halfpenny C, Scolding N (2001) Glial cells as targets for cytotoxic immune mediators. *Glia* 36: 200–11.

Bidwell JL, Wood NA, Morse HR, Olomolaiye OO, Keen LJ, Laundy GJ (1999) Human cytokine gene nucleotide sequence alignments: supplement 1. *Eur J Immunogenet* 26: 135–223.

Bidwell J, Keen L, Gallagher G, Kimberly R, Huizinga T, McDermott MF Oksenberg J, McNicholl J, Pociot F, Hardt C, D'Alfonso F (2001) Cytokine gene polymorphism in human disease: on-line databases, supplement 1. *Genes Immun* 2: 61–70.

Blatt GJ, Fitzgerald CM, Guptill JT, Booker AB, Kemper TL, Bauman ML (2001) Density and distribution of hippocampal neurotransmitter receptors in autism: an autoradiographic study. *J Autism Dev Disord* 31: 537–43.

Burger RA, Warren RP (1998) Possible immunogenetic basis for autism. *Ment Retard Dev Disabil Res Rev* 4: 137–41.

Chess S (1977) Follow-up report on autism in congenital rubella. *J Autism Child Schizophr* 7: 69–81.

Chez MG, Chin K, Hung PC (2004) Immunizations, immunology, and autism. *Semin Pediatr Neurol* 11: 214–7.

Church AJ, Dale RC, Cardoso F, Candler PM, Chapman MD, Allen ML, Klein NJ, Lees AJ, Giovannoni G (2003) CSF and serum immune parameters in Sydenham's chorea: evidence of an autoimmune syndrome? *J Neuroimmunol* 136: 149–53.

Ciranna L, Licata F, Li Volsi G, Santangelo F (2004) Alpha 2- and beta-adrenoceptors differentially modulate GABAA- and GABAB-mediated inhibition of red nucleus neuronal firing. *Exp Neurol* 185: 297–304.

Comi AM, Zimmerman AW, Frye VH, Law PA, Peeden JN (1999) Familial clustering of autoimmune disorders and evaluation of medical risk factors in autism. *J Child Neurol* 14: 388–94.

Connolly AM, Chez MG, Pestronk A, Arnold ST, Mehta S, Deuel RK (1999) Serum autoantibodies to brain in Landau-Kleffner variant, autism, and other neurologic disorders. *J Pediatr* 134: 607–13.

Connors SL, Crowell DE, Eberhart CG, Copeland J, Newschaffer CJ, Spence SJ, Zimmerman AW (2005) Beta-2 adrenergic receptor activation and genetic polymorphisms in autism: data from dizygotic twins. *J Child Neurol* 20: 876–84.

Courchesne E (1997) Brainstem, cerebellar and limbic neuroanatomical abnormalities in autism. *Curr Opin Neurobiol* 7: 269–78.

Croen LA, Grether JK, Yoshida CK, Odouli R, Van de Water J (2005) Maternal autoimmune diseases, asthma and allergies, and childhood autism spectrum disorders: a case–control study. *Arch Pediatr Adolesc Med* 159: 151–7.

Croonenberghs J, Delmeire L, Verkerk R, Lin AH, Meskal A, Neels H, Van der Planken M, Scharpe S, Deboutte D, Pison G, Maes M (2000) Peripheral markers of serotonergic and noradrenergic function in post-pubertal, caucasian males with autistic disorder. *Neuropsychopharmacology* 22: 275–83.

Dalton P, Deacon R, Blamire A, Pike M, McKinlay I, Stein J, Styles P, Vincent A (2003) Maternal neuronal antibodies associated with autism and a language disorder. *Ann Neurol* 53: 533–7.

Dame JB, Juul SE (2000) The distribution of receptors for the pro-inflammatory cytokines interleukin (IL)-6 and IL-8 in the developing human fetus. *Early Hum Dev* 58: 25–39.

DeLong GR, Bean SC, Brown FR (1981) Acquired reversible autistic syndrome in acute encephalopathic illness in children. *Arch Neurol* 38: 191–4.

Di Pucchio T, Ennas MG, Presta M, Lauro GM (1996) Basic fibroblast growth factor modulates in vitro differentiation of human fetal microglia. *Neuroreport* 7: 2813–7.

Dominguez del Toro E, Juiz JM, Smillie FL, Lindstrom J, Criado M (1997) Expression of alpha 7 neuronal nicotinic receptors during postnatal development of the rat cerebellum. *Brain Res Dev Brain Res* 98: 125–33.

Dong Y, Benveniste EN (2001) Immune function of astrocytes. *Glia* 36: 180–90.

Fatemi SH, Halt AR, Stary JM, Kanodia R, Schulz SC, Realmuto GR (2002) Glutamic acid decarboxylase 65 and 67 kDa proteins are reduced in autistic parietal and cerebellar cortices. *Biol Psychiatry* 52: 805–10.

Feng J, Sobell JL, Heston LL, Cook EH, Goldman D, Sommer SS (1998) Scanning of the dopamine D1 and D5 receptor genes by REF in neuropsychiatric patients reveals a novel missense change at a highly conserved amino acid. *Am J Med Genet* 81: 172–8.

Ferro A, Queen LR, Priest RM, Xu B, Ritter JM, Poston L, Ward JP (1999) Activation of nitric oxide synthase by beta 2-adrenoceptors in human umbilical vein endothelium in vitro. *Br J Pharmacol* 126: 1872–80.

Fields RD, Stevens-Graham B (2002) New insights into neuron–glia communication. *Science* 298: 556–62.

Fiumara A, Sciotto A, Barone R, D'Asero G, Munda S, Parano E, Pavone L (1999) Peripheral lymphocyte subsets and other immune aspects in Rett syndrome. *Pediatr Neurol* 21: 619–21.

Gillberg C (1991) Autistic syndrome with onset at age 31 years: herpes encephalitis as a possible model for childhood autism. *Dev Med Child Neurol* 33: 920–4.

Gillberg C, Coleman M (2000) *The Biology of the Autistic Syndromes, 3rd edn. Clinics in Developmental Medicine No. 153/154.* London: Mac Keith Press.

Gillberg C, Svennerholm L (1987) CSF monoamines in autistic syndromes and other pervasive developmental disorders of early childhood. *Brit J Psych* 151: 89–94.

Gonzalez E, Rovin BH, Sen L, Cooke G, Dhanda R, Mummidi S, Kulkarni H, Bamshad MJ, Telles V, Anderson SA, Walter EA, Stephan KT, Deucher M, Mangano A, Bologna R, Ahuja SS, Dolan MJ, Ahuja SK (2002) HIV-1 infection and AIDS dementia are influenced by a mutant MCP-1 allele linked to increased monocyte infiltration of tissues and MCP-1 levels. *Proc Natl Acad Sci USA* 99: 13795–800.

Graeber MB, Bise K, Mehraein P (1993) Synaptic stripping in the human facial nucleus. *Acta Neuropathol* 86: 179–81.

Gupta S, Aggarwal S, Rashanravan B, Lee T (1998) Th-1 and Th2-like cytokines in CD4+ and CD8+ cells in autism. *J Neuroimmunol* 85: 106–9.

Haukim N, Bidwell JL, Smith AJ, Keen LJ, Gallagher G, Kimberly R, Huizinga T, McDermott MF, Oksenberg J, McNicholl J, Pociot F, Hardt C, D'Alfonso F (2002) Cytokine gene polymorphism in human disease: on-line databases, supplement 2. *Genes Immun* 3: 313–30.

Hebebrand J, Hofmann D, Reichelt R, Schnarr S, Knapp M, Propping P, Fodisch HJ (1988) Early ontogeny of the central benzodiazepine receptor in human embryos and fetuses. *Life Sci* 43: 2127–36.

Hellstrom-Lindahl E, Gorbounova O, Seiger A, Mousavi M, Nordberg A (1998) Regional distribution of nicotinic receptors during prenatal development of human brain and spinal cord. *Dev Brain Res* 108: 147–60.

Hirstein W, Iversen P, Ramachandran VS (2001) Autonomic responses of autistic children to people and objects. *Proc R Soc Lond B Biol Sci* 268: 1883–8.

Kawashima H, Mori T, Kashiwagi Y, Takekuma K, Hoshika A, Wakefield A (2000) Detection and sequencing of measles virus from peripheral mononuclear cells from patients with inflammatory bowel disease and autism. *Dig Dis Sci* 45: 723–9.

Kemper TL, Bauman M (1998) Neuropathology of infantile autism. *J Neuropathol Exp Neurol* 57: 645–52.

Korvatska E, Van de Waters JW, Anders TF, Gershwin ME (2002) Genetic and immunologic considerations in autism. *Neurobiol Dis* 9: 107–25.

Lee M, Nicklaus KJ, Manning DR, Wolfe BB (1990) Ontogeny of cortical muscarinic receptor subtypes and muscarinic receptor-mediated responses in rat. *J Pharmacol Exp Ther* 252: 482–90.

Lee M, Martin-Ruiz C, Graham A, Court J, Jaros E, Perry R, Iversen P, Bauman M, Perry E (2002) Nicotinic receptor abnormalities in the cerebellar cortex in autism. *Brain* 125: 1483–95.

Levin L, Ban Y, Concepcion E, Davies TF, Greenberg DA, Tomer Y (2004) Analysis of HLA genes in families with autoimmune diabetes and thyroiditis. *Hum Immunol* 65: 640–7.

Licinio J, Alvarado I, Wong ML (2002) Autoimmunity in autism. *Mol Psychiatry* 7: 329.

Lipkin WI, Hornig M (2003) Microbiology and immunology of autism spectrum disorders. *Novartis Found Symp* 251: 129–43; discussion 144–8, 281–97.

Martineau J, Barthelemy C, Jouve J, Muh JP, Lelord G (1992) Monoamines (serotonin and catecholamines) and their derivatives in infantile autism; age related changes and drug effects. *Dev Med Child Neurol* 34: 593–603.

Meenagh A, Williams F, Ross OA, Patterson C, Gorodezky C, Hammond M, Leheny WA, Middleton D (2002) Frequency of cytokine polymorphisms in populations from western Europe, Africa, Asia, the Middle East and South America. *Hum Immunol* 63: 1055–61.

Meng SZ, Oka A, Takashima S (1999) Developmental expression of monocyte chemoattractant protein-1 in the human cerebellum and brainstem. *Brain Dev* 21: 30–5.

Micali N, Chakrabarti S, Fombonne E (2004) The broad autism phenotype: findings from an epidemiological survey. *Autism* 8: 21–37.

Ming X, Julu POO, Brimacombe M, Connor S, Daniels ML (2005) Reduced cardiac parasympathetic activity in children with autism. *Brain Dev* 27: 509–16.

Money J, Bobrow NA, Clarke FC (1971) Autism and autoimmune disease: a family study. *J Autism Child Schizophr* 1: 146–60.

Mori K, Ozaki E, Zhang B, Yang L, Yokoyama A, Takeda I, Maeda N, Sakanaka M, Tanaka J (2002) Effects of norepinephrine on rat cultured microglial cells that express alpha1, alpha2, beta1 and beta2 adrenergic receptors. *Neuropharmacology* 43: 1026–34.

Mundo E, Altamura AC, Vismara S, Zanardini R, Bignotti S, Randazzo R, Montresor C, Gennarelli M (2005) MCP-1 gene (SCYA2) and schizophrenia: a case-control association study. *Am J Med Genet B Neuropsychiatr Genet* 132: 1–4.

Murphy JV, Wheless JW, Schmoll CM (2000) Left vagal nerve stimulation in six patients with hypothalamic hamartomas. *Pediatr Neurol* 23: 167–8.

Nakayama H, Okuda H, Nakashima T (1993) Phosphorylation of rat brain nicotinic acetylcholine receptor by cAMP-dependent protein kinase in vitro. *Brain Res Mol Brain Res* 20: 171–7.

Narayan M, Srinath S, Anderson GM, Meundi DB (1993) Cerebrospinal fluid levels of homovanillic acid and 5-hydroxyindoleacetic acid in autism. *Biol Psychiatry* 33: 630–5.

Nedergaard M, Takano T, Hansen AJ (2002) Beyond the role of glutamate as a neurotransmitter. *Nat Rev Neurosci* 3: 748–55.

Neumann H (2001) Control of glial immune function by neurons. *Glia* 36: 191–9.

Newschaffer CJ, Fallin D, Lee NL (2002) Heritable and nonheritable risk factors for autism spectrum disorders. *Epidemiol Rev* 24: 137–53.

Nishimura M, Kuno S, Mizuta I, Ohta M, Maruyama H, Kaji R, Kawakami H (2003) Influence of monocyte chemoattractant protein 1 gene polymorphism on age at onset of sporadic Parkinson's disease. *Mov Disord* 18: 953–5.

Odell D, Maciulis A, Cutler A, Warren L, McMahon WM, Coon H, Stubbs G, Henley K, Torres A (2005) Confirmation of the association of the C4B null allelle in autism. *Hum Immunol* 66: 140–5.

Palkovitz RJ, Wiesenfeld AR (1980) Differential autonomic responses of autistic and normal children. *J Autism Dev Disord* 10: 347–60.

Patterson PH (2002) Maternal infection: window on neuroimmune interactions in fetal brain development and mental illness. *Curr Opin Neurobiol* 12: 115–8.

Perry EK, Smith CJ, Atack JR, Candy JM, Johnson M, Perry RH (1986) Neocortical cholinergic enzyme and receptor activities in the human fetal brain. *J Neurochem* 47: 1262–9.

Perry EK, Lee ML, Martin-Ruiz CM, Court JA, Volsen SG, Merrit J, Folly E, Iversen PE, Bauman ML, Perry RH, Wenk GL (2001) Cholinergic activity in autism: abnormalities in the cerebral cortex and basal forebrain. *Am J Psychiatry* 158: 1058–66.

Pletnikov MV, Moran TH, Carbone KM (2002) Borna disease virus infection of the neonatal rat: developmental brain injury model of autism spectrum disorders. *Front Biosci* 7: d593–607.

Plioplys AV, Greaves A, Yoshida W (1989) Anti-CNS antibodies in childhood neurologic diseases. *Neuropediatrics* 20: 93–102.

Podojil JR, Sanders VM (2003) Selective regulation of mature IgG1 transcription by CD86 and beta 2-adrenergic receptor stimulation. *J Immunol* 170: 5143–51.

Poulter MO, Barker JL, O'Carroll AM, Lolait SJ, Mahan LC (1992) Differential and transient expression of GABAA receptor alpha-subunit mRNAs in the developing rat CNS. *J Neurosci* 12: 2888–900.

Prat A, Biernacki K, Wosik K, Antel JP (2001) Glial cell influence on the human blood–brain barrier. *Glia* 36: 145–55.

Queen LR, Xu B, Horinouchi K , Fisher I, Ferro A (2000) Beta(2)-adrenoceptors activate nitric oxide synthase in human platelets. *Circ Res* 87: 39–44.

Raman IM, Tong G, Jahr CE (1996) Beta-adrenergic regulation of synaptic NMDA receptors by cAMP-dependent protein kinase. *Neuron* 16: 415–21.

Rhodes MC, Seidler FJ, Abdel-Rahman A, Tate CA, Nyska A, Rincavage HL, Slotkin TA (2003) Terbutaline is a developmental neurotoxicant: effects on neuroproteins and morphology in cerebellum, hippocampus, and somatosensory cortex. *Pharmacol Exp Ther* 308: 529–37.

Ritter LM, Unis AS, Meador-Woodruff JH (2001) Ontogeny of ionotropic glutamate receptor expression in human fetal brain. *Brain Res Dev Brain Res* 127: 123–33.

Riva MA, Molteni R, Racagni G (1998) Differential regulation of FGF-2 and FGFR-1 in rat cortical astrocytes by dexamethasone and isoproterenol. *Brain Res Mol Brain Res* 57: 38–45.

Robinson PD, Schutz CK, Macciardi F, White BN, Holden JJA (2001) Genetically determined low maternal serum dopamine ≤-hydroxylase levels and the etiology of autism spectrum disorders. *Am J Med Genet* 100: 30–6.

Rose NR, Bona C (1993) Defining criteria for autoimmune diseases (Witebsky's postulates revisited). *Immunol Today* 14: 426–30.

Rosenberg GA (2002) Matrix metalloproteinases in neuroinflammation. *Glia* 39: 279–91.

Saitow F, Satake S, Yamada J, Konishi S (2000) _-adrenergic receptor-mediated presynaptic facilitation of inhibitory GABAergic transmission at cerebellar interneuron-Purkinje cell synapses. J Neurophysiol 84: 2016-2025.

Saitow F, Suzuki H, Konishi S (2005) β-adrenoceptor-mediated long-term upregulation of the release machinery at rat cerebellar GABAergic synapse. *J Physiol* 565: 487–502.

Salero-Coca E, Vergara P, Segovia J (1995) Intracellular increases of cAMP induce opposite effects in glutamic acid decarboxylase (GAD 67) distribution and glial fibrillary acidic protein immunoreactivities in C6 cells. *Neurosci Lett* 191: 9–12.

Schroer RJ, Phelan MC, Michaelis RC, Crawford EC, Skinner SA, Cuccaro M, Simensen RJ, Bishop J, Skinner C, Fender D, Steveson RE (1998) Autism and maternally derived aberrations of chromosome 15q. *Am J Med Genet* 76: 327–36.

Shi L, Fatemi SH, Sidwell RW, Patterson PH (2003) Maternal influenza infection causes marked behavioral and pharmacological changes in the offspring. *J Neurosci* 23: 297–302.

Silva SC, Correia C, Fesel C, Barreto M, Coutinho AM, Marques C, Miguel TS, Ataide A, Bento C, Borges L, Oliveira G, Vicente AM (2004) Autoantibody repertoires to brain tissue in autism nuclear families. *J Neuroimmunol* 152: 176–82.

Singer HS (2005) Tourette's syndrome: from behaviour to biology. *Lancet Neurol* 4: 149–59.

Singh VK, Rivas WH (2004) Prevalence of serum antibodies to caudate nucleus in autistic children. *Neurosci Lett* 355: 53–6.

Singh VK, Warren RP, Odell JD, Warren WL, Cole P (1993) Antibodies to myelin basic protein in children with autistic behavior. *Brain Behav Immun* 7: 97–103.

Singh VK, Warren R, Averett R, Ghaziuddin M (1997) Circulating autoantibodies to neuronal and glial filament proteins in autism. *Pediatr Neurol* 17: 88–90.

Singh VK, Lin SX, Yang VC (1998) Serological association of measles virus and human herpesvirus-6 with brain autoantibodies in autism. *Clin Immunol Immunopathol* 89: 105–8.

Slotkin TA, Lau C, Seidler FJ (1994) Beta-adrenergic overexpression in the fetal rat: distribution, receptor subtypes, and coupling to adenylate cyclase activity via G-proteins. *Toxicol Appl Pharmacol* 129: 223–34.

Slotkin TA, Auman JT, Seidler FJ (2003) Ontogenesis of beta-adrenoceptor signaling: implications for perinatal physiology and for fetal effects of tocolytic drugs. *J Pharmacol Exp Ther* 306: 1–7.

Sogut S, Zoroglu SS, Ozyurt H, Yilmaz HR, Ozugurlu F, Sivasli E, Yetkin O, Yanik M, Tutkun H, Savas HA, Tarakcioglu M, Akyol O (2003) Changes in nitric oxide levels and antioxidant enzyme activities may have a role in the pathophysiological mechanisms involved in autism. *Clin Chim Acta* 331: 111–7.

Stubbs EG, Crawford ML (1977) Depressed lymphocyte responsiveness in autistic children. *J Autism Child Schizophr* 7: 49–55.

Sundstrom E, Kolare S, Souverbie F, Samuelsson E-B, Pschera H, Lunell N-O, Seiger A (1993) Neurochemical differentiation of human bulbospinal monoaminergic neurons during the first trimester. *Dev Brain Res* 75: 1–12.

Sweeten TL, Bowyer SL, Posey DJ, Halberstadt GM, McDougle CJ (2003) Increased prevalence of familial autoimmunity in probands with pervasive developmental disorders. *Pediatrics* 112: e420.

Sweeten TL, Posey DJ, McDougle CJ (2004a) Brief report: autistic disorder in three children with cytomegalovirus infection. *J Autism Dev Disord* 34: 583–6.

Sweeten TL, Posey DJ, Shankar S, McDougle CJ (2004b) High nitric oxide production in autistic disorder: a possible role for interferon-gamma. *Biol Psychiatry* 55: 434–7.

Thirumalai SS, Shubin RA, Robinson R (2002) Rapid eye movement sleep behavior disorder in children with autism. *J Child Neurol* 17: 173–8.

Todd RD, Hickok JM, Anderson GM, Cohen DJ (1988) Antibrain antibodies in infantile autism. *Biol Psychiatry* 23: 644–7.

Torres AR, Maciulis A, Stubbs EG, Cutler A, Odell D (2002) The transmission disequilibrium test suggests that HLA-DR4 and DR13 are linked to autism spectrum disorder. *Hum Immunol* 63: 311–6.

Trajkovski V, Ajdinski L, Spiroski M (2004) Plasma concentration of immunoglobulin classes and subclasses in children with autism in the Republic of Macedonia: retrospective study. *Croat Med J* 45: 746–9.

Uhlmann V, Martin CM, Sheils O, Pilkington L, Silva I, Killalea A, Murch SB, Walker-Smith J, Thomson M, Wakefield AJ, O'Leary JJ (2002) Potential viral pathogenic mechanism for new variant inflammatory bowel disease. *Mol Pathol* 55: 84–90.

Van Engeland H (1984) The electrodermal orienting response to auditive stimuli in autistic children, normal children, mentally retarded children, and child psychiatric patients. *J Autism Dev Disord* 14: 261–79.

Vargas DL, Nascimbene C, Krishnan C, Zimmerman AW, Pardo CA (2005) Neuroglial activation and neuroinflammation in the brain of patients with autism. *Ann Neurol* 57: 67–81.

Verney C, Zecevic N, Ezan P (2001) Expression of calbindin D28K in the dopaminergic meso-telencephalic system in embryonic and fetal human brain. *J Comp Neurol* 429: 45–58.

Vincent A, Dalton P, Clover L, Palace J, Lang B (2003) Antibodies to neuronal targets in neurological and psychiatric diseases. *Ann NY Acad Sci* 992: 48–55.

Wagner JP, Seidler FJ, Slotkin TA (1995) Role of presynaptic input in the ontogeny of adrenergic cell signaling in rat brain: beta receptors, adenylate cyclase and c-fos protooncogene expression. *J Pharmacol Exp Ther* 273: 415–26.

Wakefield AJ, Anthony A, Murch SH, Thomson M, Montgomery SM, Davies S, O'Leary JJ, Berelowitz M, Walker-Smith JA (2000) Enterocolitis in children with developmental disorders.

Am J Gastroenterol 95: 2285–95.

Warren RP, Margaretten NC, Pace NC, Foster A (1986) Immune abnormalities in patients with autism. *J Autism Dev Disord* 16: 189–97.

Warren RP, Foster A, Margaretten NC (1987) Reduced natural killer cell activity in autism. *J Am Acad Child Adolesc Psychiatry* 26: 333–5.

Warren RP, Cole P, Odell JD, Pingree CB, Warren WL, White E, Yonk J, Singh VK (1990a) Detection of maternal antibodies in infantile autism. *J Am Acad Child Adolesc Psychiatry* 29: 873–7.

Warren RP, Yonk LJ, Burger RA, Cole P, Odell JD, Warren WL, White E, Singh VK (1990b) Deficiency of suppressor-inducer (CD4+CD45RA+) T cells in autism. *Immunol Invest* 19: 245–51.

Whalen MM, Bankhurst AD (1990) Effects of beta-adrenergic receptor activation, cholera toxin and forskolin on human natural killer cell function. *Biochem J* 272: 327–31.

Wierzba-Bobrowicz T, Kosno-Kruszewska E, Gwiazda E, Lechowicz W (2000a) Major histo-compatability complex class II (MHC II) expression during the development of human fetal cerebral occipital lobe, cerebellum, and hematopoietic organs. *Folia Neuropathol* 38: 111–8.

Wierzba-Bobrowicz T, Schmidt-Sidor B, Gwiazda E, Lechowicz W, Kosno-Kruszewska E (2000b) Major histocompatibility complex class II expression in the frontal and temporal lobes in the human fetus during development. *Folia Neuropathol* 38: 73–7.

Wordsworth BP, Lanchbury JS, Sakkas LI, Welsh KI, Panayi GS, Bell JI (1989) HLA-DR4 sub-type frequencies in rheumatoid arthritis indicate that DRB1 is the major susceptibility locus within the HLA class II region. *Proc Natl Acad Sci USA* 86: 10049–53.

Yamashita Y, Fujimoto C, Nakajima E, Isagai T, Matsuishi T (2003) Possible association between congenital cytomegalovirus infection and autistic disorder. *J Autism Dev Disord* 33: 455–9.

Zimmerman AW (2005) The immune system. In: Bauman ML, Kemper TL, eds. *The Neurobiology of Autism, 2nd edn.* Baltimore: Johns Hopkins University Press, pp. 371–86.

Zola H, Ridings J, Elliott S, Nobbs S, Weedon H, Wheatland L, Haslam R, Robertson D, Macardle PJ (1998) Interleukin 2 receptor regulation and IL-2 function in the human infant. *Hum Immunol* 59: 615–24.

10
ELECTROPHYSIOLOGY AND EPILEPSY IN AUTISM

Kent R Kelley and Solomon L Moshé

Contemporary electrophysiologic tools contribute a great deal to investigations of the pathophysiology of autism. It was a third of a century ago that awareness of the increased prevalence of epilepsy in autism provided persuasive evidence that an abnormal brain rather than an inadequately nurturing environment causes autism in young children. Vexing uncertainty remains about the relationship of epilepsy to autism. Is autism in some children a consequence of some particularly malignant forms of epilepsy? Do subclinical epileptiform discharges in the EEG in the absence of clinical seizures play a role in the maintenance or the development of autism; in other words, are they causal? Or are autism, epilepsy and epileptiform discharges but the consequences of damage or dysfunction in the brain caused by a subset of their etiologies? Even more vexing questions are what role, if any, epilepsy plays in the toddler whose language regresses and who becomes autistic, or in the older child who becomes demented, mute, and autistic without evidence of a degenerative disease of the brain. Not one of these questions has been answered satisfactorily to date, which means that there is little or no empirical evidence to guide treatment decisions, especially in the absence of overt seizures. The heterogeneous nature of autism and of epilepsy has hindered research in this area. Most available clinical studies are weakened by the small number of children studied, their clinical heterogeneity, the frequent lack of controls, and the lack of specificity of the techniques used to study them.

We start this chapter with a brief review of the contributions of neurophysiologic tools to clinical diagnosis in autism and to the understanding of its pathophysiology, especially regarding auditory and language function. We then discuss at greater length the thorny questions just raised about EEG abnormalities and epilepsy in autism.

AUDIOLOGY AND EVOKED POTENTIAL STUDIES
BRAINSTEM AUDITORY EVOKED POTENTIAL STUDIES
The committee on Infant Hearing of the American Speech–Language–Hearing Association recommends that all children with developmental delays, especially in the domains of social and language development, have a formal audiologic hearing evaluation (ASHA

1991). The Autism Practice Parameter guideline of the American Academy of Neurology and the Child Neurology Society recommends prompt referral for formal audiologic evaluation, including behavioral audiologic measures, assessment of middle ear function, and electrophysiological testing in children who do not speak fluently (Filipek et al. 2000). In addition to the peripheral hearing disorders that are seen in a small minority of children with autism (Jure et al. 1991), a series of studies using brainstem auditory evoked responses (BAERs) in the 1970s and 1980s suggested that symptoms of early infantile autism might result from abnormalities in processing sensory input at the level of the brainstem, or that some children with autism might have central processing deficits in addition to peripheral hearing losses (Taylor et al. 1982). Results, however, were variable and inconsistent (Rosenblum et al. 1980, Garreau et al. 1984, Klin 1993).

COGNITIVE POTENTIALS

A number of studies of auditory event related potentials (ERPs) support the hypothesis that auditory language processing is aberrant in children with autism (Klin 1993, Klein et al. 1995, Dunn and Bates 2005). The N1c is a component of the obligatory auditory ERP and measures function of the lateral surface of the superior temporal gyrus. In some 4- to 8-year-old children with autism, in response to pure tones or words, the amplitude of the N1c is diminished and its latency prolonged (Bruneau et al. 1999). A more robust age-specific effect was identified with measurements of N1c amplitudes in response to the intensity of the stimulus. In normal children, increasing the intensity of the stimulus increases the N1c amplitude, more over the left temporal gyrus than the right. In 4- to 8-year-old children with autism this expected increase in amplitude does not occur on the left side, resulting in a larger N1c on the right. This is the opposite of what is observed in normal children (Bruneau et al. 2003). Dunn et al. (1999) suggested that the lack of intensity effect, in combination with N1 prolongation, may reflect slower processing of linguistic stimuli in children with autism (mean age 8–10 years) due to differing maturational rates and time-to-maturity of subcomponents of the ERP. Recently, Dunn and Bates (2005) found that the latency of the early N1c in response to in-category words is age specific. It was prolonged in 8- and 9-year-old children with autism, but not in the 11–12 years age group. They concluded that the speed of early cortical processing of auditory verbal stimuli improves with age in autism and that the "aberrant contextual processing of words is not an immediate consequence of slowed early cortical auditory processing". They then studied the response to in- and out-of-category words as determined by the amplitude of the N4 component. In normal children, it is enhanced with out-of-category words. In the 8- and 9-year-old children with autism, the N4 was not affected by in- versus out-of-category words, while in the 11-year-olds there was a significant attenuation of the N4 to all stimuli, "as if all words were expected." Based on these data, Dunn and Bates suggest that the persistence of abnormalities in N4 in response to context-dependent words identifies specific abnormalities in cognition in autism that "may in turn implicate categorical organization within the lexicon".

Magnetoencephalography (MEG)

MEG provides a means for evaluating neural responses from the primary auditory cortex (Heschl's gyrus) of each hemisphere independently. Because of the horizontal orientation of Heschl's gyrus, scalp recorded auditory ERPs project to the vertex, which makes it very difficult to distinguish the ERPs of the two cerebral hemispheres. The magnetic analog of the electric N1, the M100 (or N1m) detected by MEG, is primarily sensitive to sulcal neural activity and is generated mainly in supratemporal cortical fields, with a source that localizes it to auditory cortex. Comparison of M100 frequency dependence in children with autism and normal controls indicates that children with autism have a much reduced range of modulation in right hemisphere sites (Gage et al. 2003). These M100 findings indicate that frequency encoding mechanisms may follow a different maturational path in children with autism than in controls; they also suggest that hemispheric asymmetries and different rates of maturation may be critical to the disordered auditory processing of some children with autism and may account for their inadequate decoding of the phonology of speech (Rapin and Dunn 2003, Tager-Flusberg and Joseph 2003). Combined ERP and MEG results therefore suggest that there are developmental electrophysiologic abnormalities related to abnormal brain maturation in the processing of words and simple nonverbal auditory stimuli that may account for some of the subtypes of language disorders in children with autism.

Coherence Studies

Central coherence has been defined as "the everyday tendency to process incoming information in its context – that is pulling information together for higher level meaning, often at the expense of memory of detail" (Brock et al. 2002). Frith (1989) proposed a theory of weak central coherence in autism characterized by an unusual tendency toward piecemeal rather than configurational processing, and a reduction in the normal tendency to process information in context, i.e. autistic children perceive the details but not the bigger picture. The hypothesis is that the mechanisms that give rise to "weak central coherence" effects may be perceptual; failure to utilize context in language processing results from a reduction in the integration of specialized local neural networks due to a deficit in the temporal binding reflected in the high frequency 30–100 Hz gamma brain activity. Lack of central coherence might also mean that individuals with autism fail to integrate information about the environment presented to the brain via the different sensory modalities.

Brock et al. (2002) have suggested that temporal binding deficits, i.e. the failure of integration between different brain regions leading to difficulties in integration of information into hierarchies, might contribute to executive dysfunction in autism, and to some of the deficits in socialization and communication. The temporal binding hypothesis assumes that local networks are not temporally correlated and that each of the local networks processes information in relative isolation. The hypothesis is potentially testable by assessing EEG coherence and measuring late auditory or visual ERPs; this work is just emerging (Kutas and Federmeir 2000, Braeutigam et al. 2001, Townsend et al. 2001, Dunn and Bates 2005).

DEFINITIONS AND CLINICAL STUDIES OF EPILEPSY IN AUTISM
DEFINITIONS
Hughlings Jackson defined a seizure as the result of occasional, excessive, and disorderly discharge of gray matter (see Klass and Daly 1979). Clinically, seizures are defined as paroxysmal, stereotyped, relatively brief interruptions of ongoing behavior, associated with electrographic seizure patterns. *Non-convulsive "subclinical" seizures* refer to EEG abnormalities, seemingly ictal electrographic patterns, without clinically recognizable cognitive, behavioral or motor functions or apparent impairment of consciousness. The proper classification of a seizure as subclinical requires a concurrent EEG, close observation, and behavioral and cognitive testing. *Interictal epileptiform activity* is paroxysmal electrographic activity containing spikes or sharp waves that interrupts the background. Typical epileptiform activities include spike discharges (defined as lasting less than 70 milliseconds) and sharp discharges (70–200 ms) that are followed by an after-going slow wave. The term *autistic epileptic regression* has been used to define children with autism, a history of regression and epilepsy. The term *autistic regression with an epileptiform EEG* is used to describe those children with autism but without epilepsy who have an epileptiform EEG.

PREVALENCE OF EPILEPSY IN AUTISM
Epilepsy is common in children and adults with autism, but to determine its prevalence with any precision is difficult. Part of this difficulty has to do with the variability in the definitions of epilepsy adopted by different investigators; a probably much larger part stems from various investigators' definitions of autism, depending on whether they included only classic autistic disorder – the more severely affected end of the autism spectrum – or the entire spectrum. Epilepsy is more prevalent in children with autism combined with cerebral palsy (27%) and cerebral palsy plus severe mental retardation (67%) than in those without (Tuchman et al. 1991b). Although approximately 1 in 4 children aged 6–13 years with epilepsy and mental retardation have autism (Riikonen and Amnell 1981), this association and the relationship of epileptiform activity to autism raise many questions.

Age is another variable that influences prevalence estimates of epilepsy in autism. Prevalence peaks in early childhood and again in adolescence (Olsson et al. 1988, Volkmar and Nelson 1990, McDermott et al. 2005). The incidence of epilepsy increases with age in children with idiopathic autism: quoted as 24% in a group of children of mean age 12 years (Rossi et al. 1995), it rose to 38% in a group of teens (mean age 17 years) (Rossi et al. 2000). The cumulative risk of epilepsy in adults with autism is estimated at 20–35% (Tuchman et al. 1991b). In children with idiopathic autism without associated disabilities and without a family history of epilepsy or other risk factors for epilepsy, the prevalence of epilepsy is as low as 6%, but still much higher than in the general population (Tuchman et al. 1991b). A recent prospective follow-up study of 120 adults with autism diagnosed in childhood in Göteborg found that 38% had had epilepsy at some time and 16% were in remission (Danielsson et al. 2005).

Seizure types associated with autism depend on age and etiology; all seizure types have been reported (Steffenburg et al. 1991, Tuchman et al. 1991b). It should be noted that children with autism have many seizure-like behaviors that are not epileptic, and video-EEG is recommended to confirm that these behaviors are indeed epileptic (see Chapter 11 for further discussion of this issue).

EPILEPTIC SYNDROMES ASSOCIATED WITH AUTISM

The term *epileptic encephalopathy* describes a clinically defined disorder of cerebral function characterized by an age dependency, typical seizure types and EEG abnormalities, and failure or loss of cognition with associated neuropsychiatric disturbances, without necessarily implying that the epilepsy is causative. Epileptic encephalopathies can result from various structural, metabolic and genetic etiologies. The International League Against Epilepsy has defined an epileptic encephalopathy as "a condition in which the epileptiform abnormalities themselves are believed to contribute to the progressive disturbance in cerebral function" (Engel 2001). This definition is debatable because the core question of cause and effect remains unresolved, that is, are the developmental and behavioral problems, seizures and EEG abnormalities all secondary to the underlying brain dysfunction, or are the epileptiform activity and seizures primary or contributory to the other deficits, which would mean that the natural history may be modifiable by treatment? Furthermore, there is the critical question of the effects of age of onset and the duration of the epileptic encephalopathy on neurodevelopment and the appearance of autistic features. These issues, and the debated question of whether epileptiform activity, whether it is interictal or recorded in the EEG of some children who have no clinical seizures, may of itself be responsible for the encephalopathy, are discussed in greater detail in Chapter 11.

West syndrome (infantile spasms) is paradigmatic of an epileptic encephalopathy that occurs in infancy. West syndrome is characterized by a unique high-voltage, multifocal and chaotic EEG pattern – hypsarrhythmia, a unique seizure type – infantile spasms that occur in clusters, and profound neurodevelopmental problems. West syndrome has a variety of structural and metabolic causes and is common in tuberous sclerosis. The onset of hypsarrhythmia and spasms is frequently associated with neurodevelopmental regression, thus implicating a role of the epileptic process in this regression. Indeed, there is a small group of infants without demonstrable etiology, in whom the onset of spasms and hypsarrhythmia is temporally associated with developmental regression, who, if promptly and successfully treated, go on to have normal development and subsequent recovery with resolution of seizures and normalization of EEG (Kivity et al. 2004).

Landau–Kleffner syndrome (LKS) or acquired epileptic aphasia is another age

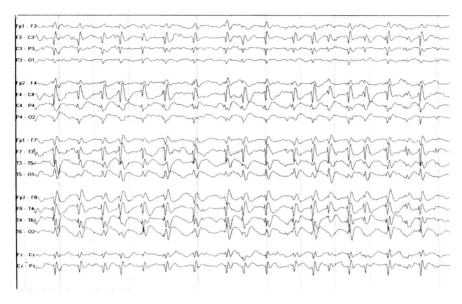

Fig. 10.1. EEG of 6-year-old boy with continuous bisynchronous spike and wave discharges in slow sleep. Longitudinal bipolar montage, 30 mm/s, sensitivity 30 mV/mm.

dependent epileptic encephalopathy that occurs typically in mid-childhood. LKS is characterized by an epileptiform EEG, rare seizures, and an acquired aphasia – predominantly receptive – which leads to secondary impairment of expressive language. There may be associated behavioral disturbances, especially frustration, unless the child learns to use the visual modality to communicate. The EEG abnormalities include mid-temporal, temporo-parietal (perisylvian) spikes, sharps and slow waves – typically bilateral and independent (Tuchman and Rapin 2002) – and generalized spike-waves, initially at 3–4 Hz with later slowing to 1.5–3 Hz (Niedermeyer 1999). Spikes are characteristically increased in drowsiness and sleep, often to a degree that meets the criteria of continuous spike-wave of slow sleep (CSWS; see below). Seizures are usually easy to treat with standard antiepileptic drugs. The epileptiform changes, along with the clinical seizures if any, resolve spontaneously before or during adolescence. Children with LKS do not have an identifiable etiology, although MRI volumetric analysis in 4 children with typical LKS disclosed volume reduction in superior temporal areas bilaterally, areas that are concerned with receptive language processing (Takeoka et al. 2004).

Continuous spikes and waves during slow sleep (CSWS), also known as *electrographic status epilepticus of sleep (ESES)*, is a third example of an epileptic encephalopathy often associated with autism. CSWS is a transitory (months to years), age dependent syndrome of childhood (onset 1–10 years, peak 4–5 years) characterized by spike and wave discharges predominantly in non-REM sleep (Fig. 10.1), mixed seizure types, and associated

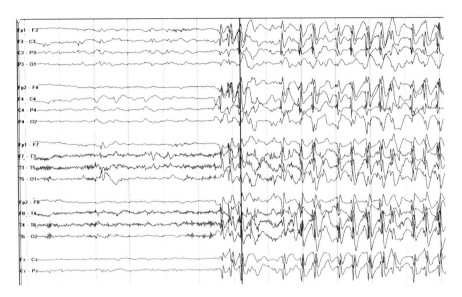

Fig. 10.2. EEG of the same boy as in Figure 10.1, recorded during a cluster of clinical negative myoclonus and cognitive regression. Longitudinal bipolar montage, 30 mm/s, sensitivity 20 mV/mm.

neurodevelopmental and behavioral disorders. There is often global deterioration of language (especially expressive), temporal and spatial disorientation, short term memory problems, and cognitive and behavioral changes, including dementia (Rousselle and Revol 1995, McVicar and Shinnar 2004). Behavioral disturbances are present in almost all the children and include decreased attention, hyperactivity, aggressiveness, difficulty in interpersonal interactions, and psychosis in 5% (Rousselle and Revol 1995), abnormalities that are analogous to those in children with autistic disorder (Ballaban-Gil and Tuchman 2000), in which case it fulfills criteria for disintegrative disorder. In addition, stereotypies, hyperorality, pain insensitivity, self-mutilation, echolalia and echopraxia have been noted (for a review, see Galanopoulou et al. 2000). Seizure types include partial or generalized seizures, and, at the time of neuropsychological deterioration, there may be an increase and change in seizure types to atypical absence and seizures with falls (negative myoclonus, Fig. 10.2), but not tonic seizures. The EEG typically shows focal or multifocal spikes and slow spikes while awake. As the child falls asleep, there is a marked activation consisting of continuous, diffuse, bilateral, usually slow spike-waves (1.5–2 Hz), which appear throughout all slow sleep stages and interrupt the normal cycling of sleep stages. It has been suggested, however, that the persistence of spike-wave activity during REM sleep in LKS distinguishes LKS from CSWS (Genton et al. 1990). The epileptiform activity is generally bilateral and symmetrical, but may be asymmetrical in children with structural lesions and during transitions in sleep stages. More than a third of children with

CSWS have abnormal neuroimaging, including atrophy and cortical malformations (Galanopoulou et al. 2000, Guzzetta et al. 2005), which is not the case with LKS.

The clinical and EEG features of CSWS and LKS may overlap with the syndrome of *benign rolandic epilepsy (BRE)/benign childhood epilepsy with centro-temporal spikes (BCECTS)*. This is a childhood epilepsy syndrome characterized by rare nocturnal seizures with peri-oral manifestations, a characteristic stereotyped blunt "centro-temporal" sharp-wave discharge that increases in frequency in sleep, and normal cognitive and behavioral development. The rolandic spike is a genetic trait (Niedermeyer 1999, Vadlamudi et al. 2004) and may occur in 1–2.5% of normal children (Eeg-Olofsson et al. 1971, Cavazutti et al. 1980). Many children with BRE do well in terms of the epilepsy, cognitively and behaviorally, regardless of treatment (Peters et al. 2001). There is, however, a spectrum; some children with rolandic seizures may have transient language and behavioral disorders, while others may have mental retardation or selective deficits of development (Doose 1989). Verbal dysfunction as well as impaired visuo-motor coordination, specific learning disabilities and attention deficits have been reported (Weglage et al. 1997). A few children with initially normal development and typical nocturnal seizures later develop partial or generalized atonic seizures and myoclonus in clusters and have a deterioration of school function. For these cases, the term "atypical benign focal epilepsy" has been suggested (Aicardi 1979, 2002). These children have the mixed seizure types of the Lennox–Gastaut syndrome and often have continuous spike wave in sleep. In addition, Deonna et al. (1986) described children with atypical rolandic seizures consisting of minor motor seizures of the myoclonic–astatic type associated with diffuse slow spike-waves on the EEG and the maintenance of a normal neurological function, although transient mental deterioration occurred during the active seizure periods (see also Chapter 11). There are also children who may start with the typical clinical and EEG features of rolandic seizures, but then develop a more malignant course of reversible or persistent serious epileptic events including status epilepticus and language, cognitive or behavioral impairments, even after they become seizure free (Fejerman et al. 2000, Hahn et al. 2001). The recognition that EEG discharges may influence cognition and behavior and may be related to autism has prompted a series of studies to assess EEG changes in autism.

CLINICAL EEG AND MEG IN AUTISM

EEG epileptiform activity is more common in both children and adults with autism spectrum disorders (ASDs) than in the general population, even in those without clinical seizures. Between 8% and 20% of children with autism without an identified cause and without epilepsy have epileptiform activity (Tuchman et al. 1991b, Tuchman and Rapin 1997). In children with autism and epilepsy, it is approximately double that, especially in children with "syndromic" autism (Rossi et al. 1995). In general, the frequency of epileptiform activity depends on the conditions under which the EEG was obtained, the age of the child, the underlying etiology, and the coexistence of mental retardation and epilepsy.

Technical factors such as the length of EEG study and whether sleep was recorded during diurnal and/or nocturnal sleep with slow-wave sleep are important (Shinnar et al. 1994). A large study of 894 patients with autism spectrum disorders (ASDs) found epileptiform activity in 19% on overnight EEG, but no CSWS/ESES (Pearl et al. 2001). The use of MEG to detect epileptiform activity may be complementary to, but is not superior to EEG (Huiskamp et al. 2004, Iwasaki et al. 2005). The frequency of epileptiform activity in idiopathic autism is age-dependent and decreases with age from 19% in peri-pubertal children to 6.7% in young adults (Rossi et al. 1995, 2000). This is in contrast to the overall increase in the prevalence of epilepsy with increasing age in adults with autism found by the same authors.

It is also likely that genetics has an important primary role in the development of epileptiform activity and epilepsy in autism. Examples of disorders associated with epilepsy, EEG abnormalities and autism are tuberous sclerosis complex (Curatolo et al. 2004), fragile-X syndrome (Berry-Kravis 2002), and Rett syndrome. In addition, autism and cognitive regression have been reported within some families with generalized epilepsy, febrile seizure plus, and defects in the sodium channels SCN1A and SCN2A (Weiss et al. 2003, Dixon-Salazar et al. 2004, Kamiya et al. 2004) (see Chapter 11 for further discussion).

Epileptiform activity is particularly common in a subgroup of children with language and/or autistic regression. Tuchman and Rapin (1997) reported that extended sleep EEGs identified epileptiform activity in more than twice the number of children with autism and regression without epilepsy, as compared to those without regression. Because of the overlap of epilepsy, mental retardation and autistic regression, and because language regression also occurs in younger children, frequently in the context of a more global autistic regression, the term *autistic regression with epileptiform EEG* has been proposed (Tuchman 1999). However, young children with an isolated language regression had three times more frequently the epileptiform activity and more continuous spike-wave in sleep than those children with combined language and autistic regression (McVicar et al. 2005).

The association of autistic regression with epilepsy, as opposed to epileptiform activity, is not clear. In one study of 77 children, autistic regression was more frequent in children with epilepsy than in non-epileptic patients (Hrdlicka et al. 2004). Those authors also found that abnormal development during the first year of life was significantly associated with epileptiform activity and that epilepsy correlated significantly with mental retardation. A larger study of 145 children, however, found that autistic regression is more common in children without seizures, if the regression occurs in children less than 36 months of age (Tuchman et al. 1991a). A third study found that there was no difference in the proportion of children with regression, whether or not they had epilepsy (Tuchman and Rapin 1997), although they did find that regression was associated with epileptiform activity.

There are few data regarding epileptiform activity and epilepsy in disintegrative disorders. Kurita et al. (1992) suggested in a report on a series of 18 children that EEG abnormalities were significantly more common in the histories of those with disintegrative disorder than those with infantile autism. Mouridsen et al. (1999) compared 13 individuals with disintegrative disorder and 39 with a history of infantile autism matched for sex, age, IQ and socioeconomic status, followed for more than 20 years. The prevalence of epilepsy was higher (77%) in those with disintegrative disorder than in those with autism (33%).

NEUROCOGNITIVE CONSEQUENCES OF EPILEPSY AND EEG EPILEPTIFORM ACTIVITY

The neurocognitive effects of epileptiform activity and seizures are controversial because they may derive from the underlying etiology and epilepsy syndrome, the direct effect of the seizures themselves or the transient effects of epileptiform activity. Focal spikes may be associated with transient functional impairment of the underlying cortical area (Aarts et al. 1984, Kasteleijn-Nolst et al. 1988, Siebelink et al. 1988). Shewmon and Erwin (1988) suggested that it is the inhibition associated with the aftergoing slow wave rather than the spike itself that causes the transitory functional impairment. Aldenkamp and Arends (2004) evaluated the contribution of short nonconvulsive seizures and the location and duration of the epileptiform discharges. Short nonconvulsive seizures impaired alertness and information processing speed, in addition to short-term memory. In patients with frequent epileptiform activity there was only a relatively mild additional effect on attentional processes and speed of information processing. Their subsequent analysis of lateralization and localization of epileptiform discharges did not uncover any further specific differences on the cognitive tests.

The timing during critical windows of development and the duration of the epileptiform activity are almost certainly important (Rouselle and Revol 1995). While most investigators think that early and effective treatment of infantile spasms improves developmental outcome, the data are limited (Kivity et al. 2004). Similarly, case series seem to indicate that a duration of CSWS that exceeds 3 years in LKS correlates with poor language recovery (Robinson et al. 2001). One study reported that the "most striking effect" of multiple subpial transections in 5 children with LKS was on behavior (attention was improved and aggressiveness was decreased) and seizures, and less on language recovery (Irwin et al. 2001). This observation has not been duplicated.

TREATMENT

Evidence upon which to base a rational treatment is limited. To date results are inconsistent due to the small numbers of children studied. There is a great need for further clinical studies to better characterize the electrophysiologic abnormalities and assess the efficacy of controlled treatments on the behaviors, seizures and EEG epileptiform discharges. The treatment of epileptiform activity must be considered within the broader context of the individual needs of the child with autism (Tuchman 2004). Treatment is discussed further in the following chapter.

ACKNOWLEDGMENTS
The authors are supported by grants NS-20253 and NS-43209 from the Heffer Family Medical Foundation. SLM is the recipient of the Martin A and Emily L Fisher fellowship in Neurology and Pediatrics.

REFERENCES
Aarts JHP, Binnie CD, Smit AM, Wilkens AJ (1984) Selective cognitive impairment during focal and generalized epileptiform EEG activity. *Brain* 107: 293–308.

Aicardi J (1979) Benign epilepsy of childhood with rolandic spikes. *Brain Dev* 1: 71–3.

Aicardi J (1996) *Epilepsy in Children, 2nd edn. International Review of Child Neurology Series.* Philadelphia: Lippincott-Raven.

Aicardi J (2002) Atypical semiology of rolandic epilepsy in some related syndromes. *Epileptic Disord Suppl* 1: S5-S9.

Aldenkamp A, Arends J (2004) The relative influence of epileptic EEG discharges, short nonconvulsive seizures, and type of epilepsy on cognitive function. *Epilepsia* 45: 54–63.

ASHA (1991) Guidelines for the audiologic assessment of children from birth through 36 months of age. Committee on Infant Hearing American Speech–Language–Hearing Association. *ASHA Suppl* Mar (5): 37–43.

Ballaban-Gil K, Tuchman R (2000) Epilepsy and epileptiform EEG: association with autism and language disorders. *Ment Retard Dev Dis Res Rev* 6: 300–8.

Berry-Kravis E (2002) Epilepsy in fragile X syndrome. *Dev Med Child Neurol* 44: 724–8.

Braeutigam S, Bailey AJ, Swithenby SJ (2001) Phase-locked gamma band response to semantic violation stimuli. *Cogn Brain Res* 10: 365–77.

Brock J, Brown CC, Boucher J, Rippon G (2002) The temporal binding deficit hypothesis of autism. *Dev Psychopathol* 4: 209–24.

Bruneau N, Roux S, Adrien JL, Bartelemy C (1999) Auditory associative cortex dysfunction in children with autism: evidence from late auditory evoked potentials (N1 wave-T complex). *Clin Neurophysiol* 10: 1927–34.

Bruneau N, Bonnet-Brilhault F, Gomot M, Adrien JL, Barthelemy C (2003) Cortical auditory processing and communication in children with autism: electrophysiological/behavioral relations. *Int J Psychophysiol* 51: 17–25.

Cavazutti GB, Cappella L, Nailn A (1980) Longitudinal study of epileptiform EEG patterns in normal children. *Epilepsia* 21: 43–55.

Curatolo P, Porfirio MC, Manzi B, Seri S (2004) Autism in tuberous sclerosis. *Eur J Paediatr Neurol* 8: 327–32.

Danielsson S, Gillberg IC, Billstedt E, Gillberg C, Olsson I (2005) Epilepsy in young adults with autism: a prospective population-based follow-up study of 120 individuals diagnosed in childhood. *Epilepsia* 46: 918–23.

Deonna T, Ziegler AL, Despland PA (1986) Combined myoclonic-astatic and "benign" focal epilepsy of childhood ("atypical benign partial epilepsy of childhood"). A separate syndrome? *Neuropediatrics* 17: 144–51.

Dixon-Salazar TJ, Keeler LC, Trauner DA, Gleeson JG (2004) Autism in several members of a family with generalized epilepsy with febrile seizures plus. *J Child Neurol* 19: 597–603.

Doose H (1989) Symptomatology in children with focal sharp waves of genetic origin. *Eur J Pediatr* 149: 210–5.

Dunn M, Vaughn HG, Kreutzer J, Kurtzberg D (1999) Electrophysiologic correlates of semantic classification in autistic and normal children. *Dev Neuropyschol* 16: 75–99.

Dunn MA, Bates JC (2005) Developmental change in neural processing of words by children with autism. *J Autism Dev Disord* 35: 361–76.

Eeg-Olofsson O, Petersen I, Sellden U (1971) The development of the electroencephalogram in normal children from the age 1 through 15 years: paroxysmal activity. *Neuropediatrics* 2: 375–404.

Engel J (2001) A proposed diagnostic scheme for people with epileptic seizures and epilepsy: report of the ILAE Task Force on Classification and Terminology. *Epilepsia* 42: 796–803.

Fejerman N, Caraballo R, Tenembaum SN (2000) Atypical evolutions of benign localization-related epilepsies in children: are they predictable? *Epilepsia* 41: 380–90.

Filipek PA, Accardo PJ, Ashwal S, Baranek GT, Cook EH Jr, Dawson G, Gordon B, Gravel JS, Johnson CP, Kallen RJ, Levy SE, Minshew NJ, Ozonoff S, Prizant BM, Rapin I, Rogers SJ, Stone WL, Teplin SW, Tuchman RF, Volkmar FR (2000) Practice parameter: screening and diagnosis of autism: report of the Quality Standards Subcommittee of the American Academy of Neurology and the Child Neurology Society. *Neurology* 55: 468–79.

Frith U (1989) *Autism: Explaining the Enigma.* Oxford: Blackwell.

Gage NM, Siegel B, Callen M, Roberts TP (2003) Cortical sound processing in children with autism disorder: an MEG investigation. *Neuroreport* 14: 2047–51.

Galanopoulou A, Bojko A, Lado F, Moshé SL (2000) The spectrum of neuropsychiatric abnormalities associated with electrical status epilepticus in sleep. *Brain Dev* 22: 279–95.

Garreau B, Tanguay P, Roux S, Lelord G (1984) Brain stem auditory evoked potentials in the normal and autistic child. *Rev Electroencephalogr Neurophysiol Clin* 14: 25–31.

Genton P, Ogihara M, Samoggia G, Guerrini R, Roger J (1990) Activation élective des paroxysmes temporax à l'endormissement et pendant le sommeil dans un cas de synfrome de Landau–Kleffner. *Rev EEG Neurophysiol Clin* 20: 529.

Guzzetta F, Battaglia D, Veredice C, Donvito V, Pane M, Lettori D, Chiricozza F, Chieffo D, Tartaglione T, Dravet C (2005) Early thalamic injury associated with epilepsy and continuous spike-wave during slow sleep. *Epilepsia* 46: 889–900.

Hahn A, Pistohl J, Neubauer BA, Stephani U (2001) Atypical "benign" partial epilepsy or pseudo-Lennox syndrome. Part I: Symptomatology and long-term prognosis. *Neuropediatrics* 32: 1–8.

Hrdlicka M, Komarek V, Propper L, Kulisek R, Zumrova A, Faladova L, Havlovicova M, Sedlacek Z, Blatny M, Urbanek T (2004) Not EEG abnormalities but epilepsy is associated with autistic regression and mental functioning in childhood autism. *Eur Child Adolesc Psychiatry* 13: 209–13.

Huiskamp G, van Der Meij W, van Huffelen A, van Nieuwenenhuizen O (2004) High resolution spatio-temporal EEG-MEG analysis of rolandic spikes. *J Clin Neurophysiol* 21: 84–95.

Irwin K, Birch V, Lees J, Polkey C, Alarcon G, Binnie C, Smedley M, Baird G, Robinson RO (2001) Multiple subpial transection in Landau-Kleffner syndrome. *Dev Med Child Neurol* 43: 248–52.

Iwasaki M, Pestana E, Burgess RC, Luders HO, Shamoto H, Nakasato N (2005) Detection of epileptiform activity by human interpreters: blinded comparison between electroencephalography and magnetoencephalography. *Epilepsia* 46: 59–68.

Jure R, Rapin I, Tuchman RF (1991) Hearing impaired autistic children. *Dev Med Child Neurol* 33: 1062–72.

Kamiya K, Kaneda M, Sugawara T, Mazaki E, Okamura N, Montal M, Makita N, Tanaka M, Fukushima K, Fujiwara T, Inoue Y, Yamakawa K (2004) A nonsense mutation of the sodium channel gene SCN2A in a patient with intractable epilepsy and mental decline. *J Neurosci* 24: 2690–8.

Kasteleijn-Nolst Trenite DG, Bakker DJ, Binnie CD, Buerman A, Van Raaij M (1988) Psychological effect of subclinical epileptiform EEG discharges. I. Scholastic. *Epilepsy Res* 2: 111–6.

Kivity S, Lerman P, Ariel R, Danziger Y, Mimouni M, Shinnar S (2004) Long-term cognitive outcomes of a cohort of children with cryptogenic infantile spasms treated with high-dose adrenocorticotropic hormone. *Epilepsia* 45: 255–62.

Klass DW, Daly DD (1979) *Current Practice of Clinical Electroencephalography.* New York: Raven Press.

Klein SK, Kurtzberg D, Brattson A, Kreuzer JA, Stapells DR, Dunn MA, Rapin I, Vaughn HG (1995) Electrophysiologic manifestations of impaired temporal lobe auditory processing in verbal auditory processing. *Brain Lang* 51: 383–405.

Klin A (1993) Auditory brainstem responses in autism: brainstem dysfunction or peripheral hearing loss? *J Autism Dev Disord* 23: 15–35.

Kurita H, Kita M, Miyake Y (1992) A comparative study of development and symptoms among disintegrative psychosis and infantile autism with and without speech loss. *J Autism Dev Disord* 22: 175–88.

Kutas M, Federmeir KD (2000) Electrophysiology reveals semantic memory use in language comprehension. *Trends Cogn Sci* 4: 463–70.

McDermott S, Moran R, Platt T, Wood H, Isaac T, Dasari S (2005) Prevalence of epilepsy in adults with mental retardation and related disabilities in primary care. *Am J Ment Retard* 110: 48–56.

McVicar K, Shinnar S (2004) Landau–Kleffner syndrome, electrical status epilepticus in slow sleep and language regression in children. *Ment Retard Dev Disabil Res Rev* 10: 144–9.

McVicar KA, Ballaban-Gil K, Rapin I, Moshe SL, Shinnar S (2005) Epileptiform EEG abnormalities in children with language regression. *Neurology* 65: 129–31.

Mouridsen SE, Rich B, Isager T (1999) Epilepsy in disintegrative psychosis and infantile autism: a long-term validation study. *Dev Med Child Neurol* 41: 110–4.

Niedermeyer E (1999) Epileptic seizure disorders. In: Niedermeyer E, Da Silva FL, eds. *Electroencephalography, 4th edn.* Baltimore: Williams & Wilkins, pp. 534–5.

Olsson I, Steffenburg S, Gillberg C (1988) Epilepsy in autism and autisticlike conditions. A population-based study. *Arch Neurol* 45: 666–8.

Pearl PL, Conry JA, Reigle S, Stahl AM, Allen E, Rich S, Mott SH, Weinstein SL, Gaillard ND (2001) Lack of utility of EEG monitoring in autistic syndrome patients for the identification of Landau-Kleffner syndrome. *Ann Neurol* 50 suppl: S115.

Peters JM, Camfield CS, Camfield PR (2001) Population study of benign rolandic epilepsy: is treatment needed? *Neurology* 57: 537–9.

Rapin I, Dunn M (2003) Update on the language disorders of individuals on the autistic spectrum. *Brain Dev* 25: 66–172.

Riikonen R, Amnell G (1981) Pyschiatric disorders in children with earlier infantile spasms. *Dev Med Child Neurol* 23: 747–60.

Robinson RO, Baird G, Robinson G, Simonoff E (2001) Landau–Kleffner syndrome: course and correlates with outcome. *Dev Med Child Neurol* 43: 243–7.

Rosenblum SM, Arick JR, Krug DA, Stubbs EG, Young NB, Pelson RO (1980) Auditory brainstem evoked responses in autistic children. *J Autism Dev Disord* 10: 215–25.

Rossi PG, Parmeggiani A, Bach V, Santucci M, Visconti P (1995) EEG features and epilepsy in patients with autism. *Brain Dev* 17: 169–74.

Rossi PG, Posar A, Parmeggiani A (2000) Epilepsy in adolescents and young adults with autistic disorder. *Brain Dev* 22: 102–6.

Rousselle C, Revol M (1995) Relations between cognitive functions and continuous spikes and waves during slow sleep. In: Beaumanoir A, Bureau M, Deonna T, Mira L, Tassinari CA, eds. *Continuous Spikes and Waves During Slow Sleep: Acquired Epileptic Aphasia and Related Conditions.* London: John Libbey, pp. 123–33.

Shewmon DA, Erwin RJ (1988) Focal spike-induced cerebral dysfunction is related to the after-coming slow wave. *Ann Neurol* 23: 131–7.

Shinnar S, Kang H, Berg AT, Goldensohn ES, Hauser WA, Moshe SL (1994) EEG abnormalities in children with a first unprovoked seizure. *Epilepsia* 35: 471–6.

Siebelink BM, Bakker DJ, Binnie CD, Kasteleijn-Nolst Trenite DGA (1988) Psychological effect of subclinical epileptiform EEG discharges. II: General intelligence test. *Epilepsy Res* 2: 117–21.

Steffenburg S, Gillberg C, Steffenburg U (1991) Pyschiatric disorders in children and adolescents with mental retardation and active epilepsy. *Arch Neurol* 53: 904–12.

Takeoka M, Riviello JJ, Duffy FH, Kim F, Kennedy DN, Makris N, Caviness VS, Holmes GL (2004) Bilateral volume reduction of the superior temporal areas in Landau–Kleffner syndrome. *Neurology* 63: 1289–92.

Tager-Flusberg H, Joseph H (2003) Identifying neurocognitive phenotypes in autism. *Philos Trans R Soc Lond B Biol Sci* 358: 303–24.

Taylor MJ, Rosenblatt B, Linschoten L (1982) Auditory brainstem response abnormalities in autistic children. *Can J Neurol Sci* 9: 429–33.

Townsend J, Westerfield M, Leaver E, Makeig S, Jung T, Pierce K, Courchesne E (2001) Event-related brain response abnormalities in autism: evidence for impaired cerebello-frontal spatial attention networks. *Brain Res Cogn Brain Res* 11: 127–45.

Tuchman RF (1999) Epileptiform disorders with cognitive symptoms. In: Swaiman KF, Ashwal S, eds. *Pediatric Neurology: Principles and Practice, 3rd edn.* St Louis: Mosby, pp. 661–7.

Tuchman R (2004) AEDs and psychotropic drugs in children with autism and epilepsy. *Ment Retard Dev Dis Res Rev* 10: 135–8.

Tuchman RF, Rapin I (1997) Regression in pervasive developmental disorders: seizures and epileptiform electroencephalogram correlates. *Pediatrics* 22: 560–6.

Tuchman R, Rapin I (2002) Epilepsy in autism. *Lancet Neurol* 1: 352–8.

Tuchman RF, Rapin I, Shinnar S (1991a) Autistic and dysphasic children. I: Clinical characteristics. *Pediatrics* 88: 1211–8.

Tuchman RF, Rapin I, Shinnar S (1991b) Autistic and dysphasic children. II. Epilepsy. *Pediatrics* 88: 1219–25.

Vadlamudi L, Harvey AS, Connellan MM, Milne RL, Hopper JL, Scheffer IE, Berkovic SF (2004) Is benign rolandic epilepsy genetically determined? *Ann Neurol* 56: 129–32.

Volkmar FR, Nelson DS (1990) Seizure disorders in autism. *J Am Acad Child Adolesc Psychiatry* 29: 127–9.

Weglage J, Demsky A, Pietsch M, Kurlmann G (1997) Neuropyschological, intellectual, and behavioral findings in patients with centrotemporal spikes with and without seizures. *Dev Med Child Neurol* 39: 646–51.

Weiss LA, Escayg A, Kearney JA, Trudeau M, MacDonald BT, Mori M, Reichert J (2003) Sodium channels SCN1A, SCN2A and SCN3A in familial autism. *Mol Psychiatry* 8: 186–94.

11

AUTISM, EPILEPSY AND EEG EPILEPTIFORM ACTIVITY

Eliane Roulet-Perez and Thierry Deonna

Autism is a behavioral phenotype associated with or caused by many different brain disorders of known or unknown etiology. The increased prevalence (5–40%) of epilepsy in patients with this disorder (Tuchman and Rapin 2002) is hardly surprising, especially in the face of other impairments like mental retardation or motor deficits (see Chapter 10). Moreover, autistic features, together with various other cognitive and neurological impairments, are reported in patients with certain epileptic disorders or syndromes (Besag 2004), suggesting that electrophysiological abnormalities may, in some cases, interfere with the function and development of neural networks supporting communication and social behaviors. Consequently, autistic behaviors may represent one of the many possible behavioral and cognitive disorders of epileptic origin in children (Deonna and Roulet-Perez 2005). When assessing an autistic child who presents with epileptic seizures or in whom epileptic discharges are found on an EEG, it is necessary to keep in mind that autism and epilepsy may occur together for different reasons (Table 11.1):

(1) *Both conditions are entirely independent* and co-occur in a child who has acquired or inherited them together by chance (e.g. there is history of typical childhood absence epilepsy on the maternal side and of an autism spectrum disorder (ASD) on the paternal side);

(2) *The autistic phenotype and the epilepsy are associated*, both being independent consequences of the same genetic disorder (e.g. fragile-X syndrome) or of the same acquired early cerebral insult (e.g. congenital rubella). In such cases, the epileptic seizures or epileptiform discharges are the markers of an underlying cerebral pathology that modifies the threshold of neuronal excitability, either focally or diffusely, but they have no direct causal role in the autistic behaviors. This is probably the most frequent situation, keeping in mind that severe or frequent seizures may worsen some aspects of cognitive and motor function of an autistic child, as can happen in non-autistic intellectually disabled children (Laan et al. 1997, Deonna and Roulet-Perez 2005). Interestingly, some children who have an autistic phenotype associated with mental retardation and, in some cases, with epilepsy, have cytogenetic abnormalities (for example of chromosome 15q11-q13 or 7q22q33) in regions containing genes that play

TABLE 11.1
ASD and epilepsy: why together?

(1) Both are independent, co-occur by chance, e.g.
   • childhhood absence epilepsy and ASD

(2) Both are consequences of a common cerebral pathology, e.g.
   • early aquired cerebral insult (e.g. congenital rubella)
   • genetic syndrome (e.g. fragile-X syndrome)

(3) ASD is a consequence of epilepsy that starts in or spreads to developing networks involved in communication and social behavior, e.g. the limbic system
   • repeated ictal and postictal states due to congenital epileptogenic lesion
   • prolonged status epilepticus leading to bilateral hippocampal sclerosis
   • sustained bilateral epileptic discharges (mainly frontal or temporal regions)

(4) ASD results from a withdrawal reaction in a child with acquired epileptic aphasia (Landau–Kleffner syndrome)

a role in the expression of neurotransmitter receptors or in the structural development of the brain (Muhle et al. 2004). The respective roles of these genes in the pathogenesis of the epilepsy, of the autistic phenotype, and of the mental deficiency are not well understood;

(3) *An epileptic process interferes directly with the function of specific networks involved in the development of human communication and social behavior.* In these cases, the underlying pathology (which is of either known – e.g. a focal cortical dysplasia or hypothalamic hamartoma – or unknown origin) is not directly responsible for the autistic phenotype but for the epilepsy it triggers. The epileptic process then spreads to structures thought to be dysfunctional in ASD like orbitofrontal cortex, anterior cingulate gyrus or amygdala that belong to the limbic system, and other related circuits (dorsomedial frontal cortex/anterior cingulate circuit) (Deonna et al. 1993, Mundy 2003, Tuchman 2003, Allman et al. 2005), possibly at a critical period of their maturation, and generates the autistic symptoms. These networks may already be abnormal for some reason (genetic or early damage) and thus be at the origin of a mild ASD or cognitive delay, and later trigger an epilepsy that aggravates the symptoms;

(4) In a vulnerable child, an autistic phenotype may result from *the child's withdrawal reaction when an epileptic process interferes with a specific sensory or cognitive function* (e.g. the sound decoding system in verbal auditory agnosia) that is important for communication, even if the function is not directly related to the emotional and social behavioral processing systems. The child is suddenly deprived of a meaningful language input from his/her surroundings. In this case, the child may benefit greatly from the introduction, besides medical therapy, of substitutive communication means like simplified sign language or other visually mediated codes (Roulet Perez et al. 2001).

This chapter focuses on situations in which a direct link between epilepsy and autism may exist, and the following points will be addressed:

(1) Can seizure types and localization found in children with an ASD indicate which regions of the brain are affected?
(2) Does epilepsy play a role in autistic regression?
(3) Does epilepsy play a role in disintegrative disorder?
(4) What does "subclinical" or "hidden epilepsy" mean in children with ASD?
(5) How does one go about determining the role of clinical/subclinical epilepsy in autism?
(6) When is antiepileptic treatment indicated?

(1) CAN SEIZURE TYPES OR THE LOCALIZATION OF EEG ABNORMALITIES FOUND IN CHILDREN WITH AN ASD INDICATE WHICH REGIONS OF THE BRAIN ARE AFFECTED?

All seizure types and severities have been reported in patients with autism (for reviews, see Volkmar 1990, Tuchman and Rapin 2002, Levisohn 2004; and Chapter 10). This is readily understandable when the width of the spectrum and its many possible etiologies are considered. Studies directed at identifying the localization of EEG abnormalities in large samples of autistic patients will inevitably reflect this diversity and give only broad indications about the dysfunctional regions, but they will not solve the question of a possible direct role of epilepsy. For example, Hashimoto et al. (2001) found midline frontal foci in 37 out of 86 (43%) autistic patients in whom a sleep EEG disclosed epileptic activity. The dipole of these midline spikes was found in the deep frontal region, suggesting its cingulate origin. The authors argued in favor of a frontal dysfunction in autism, but also noted that other groups found different results attributable either to subject selection criteria or recording techniques.

In a retrospective study of tuberous sclerosis, Bolton et al. (2002, 2004) analyzed the factors that determined the autistic phenotype in their patients. They found that it was the presence of sustained epileptic activity originating in tubers located in the temporal lobes and starting early in life that was crucial for the development of autism, rather than the number of tubers, their precise locations in the temporal lobe, early onset epilepsy, or infantile spasms per se. These findings need to be confirmed by longitudinal prospective studies, but they illustrate the potential role of an epileptic disturbance in the genesis of an ASD in cases where an underlying lesion – cortical tuber – is present in a strategic location, e.g. situated in, or connected to, the limbic system. They also suggest that the cognitive/behavioral functions supported by the affected network must occur at a critical period of development. Asano et al. (2001) had also found that the burden of tubers and their location determined whether the children would be cognitively impaired or autistic, with or without language deficit.

(2) DOES EPILEPSY PLAY A ROLE IN AUTISTIC REGRESSION?

One-third of parents of children later diagnosed as autistic report a history of regression or stagnation in language, communication and play after seemingly normal early development occurring before age 3 years, usually between 18 and 24 months (Rapin 1991). This regression is usually followed by a plateau of variable duration (months, years), then some improvement but not complete recovery. Besides Rett syndrome and rare neurometabolic disorders that need to be considered (Pearl et al. 2003; see also Chapter 7), the search for a specific cause of this regression usually remains disappointingly negative. At this point, the question is raised of a possible disorder of epileptic origin, especially "subclinical" or "hidden" epilepsy when the child has no overt seizures. The fact that the prevalence of epilepsy increases with increasing age in children with autism is an epidemiologic argument against its role in a regression that occurs early in development. In addition, the retrospective comparison between EEG tracings of autistic children with and without a history of regression revealed no significant difference (Rapin 1995, Tuchman and Rapin 1997, Baird and Robinson 2000). In a recently published study of EEG abnormalities in children with language regression and no identified encephalopathy, 103 patients had a combined language and autistic regression but only 8 had seizures, and less than a third (n=29) had epileptiform discharges on 24-hour EEG records (McVicar et al. 2005). The delay between the regression and the EEG monitoring was not stated, but had epilepsy had a clear causal role in the autistic regression of this population, the rate of abnormalities should have been much higher. It now seems clear that the early regression reported in children later diagnosed with classic "idiopathic" autism is not of epileptic origin. This statement does not exclude epilepsy as the cause of the regression in individual cases with unusual clinical features such as dissociated or successively appearing deficits and fluctuations (Zappella 2005). Table 11.2 summarizes data from 11 prospective studies (single cases or small groups) in which the authors assumed that the ASD was of epileptic origin and provided enough clinical data to discern whether this was likely. They tried to correlate the autistic behavior or regression and its fluctuations with the epileptic activity, using EEG records and clinical evolution before and after medical or surgical treatment. Among 24 studied children, only 8 had an ASD that could clearly be related causally to the epilepsy, showing that these cases exist but are not frequent and are difficult to document. These data suggest that epilepsy is always a consideration in the work-up of a child with an autistic regression, even though it will end up discarded in the majority of cases. There are three situations to consider:

(a) *Autistic and developmental regression is the presenting symptom in a child in whom epilepsy can be documented unequivocally with the appropriate work-up*

These children present with a developmental problem or sometimes with a first seizure, but their history reveals recent developmental regression or stagnation, in some cases with important behavioral fluctuations. Video-EEG records may disclose (although by no means in every child) complex partial seizures of frontal or temporal origin, or late infantile spasms (Bednarek et al. 1998) with or without underlying brain lesions. Focal or generalized interictal epileptic discharges are usually also evident during wakefulness or the sleep state. Making the caregivers aware of the video-EEG findings or a review of

TABLE 11.2

Summary of 11 published longitudinal case studies* of autistic behavior or regression claimed to be of epileptic origin

Number of studies	11
Number of children	24
Mention of developmental regression	19 (3 with a second phase of regression)
Duration of follow-up	1–2 years, 9 cases; 2–5 years, 8 cases; >5 years, 4 cases
Prospective evaluation	15/24
Specific pathology	8 (tuberous sclerosis 4; congenital tumour 3; cortical dysplasia 1)
Diagnosis of epileptic syndrome	7 "early Landau–Kleffner syndrome"
Seizure types	Infantile spasms 4; others 12; possible seizures 3; no seizure 5
Video-EEG analyzed autistic behaviors	None
Epilepsy surgery	14
Evaluation of improvement with treatment	7 clinical judgment only; 17 with tests and questionnaires
Causal relation between autistic behavior and epileptic activity	8 clear; 6 probable or possible; 10 doubtful

*Gillberg and Schaumann (1983), Hoon and Reiss (1992), Deonna et al. (1993, 1995), Dalla Bernardina et al. (1994), Plioplys (1994), Gillberg et al. (1996), Neville et al. (1997), Nass et al. (1999), Szabo et al. (1999), Jacobs et al. (2001).

family videos can sometimes reveal that the child had had for a long time prior to diagnosis subtle epileptic episodes manifest as minor forms of the more characteristic recorded seizures (Deonna et al. 1995, Fohlen et al. 2004). In such children the fluctuating abnormal behaviors result from repeated ictal and postictal disturbances that start in, or spread to, the frontal or temporal parts of the limbic system that support developing, and therefore vulnerable, social and emotional functions. It is important not to use the label of autism for a child who appears "disconnected" by frequent seizures, or who lacks initiative or shows no sign of visual or social interest. The term "autistic epileptic regression" should be restricted to those children in whom alterations in communication, play and behavior contrast with preserved vigilance, motricity and other sensory and cognitive (e.g. visuospatial) functions, and which are correlated in time with the epileptic disorder.

The evolution of some young children with the syndrome of gelastic epilepsy and hypothalamic hamartoma provides a good model of epileptic autistic and cognitive regression due to epileptic spread or secondary epileptogenesis (Berkovic 2003). Unfortunately, children with this disorder have only rarely been examined from the neuropsychological point of view with equal care to that given to the electrophysiological investigation (Deonna and Ziegler 2000, Perez-Jimenez et al. 2003). Table 11.3 gives some other

TABLE 11.3

Epileptic disorders and specific pathologies potentially associated with an epileptic autistic regression

Epileptic spasms ("late infantile spasms")

Early symptomatic partial complex seizures (frontal or temporal)

Acquired epileptic aphasia (Landau–Kleffner syndrome): early or more extended variants

Frontal epilepsy with continuous spike-waves during slow sleep ("acquired epileptic frontal syndrome")

Tuberous sclerosis (epileptogenic tubers in temporal lobes)

Hypothalamic hamartoma and epilepsy (early onset)

examples of epileptic disorders or specific brain pathologies in which an epileptic autistic regression can occur and which provide useful models for correlative studies.

    (b) Autistic and cognitive regression following repeated or prolonged seizures (status epilepticus)

A severe regression with loss of language, social interaction and purposeful activities was first reported in two previously normal children at ages 23 and 30 months after an afebrile status epilepticus (DeLong and Heinz 1997). The EEG was normal 1 month after the status in the first child and showed asynchronous bitemporal epileptic discharges in the second. In both cases, a brain MRI showed bilateral hippocampal sclerosis. We had the opportunity to study a similar case, with the difference that in ours the child had a mild developmental delay and a seizure disorder prior to the acute dramatic regression that followed a febrile status. It is of course possible that an encephalitis, notably one due to herpes virus with its known tropism for limbic structures, was responsible for the findings, although there was no evidence for it during the acute period and the MRI showed no abnormalities besides the bilateral lesions in the hippoccampal region. This type of pathology can best be considered postepileptic, irrespective of the underlying cause of the epilepsy. Hippocampal swelling has indeed been found in some children with febrile status epilepticus with focal features provided an MRI was obtained shortly after the acute event (Van Landingham et al. 1998). To our knowledge, this type of regression is never purely autistic but cognitive as well, although the clinical picture may vary depending on the child's age and the severity of the acute event. Bilateral damage appears to be required, but the critical structures or networks that must be affected (hippocampus only versus extension to amygdala, parahippocampal structures, or others) for the regression to occur have yet to be identified.

    (c) An autistic and developmental regression has occurred and the child has epileptic discharges in the EEG but no clinical seizures

The main question here is whether the regression might be an early manifestation of certain epileptic disorders like the Landau–Kleffner syndrome (LKS) or epilepsy with continuous spike-waves during slow sleep (CSWS), which can sometimes be very active in the EEG without recognized seizures. These syndromes (see Chapter 10) are exceedingly rare under 3 years of age. If they present earlier (Uldall et al. 2000), evidence of loss of language and social skills is difficult to document since it is the emergence of these skills that is interfered with. The clinical picture will not be that of a primary ASD, but of a combination of language or/and mental regression or stagnation with autistic features that may fluctuate and change in nature and pattern over time (initially deafness or loss of first words with preserved communication, and later autistic features and other deficits).

Specialists rarely see these cases during the regressive phase; consequently they are seldom documented convincingly. We still await further detailed longitudinal studies. In LKS or epilepsy with CSWS (see Chapter 10), the epileptic dysfunction that is manifest on the surface EEG with sustained, usually bilateral, temporal or frontal discharges activated by sleep is thought to interfere with developing language and cognitive–behavioral functions, and its interruption by drug treatment may bring significant improvement. The problem of "hidden" epilepsy and its clinical implications in practice are further considered below (sections 4, 5 and 6).

(3) DOES EPILEPSY PLAY A ROLE IN A DISINTEGRATIVE DISORDER?

Occasionally the cognitive and behavioral regression in children with an ASD (5–8%, Rapin 1995) occurs later than the usual 18–36 months, that is, between the third and sixth, or even up to the 10th year, when language is already developed. This situation was previously referred to as disintegrative psychosis (Hill and Rosenbloom 1986) or Heller syndrome, and is now designated as childhood disintegrative disorder (DD). The distinction between an autistic regression and a DD is thus based only on age and does not imply a specific cause. The epilepsy seems more prominent, the cognitive regression more profound, and the outcome more dismal than in the more numerous children with earlier regression classified as autistic (Mouridsen et al. 1999). These differences are probably accounted for by differences in etiologies and maturational stages of the underlying brain networks. Regarding the possible causal link between DD and epilepsy, the same three situations discussed above may pertain, namely (a) DD as the first manifestation of an epilepsy – especially a frontal epilepsy – that was not recognized earlier as such; (b) DD after prolonged status involving both mesial temporal lobes; and (c) the discovery of sustained epileptic discharges in the EEG of a child with DD but no epileptic seizures.

In this age group, the answer to the question of whether LKS or epilepsy with CSWS can, in some cases, be at the origin of a regression of communication, sociability and play is clearly "yes" in our view. A child with LKS can present a severe behavioral deterioration, besides the auditory agnosia, when the epileptic activity involves, besides the usual perisylvian localizations, other mainly frontal regions, via spread, migration or generation of new foci. In addition, a subgroup of patients with epilepsy and CSWS can present a unique and impressive behavioral and cognitive regression with aberrant thought processes, loss of creative play, repetitive activities, inattention and hyperactivity, but with preserved language and rote memory (Roulet-Perez et al. 1993). We originally coined the term "acquired epileptic frontal syndrome with CSWS" for these children who had a cryptogenic or idiopathic partial epilepsy with a frontal focus and CSWS, without the seizures necessarily being at the forefront. Early development was considered normal. We wondered in 1993 whether some children labeled with the DD diagnosis might have had this particular epileptic syndrome. We had not found another clearly similar case until 1996, when Kyllerman described a 6-year-old child with epilepsy and CSWS who underwent a mental and behavioral regression (which he labeled psychosis) that seemed to correspond to our acquired frontal syndrome or to what other investigators had called DD (Kyllerman et al. 1996, Deonna et al. 2003). There is no doubt that other cases of frontal epilepsy besides frontal epilepsy with CSWS may present with a behavioral regression compatible with DD, that is until the diagnosis of epilepsy is made and recovery takes place with treatment; most of these cases will probably not be reported as DD.

This does not mean that an epileptic disorder is responsible for the regression of every child diagnosed with DD who has epileptic discharges in the EEG, but rather that this hypothesis needs to be considered when seeking the cause of such cases. The DD, like the autistic regression, can be referred to as "idiopathic" or "primary" when no etiology is found, or as of epileptic origin when, for example, it is associated with a frontal epilepsy with CSWS, provided the conditions for the latter diagnosis are fulfilled (see Chapter 10). A further task for pediatric neurologists, psychiatrists and neuropsychologists will be to document more closely the nature and evolution of the cognitive and behavioral impairments found in these exceptional cases and to find out whether they can be distinguished on the basis of their clinical characteristics.

(4) WHAT DOES "SUBCLINICAL" OR "HIDDEN" EPILEPSY MEAN IN CHILDREN WITH ASD?

The term "subclinical epilepsy" is ambiguous because it can apply either to subtle seizures that are at the limit of clinical observation or to epileptic discharges in the EEG of a child who does not have clinical seizures, the clinical relevance of which is uncertain. The same is true of the term "hidden epilepsy". These different meanings need to be distinguished (Table 11.4).

(a) *Seizures are not recognized because short periods of unresponsiveness, brief axial spasms, or more complex stereotypic movements of the limbs can easily be missed in the context of a disturbed child, or are interpreted as one more of the child's strange behaviors* (Deonna et al. 2002, Fohlen et al. 2004). These seizures can be identified as such when a formal video-EEG with a sleep record discloses a correlation between clinical manifestations and epileptic discharges;

(b) *Seizures are evident clinically, but the interictal waking and sleep EEG does not show clear-cut epileptiform abnormalities because the epilepsy arises in deep structures (orbito- or mesiofrontal, mesiotemporal, hypothalamic regions).* In these difficult cases, prolonged video-EEG records are required, as well as a high resolution MRI that may show a focal cortical dysplasia.

TABLE 11.4
"Hidden epilepsy": different possible meanings

(1) Epileptic seizure not recognized as such, mistaken for autistic behaviors

(2) Seizures suspected clinically, but epileptic activity coming from deep structures not found on EEG

(3) No epileptic seizures but epileptic discharges (various locations and intensities) visible on EEG

(c) There are no clinical seizures, but epileptic discharges, focal, multifocal, or generalized, are recorded in the EEG. The difficult question, which has been the source of much controversy, is the interpretation of this finding: are the epileptiform discharges a "by-product" of the brain dysfunction responsible for the ASD or are they at the origin of – or at least significant contributors to – the clinical problem? There is no satisfactory answer to this question, which has to be considered in the context of each individual case (see section 5 below).

(d) When no suspect clinical manifestations are reported or observed and only dubious or sporadic epileptiform discharges are seen in a prolonged video-EEG that includes a full sleep record, an active epileptic disorder as cause of the ASD can be discarded.

(5) HOW DOES ONE GO ABOUT DETERMINING THE ROLE OF CLINICAL/SUBCLINICAL EPILEPSY IN AUTISM?

This question often arises in clinical practice and has to be answered in the context of each child's individual case.

(a) Child with a previously diagnosed ASD and new onset seizures
This situation can occur at any time during childhood and adolescence, and increases in frequency with age, depending of course on the underlying etiology. In this situation, the probability that the epilepsy contributes to the ASD is very low, unless the timing of the behavioral deterioration and the onset of seizures are correlated. Occasionally the onset of the seizures may suggest a new previously unsuspected and uninvestigated diagnosis (for example a cytogenetic abnormality). The cause of the epilepsy should be investigated as it would in any child with mental retardation and no ASD.

(b) Child with known epilepsy in whom an autistic regression or DD becomes apparent
In such cases, the probability that the epilepsy may be responsible for the regression is high. It is mandatory to look for a worsening of the epilepsy, for example for the appearance of late onset infantile spasms, the emergence of a new focus or its spread to the temporal or frontal regions, or the development of CSWS. It is important to consider worsening of the epilepsy by the prescription of an inappropriate medication, as well as a psychotic reaction induced by an antiepileptic or other drug. One also needs to look carefully for a previously missed lesion (e.g. a small hypothalamic hamartoma).

(c) Child presenting with ongoing or recent language and behavioral regression with
autistic features found to have clinical epilepsy or EEG epileptic discharges

Younger children usually come to medical attention later in the course of their regression
(or after it) than older children in whom loss of skills, especially language, is easier to
recognize. Rarely, infantile neurometabolic disorders present with an isolated autistic and
cognitive regression without other neurologic or somatic features. Rett syndrome must
always be considered because its course may be atypical (for example with a prolonged
period of preserved hand use and late onset of hand stereotypies). An undiagnosed epilepsy
with difficult to recognize seizures, or an epileptic disorder without clinical seizures but
with sustained epileptic discharges, must be looked for, especially when regression
occurred after 2 years of age or its pattern or evolution appears unusual (for example,
absence of response to sounds preceding the behavioral changes, or severe inattention,
abnormal thought and repetitive behaviors with preserved eye contact and language) or
is associated with behavioral fluctuations. A video-EEG with a sleep record is clearly
indicated in a child with an ongoing or recent regression; it is not mandatory in a child
with typical autism seen well after a regression that had occurred at 18–24 months whose
nonverbal skills are preserved and who has no dysmorphic features. It is very important
not to label every child in whom epileptic discharges are detected during sleep as having
LKS or epilepsy with CSWS. There are atypical cases that do not fit any of the established
classifications and are particularly challenging; the best plan is to describe them in detail
without attempting to classify them at all cost (O'Regan et al. 1998).

Of interest here are the cases of 2 boys, briefly mentioned by McVicar et al. (2005),
who had a regression at 5½ and 10 years of age with features of LKS "superimposed upon
a previous diagnosis of autism", one child having classic verbal auditory agnosia and
CSWS. One wonders of course whether the etiology of the autistic disorder was epileptic or "developmental" in these boys. Above all, these unusual cases show that different
clinical pictures can succeed each other at different ages and in various orders (sometimes
verbal auditory agnosia precedes the autistic regression); they are thus excellent examples
of the complexity of the problem, at pathophysiological, conceptual, and classification
levels.

(d) Young child with a developmental disorder with autistic features but no regression in
whom paroxysmal EEG abnormalities are discovered

In such cases, the probability is very high that the epileptic discharges are only associated
with, or markers of, the underlying brain pathology responsible for the developmental
disorder and may be secondary to common genetic factors (see Chapter 10). When
epileptic discharges are very frequent, bilateral, focal, multifocal or even generalized, and
there is no detectable underlying brain lesion in an otherwise neurologically normal and
non-dysmorphic child, it may be that these discharges interfered with language and social
skills so early that they prevented their emergence. This interpretation is speculative
inasmuch as to the best of our knowledge no adequate longitudinal study of such cases
supports it convincingly. Our personal experience with a few of these children was

frustrating because the epileptic discharges were exceedingly resistant to treatment and were not correlated with significant developmental changes.

(6) WHEN IS ANTIEPILEPTIC TREATMENT INDICATED?

Deciding whether to treat or not to treat the epileptic disorder in a child with an ASD is based on which of the previously discussed situations applies:

(a) The child's epilepsy and the ASD are only associated

Antiepileptic drugs may or may not be prescribed depending on the seizure type and frequency, and the impact of the seizures on the child's behavior and everyday life, as would be the case for any child with epilepsy and a developmental disorder of known or unknown etiology. Epileptiform discharges without seizures need not be treated.

(b) The child's autistic regression or DD (on the basis of previously normal or already altered development) is correlated with the epileptic disorder, making a causal link highly probable

This situation would encompass children with either seizures or only sustained epileptic discharges in their EEG who, like those with typical LKS, experience language regression, but who, because of their autistic features, may be considered LKS variants. In these children, as well as in cases with frontal epilepsy and CSWS, aggressive medical treatment with antiepileptic drugs and/or steroids is indicated. Surgery needs to be considered promptly in children with epileptic autistic regression, refractory seizures and a focal lesion (Neville et al. 1997). Some children with severe LKS and behavioral disorders who failed medical therapy seem to have benefited from subpial transections (Neville et al. 1997, Grote et al. 1999, Irwin et al. 2001). Return to normality cannot be expected, but the procedure may bring about significant improvement in seizure control and behavior, even if not in language and cognitive skills. The appropriate timing of the surgical intervention and its long versus short term effects on neuropsychological outcome remain to be studied, as well as its possible application to other situations, for example cryptogenic frontal epilepsy with CSWS. When considering epilepsy surgery in a child with an autistic regression, it is crucial to separate indications for control of refractory seizures from indications that mainly target cognitive and behavioral improvement. There is hardly any experience with the latter, and there is still no published study with prospectively obtained pre- and postoperative data that shows convincing results (Lewine et al. 1999, Nass et al. 1999). In our opinion, this type of surgery should be considered only with great caution in tertiary centers with special expertise in the care of childhood epilepsy and in developmental assessment, because a standard presurgical epilepsy work-up is clearly insufficient for such unusual cases.

(c) Dubious cases

These encompass mainly children with an ASD and epileptic discharges who have no seizures, because those who have seizures will usually require standard antiepileptic medication. The histories of such children usually reveal cognitive stagnation rather than regression. The abnormal electrical activity may be quite sustained and involve both hemispheres. It seems to us that the best option is to carry out a detailed baseline neuro-psychological evaluation, if possible video-taped, that includes appropriate questionnaires on autistic and other behaviors. This evaluation must then be repeated after an interval (e.g. 3–6 months) with an EEG recorded under the same conditions, in order to be able to appreciate the dynamics of the developmental problem and of the EEG abnormalities. Depending on the evolution, a trial with an antiepileptic drug directed at stopping the discharges can be offered, with the understanding that serial neuropsychological and EEG follow-ups and regular reconsideration of the effects of the treatment will be required. In judging the effect of the treatment, it should be kept in mind that antiepileptic drugs may have a direct psychotropic effect on the autistic symptoms (Tuchman 2004). Escalation of antiepileptic drug dosage and the use of steroids have little place except in carefully considered situations.

CONCLUSION

The possibility of an epileptic disorder must be considered in every child with an ASD, especially if there is a history of regression, even though this possibility will be discarded in the majority of cases. There is no evidence for a causal role of epilepsy in children with a typical picture of an "idiopathic" ASD, even in those with a history of regression that occurred in the second year of life. In these children, who are often first seen after 3 years of age, a screening EEG is no longer considered mandatory. One does need to keep in mind that an epileptic disorder can bring out an ASD if the underlying lesion is strategic-ally located in a network supporting social and emotional development. In view of our limited knowledge, dogmatic attitudes that state either that epileptic spikes cause autistic regression or that epileptic spikes are only markers for an abnormal brain are unwarranted. These attitudes are not helpful and make us run the risk of dismissing the truly infor-mative cases that do not conform to either of these views. There is currently no scientif-ically based evidence for the routine administration of antiepileptic therapy in autistic regression or DD. It may be that careful analysis will identify a small subgroup of children with atypical clinical features who may turn out to have an autistic regression or a DD of epileptic origin, with or without clinical seizures. Such children may benefit from antiepileptic treatment. Dubious cases must be evaluated carefully and followed diligently for a period of time prior to any attempt at treatment. They must be re-evaluated repeatedly with a critical eye. Such cases require detailed prospective studies that combine electrophysiological, structural, neuropsychological and psychiatric approaches if a consensus on a rational approach to their management is to be reached.

REFERENCES

Allman JM, Watson KK, Tetreault NA, Hakeem AY (2005) Intuition and autism: a possible role for Von Economo neurons. *Trends Cogn Sci* 9: 367–73.

Asano E, Chugani DC, Muzik O, Behen M, Janisse J, Rothermel R, Mangner TJ, Chakraborty PK, Chugani HT (2001) Autism in tuberous sclerosis complex is related to both cortical and sub-cortical dysfunction. *Neurology* 57: 1269–77.

Baird G, Robinson R (2000) Sleep EEGs in children under 48 months with autism but without epilepsy. *Dev Med Child Neurol* 42 Suppl. 85: 12 (abstract).

Bednarek N, Motte J, Soufflet C, Plouin P, Dulac O (1998) Evidence for late infantile spasms. *Epilepsia* 39: 55–60.

Berkovic SF (2003) Hypothalamic hamartoma and seizures. A treatable epileptic encephalopathy. *Epilepsia* 44: 969–73.

Besag FM (2004) Behavioral aspects of pediatric epilepsy syndromes. *Epilepsy Behav* 5 Suppl. 1: S3–13.

Bolton PF, Park RJ, Higgins JN, Griffiths PD, Pickles A (2002) Neuro-epileptic determinants of autism spectrum disorders in tuberous sclerosis complex. *Brain* 125: 1247–55.

Bolton PF (2004) Neuroepileptic correlates of autistic symptomatology in tuberous sclerosis. *Ment Retard Dev Disabil Res Rev* 10: 126–31.

Dalla Bernardina B, Fontana E, Zullini E, Avesani E, Zoccante L, Perez Jimenez A, Giardina L (1994) Unusual partial complex status with autisticlike behavior in infancy. *Epilepsia* 35 Suppl 7: 43 (abstract).

DeLong GR, Heinz ER (1997) The clinical syndrome of early life bilateral hippocampal sclerosis. *Ann Neurol* 42: 11–7.

Deonna T, Roulet-Perez E (2005) *Cognitive and Behavioural Disorders of Epileptic Origin in Children. Clinics in Developmental Medicine No. 168.* London: Mac Keith Press.

Deonna T, Ziegler AL (2000) Hypothalamic hamartoma, precocious puberty and gelastic seizures: a special model of "epileptic" developmental disorder. *Epileptic Disord* 2: 33–7.

Deonna T, Ziegler AL, Moura-Serra J, Innocenti G (1993) Autistic regression in relation to limbic pathology and epilepsy: report of two cases. *Dev Med Child Neurol* 35: 166–76.

Deonna T, Ziegler AL, Maeder IM, Ansermet F, Roulet E (1995) Reversible behavioural autistic-like regression: a manifestation of a special (new?) epileptic syndrome in a 28-month-old child. A 2-year longitudinal study. *Neurocase* 1: 91–9.

Deonna T, Fohlen,M, Jalin C, Delalande O, Ziegler AL (2002) Epileptic stereotypies in children. In: Guerrini R, Aicardi J, Andermann F, Hallett M, eds. *Epilepsy and Movement Disorders.* Cambridge: Cambridge University Press, pp. 319–32.

Deonna T, Ziegler AL, Roulet-Perez E (2003) Acquired epileptic frontal syndrome in children. In: Beaumanoir A, Andermann F, Chauvel P, Mira L, Zifkin B, eds. *Frontal Lobe Seizures and Epilepsies in Children.* Montrouge, France: John Libbey Eurotext, pp. 133–46.

Fohlen M, Bulteau C, Jalin C, Jambaque I, Delalande O (2004) Behavioural epileptic seizures: a clinical and intracranial EEG study in 8 children with frontal lobe epilepsy. *Neuropediatrics* 35: 336–45.

Gillberg C, Schaumann H (1983) Epilepsy presenting as infantile autism? Two case studies. *Neuropediatrics* 14: 206–12.

Gillberg C, Uvebrant P, Carlsson G, Heditorström A, Silfvenius H (1996) Autism and epilepsy (and tuberous sclerosis?) in two pre-adolescent boys: neuropsychiatric aspects before and after epilepsy surgery. *J Intellect Disabil Res* 40: 75–81.

Grote CL, Van Slyke P, Hoeppner JA (1999) Language outcome following multiple subpial transection for Landau–Kleffner syndrome. *Brain* 122: 561–6.

Hashimoto T, Sasaki M, Sugai K, Hanakoa S, Fukumizu M, Kato T (2001) Paroxysmal discharges on EEG in young autistic patients are frequent in frontal regions. *J Med Invest* 48: 175–80.

Hill AE, Rosenbloom L (1986) Disintegrative psychosis of childhood: teenage follow-up. *Dev Med Child Neurol* 28: 34–40.

Hoon AH, Reiss AL (1992) The mesial-temporal lobe and autism: case report and review. *Dev Med Child Neurol* 34: 252–9.

Irwin K, Birch V, Lees J, Polkey C, Alarcon G, Binnie C, Smedley M, Baird G, Robinson RO (2001) Multiple subpial transection in Landau–Kleffner syndrome. *Dev Med Child Neurol* 43: 248–52.

Jacobs R, Anderson V, Harvey AS (2001) Neuropsychological profile of a 9-year-old child with subcortical band heterotopia or "double cortex". *Dev Med Child Neurol* 43: 628–33.

Kyllerman M, Nyden A, Prauin N, Rasmussen P, Wetterquist AK, Hedström A (1996) Transient psychosis in a girl with epilepsy and continuous spikes and waves during slow sleep (CSWS). *Eur Child Adolesc Psychiatry* 5: 216–21.

Laan LA, Renier WO, Aarts WF, Buntinx IM, Burgt IJ, Stroink H, Beuten J, Zwinderman KH, van Dijk JG, Brouwer OF (1997) Evolution of epilepsy and EEG findings in Angelman syndrome. *Epilepsia* 38: 195–9.

Levisohn PM (2004) Electroencephalographic findings in autism: similarities and differnces from Landau–Kleffner syndrome. *Semin Pediatr Neurol* 11: 218–24.

Lewine JD, Andrews R, Chez M, Patil AA, Devinsky O, Smith M, Kanner A, Davis JT, Funke M, Jones G, Chong B, Provencal S, Weisend M, Lee R, Orrison WW (1999) Magnetoencephalographic patterns of epileptiform activity in children with regressive autism spectrum disorder. *Pediatrics* 104: 405–18.

McVicar KA, Ballaban-Gil K, Rapin I, Moshé SL, Shinnar S (2005) Epileptiform EEG abnormalities in children with language regression. *Neurology* 65: 129–31.

Mouridsen SE, Rich B, Isager T (1999) Epilepsy in disintegrative disorder and infantile autism: a long-term validation study. *Dev Med Child Neurol* 41: 110–4.

Muhle R, Trentacoste SV, Rapin I (2004) The genetics of autism. *Pediatrics* 113: 472–86.

Mundy P (2003) The neural basis of social impairments in autism: the role of the dorsal medial–frontal cortex and anterior cingulated system. *J Child Psychol Psychiatry* 44: 793–809.

Nass R, Gross A, Wisoff J, Devinsky O (1999) Outcome of multiple subpial transections for autistic epileptiform regression. *Pediatr Neurol* 21: 464–70.

Neville BGR, Harkness WFJ, Cross JH, Cass HC, Burch VC, Lees JA, Taylor DC (1997) Surgical treatment of severe autistic regression in childhood epilepsy. *Pediatr Neurol* 16: 137–40.

O'Regan ME, Brown JK, Goodwin GM, Clarke M (1998) Epileptic aphasia: a consequence of regional hypometabolic encephalopathy? *Dev Med Child Neurol* 40: 508–16.

Pearl PL, Gibson KM, Acosta MT, Vezina LG, Theodore WH, Rogawski MA, Novotny EJ, Gropman A, Conry JA, Berry GT, Tuchman M (2003) Clinical spectrum of succinic semialdehyde dehydrogenase deficiency. *Neurology* 60: 1413–7.

Perez-Jimenez A, Villarejo FJ, Fournier del Castillo MC, Garcia-Penas JJ, Carreno M (2003) Continuous giggling and autistic disorder associated with hypothalamic hamartoma. *Epileptic Disord* 5: 31–7.

Plioplys AV (1994) Autism: electroencephalogram abnormalities and clinical improvement with valproic acid. *Arch Pediatr Adolesc Med* 148: 220–2.

Rapin I (1991) Autistic children: Diagnosis and clinical features. *Pediatrics* 87: 751–60.

Rapin I (1995) Autistic regression and disintegrative disorder: how important the role of epilepsy? *Semin Pediatr Neurol* 2: 278–85.

Roulet-Perez E, Davidoff V, Despland PA, Deonna T (1993) Mental and behavioural deterioration of children with epilepsy and CSWS: acquired epileptic frontal syndrome. *Dev Med Child Neurol* 35: 661–74.

Roulet Perez E, Davidoff V, Prélaz AC, Morel B, Rickli F, Metz-Lutz MN, Boyes Braem P, Deonna

T (2001) Sign language in childhood epileptic aphasia (Landau–Kleffner syndrome). *Dev Med Child Neurol* 43: 739–44.

Szabo CA, Wyllie E, Dolske M, Stanford LD, Kotagal P, Comair YG (1999) Epilepsy surgery in children with pervasive developmental disorder. *Pediatr Neurol* 20: 349–53.

Tuchman R (2003) Autism. *Neurol Clin* 21: 915–32.

Tuchman R (2004) AEDs and psychotropic drugs in children with autism and epilepsy. *Ment Retard Dev Disabil Res Rev* 10: 135–8.

Tuchman R, Rapin I (1997) Regression in pervasive developmental disorders: seizures and epileptiform electroencephalographic correlates. *Pediatrics* 99: 560–6.

Tuchman R, Rapin I (2002) Epilepsy in autism. *Lancet Neuro* 1: 352–8.

Uldall P, Sahlholdt L, Alving J (2000) Landau–Kleffner syndrome with onset at 18 months and an initial diagnosis of pervasive developmental disorder. *Eur J Paediatr Neurol* 4: 81–6.

Van Landingham KE, Heinz ER, Cavazos JE, Lewis DV (1998) Magnetic resonance imaging evidence of hippocampal injury after prolonged focal febrile convulsions. *Ann Neurol* 43: 413–26.

Volkmar FR, Nelson DS (1990) Seizure disorder in autism. *J Am Acad Child Adolesc Psychiatry* 29: 127–9.

Zappella M (2005) The question of reversible autistic behavior in autism. In: Coleman M, ed. *The Neurology of Autism.* Oxford: Oxford University Press, pp. 157–72.

12

SLEEP AND AUTISM SPECTRUM DISORDERS

Beth A Malow and Susan G McGrew

Disordered sleep affects daytime health and behavioral functioning in a variety of neurologic and psychiatric conditions. Sleep disorders lead to a multitude of secondary behavioral effects that affect both the individual and the family (Christodulu and Durand 2004). Daytime sleepiness resulting from disrupted sleep often manifests itself in typically developing children as hyperactivity, inattention and aggression (Owens et al. 1998). Those with autism spectrum disorders (ASDs or "autism") may be at even higher risk for sleep disorders given the overlaps of the neurobiology of sleep and ASDs (see Chapter 15). Behaviors inherent to ASDs, such as impairments in communication and stereotypies and, even more so, aggression and hyperactivity may be exacerbated by sleepiness and interfere with the child's ability to function optimally.

NEUROBIOLOGY OF SLEEP AS RELATED TO ASDs
The complex regulation of the sleep–wake cycle involves coordinated neuronal activity in the hypothalamus, brainstem, thalamus and cortex. Several neurotransmitter systems implicated in promoting sleep and establishing a regular sleep-wake cycle are also affected by autism, and their aberrations in autism may be responsible for a component of the prevalent sleep disturbances of autism. These neurotransmitter systems include gamma-aminobutyric acid (GABA), serotonin and melatonin (see Chapter 6).

The preoptic area of the hypothalamus is a major sleep-promoting system that uses GABA as a neurotransmitter. Sleep-active neurons in the preoptic area project to brainstem regions that contain neurons involved in arousal from sleep, and inhibiting these regions in turn promotes sleep. These regions include the pedunculopontine and laterodorsal tegmental nuclei (PPT/LDT), the locus coeruleus, and the dorsal raphe (Saper et al. 2001). In autism, GABAergic interneurons appear disrupted (Levitt et al. 2004), and a genetic susceptibility region has been identified on chromosome 15q that contains GABA-related genes (McCauley et al. 2004). The expression of these autism susceptibility genes may affect sleep by interfering with the normal inhibitory function of GABA via the preoptic area neurons.

Serotonin may promote sleep by dampening systems that normally stimulate cortical activation and arousal, such as the cholinergic system. Serotonin may also be responsible for stimulating the accumulation of other sleep factors in the anterior hypothalamus (Jones 2005). Abnormalities in serotonin synthesis, metabolism or transport, reported in autism, may influence the physiological effects of serotonin on sleep promotion (Chugani 2004).

Related but separate to the promotion of sleep is the regulation of sleep–wake cycles by the circadian system. Light received via the retinohypothalamic tract to the suprachiasmatic nucleus in the anterior hypothalamus synchronizes the sleep-wake cycles to the environment. Melatonin, a sleep promoting substance released by the pineal gland, is inhibited by light (Gooley and Saper 2005). Decreased nocturnal excretion of 6-sulfatoxymelatonin, the major metabolite of melatonin, has been observed in children with ASD compared to non-autistic children (Tordjman et al. 2005).

The abnormalities in GABA, serotonin and melatonin production in ASD, along with accumulating evidence of clinical sleep and circadian disturbances (see below), provide evidence for involvement of the neurobiological networks regulating sleep in autism. Investigations linking these neurotransmitter abnormalities to the severity of sleep disturbances in ASD have yet to be investigated. Whether subsets of children with ASD who have clinical abnormalities in their sleep–wake cycle are more likely to exhibit abnormalities in sleep-related neurotransmitters remains to be determined.

PREVALENCE AND SPECTRUM OF SLEEP ABNORMALITIES IN ASDs
The prevalence of parentally reported sleep problems in typically developing children in kindergarten through fourth grade was 37% in one study (Owens et al. 2000b). In another study of typically developing 4- to 12-year-olds derived from routine pediatric practices, approximately 11% of parents surveyed reported a sleep problem in their child (Stein et al. 2001). Evidence from parental surveys and polysomnographic (sleep) studies suggests that sleep disorders are more common in children with autism, with prevalence rates ranging from 44% to 83% (Richdale 1999), and vary in type.

Symptoms of insomnia, defined as difficulty initiating or maintaining sleep, are the major sleep concerns reported by parents of children with ASD. Questionnaires and/or sleep diaries completed by parents of children with ASD and those of age-matched typical children are consistent in documenting that the children with ASD are more likely to exhibit insomnia with prolonged time to fall asleep, decreased sleep duration and continuity with increased awakenings, and, in some reports, early morning wake time (Hoshino et al. 1984, Richdale and Prior 1995, Patzold et al. 1998, Stores and Wiggs 1998, Hering et al. 1999, Richdale 1999, Honomichl et al. 2002, Wiggs and Stores 2004, Williams et al. 2004). "Difficulty falling asleep" was reported in 53% of children with ASD in one series (Williams et al. 2004). In another series of children with ASD, 55% had "difficulty falling asleep" and 26% had "difficulty staying asleep" (Wiggs and Stores, 2004). Abnormalities in development of the sleep–wake cycle, with irregular bedtime and waking times (Segawa et al. 1992) and a non-24-hour sleep–wake ("freerunning") syndrome, in which no semblance of a consistent bedtime and waking time is present (Takase et al. 1998), have also been reported (see Chapter 15 for examples of polysomnograms illustrating this problem).

Other sleep concerns these parents reported included symptoms of disordered breathing with loud snoring or noisy breathing and occasional pauses or apneas in breathing, leg movements and bruxism (tooth grinding). They also described arousals from sleep with confusion, wandering or screaming. Many mentioned daytime sleepiness, the consequence of insufficient sleep, a specific sleep disorder, or in some cases over-medication. Restless sleep, another parental concern, does not always signal a sleep disorder as it can arise from any medical or other condition that affects sleep. Bedtime resistance or night-time fears also contribute to sleep concerns in this population.

Although the degree of mental retardation tends to predict sleep abnormalities across most developmental disabilities, the level of mental retardation does not appear to affect the prevalence or severity of disordered sleep in ASD (Patzold et al. 1998, Richdale 1999). In one study, children with ASD and low IQs had more night wakings (Williams et al. 2004), although other sleep parameters were not affected. In one series, parents of younger children (less than 8 years) reported more severe sleep concerns (Richdale and Prior 1995), which was not the case in a larger series that also compared children younger and older than 8 years, with the one exception that behavioral sleep problems including limit-setting sleep disorder and sleep-onset association disorder were more common in the younger group (Wiggs and Stores 2004). This discrepancy may be due to differences in methodology as well as heterogeneity among participants.

CAUSES OF SLEEP CONCERNS IN AUTISM

Insomnia, daytime sleepiness and other types of sleep concerns have a variety of biological and behavioral causes (Table 12.1). Which of these causes are most implicated in autism is under intensive study. Challenges to answering this question include differences in the relative contribution of these causes in individual children with autism, and also that the causes of insomnia in any given child are likely to be multifactorial. Targeting effective treatment strategies is dependent on understanding the cause(s) of the disordered sleep, therefore further research is paramount.

Insomnia, defined as difficulty initiating or maintaining sleep, may result from co-existing psychiatric conditions such as anxiety or depression, as well as from the psychotropic medications often used to treat these conditions. Hyperactivity may also contribute to difficulty falling asleep. Children may lie awake for hours vocalizing or engaging in a repetitive behavior that interferes with sleep initiation. Whether these activities are the manifestations of anxiety, stereotypies, or simply habits is uncertain, although treatment with anxiolytics is often helpful. Depression may be manifested by early morning waking, and bipolar disorder by decreased need for sleep. While some psychotropic medications promote sleep through their treatment of anxiety or depression as well as through sedating effects, others like fluoxetine are highly stimulating and can interfere with sleep onset or maintenance (Schwietzer 2005). Coexisting epilepsy or its treatment

TABLE 12.1
Causes of sleep disturbance in autism

Insomnia
- Anxiety
- Depression
- Psychotropic medications
- Coexisting epilepsy
- Obstructive sleep apnea
- Periodic limb movements of sleep
- Circadian rhythm abnormalities
- Poor sleep habits
- Hypersensitivity to environmental stimuli

Daytime sleepiness
- Insufficient sleep
- Disrupted sleep from a primary sleep disorder
- Depression
- Epileptic seizures
- Medications
- Narcolepsy

Nocturnal events
- Epileptic seizures
- Non-REM arousal disorders
- REM behavior disorder
- Rhythmic movement disorder

may also disrupt sleep (Malow 2004). Medications used to treat epilepsy are usually sleep-promoting, but some like lamotrigine and felbamate may be stimulating, prolong sleep latency, and promote night wakings. Other causes of insomnia in autism include primary sleep disorders such as obstructive sleep apnea or periodic limb movements of sleep.

Circadian abnormalities have been postulated to occur in ASD, and can result in a delay in falling asleep, early morning awakening, or an irregular, shortened or lengthened sleep–wake cycle. Melatonin secretion is abnormally low in ASD (Nir et al. 1995, Tordjman et al. 2005), and exogenous melatonin given prior to bedtime decreased sleep latency in ASD in one open-label study (Paavonen et al. 2003), although it is unclear whether melatonin acted simply as a hypnotic or was resetting the circadian clock. Further study will be necessary to determine how important circadian factors are in autism.

Daytime sleepiness in typically developing children most commonly results from either inadequate sleep due to insomnia or poor sleep habits, or disrupted sleep due to primary sleep disorders such as obstructive sleep apnea. Narcolepsy is less common and may present with associated cataplexy (loss of muscle tone provoked by emotion), sleep paralysis and sleep-related hallucinations. Daytime sleepiness in children with ASD may occur from the same causes or from a coexisting conditions, including depression, epileptic seizures and medications.

Nocturnal events need to be distinguished from epileptic seizures in this population, given the increased prevalence of epilepsy in autism (Tuchman and Rapin 2002). Such events include the non-REM (rapid eye movement) arousal disorders, REM sleep behavior disorder, and rhythmic movement disorder. Nocturnal events can usually be distinguished by history, although video-EEG polysomnography in a sleep center is occasionally warranted. One of the cardinal distinguishing features of epileptic seizures is their stereotyped appearance, as well as the presence of tonic or dystonic limb posturing.

The *non-REM arousal disorders* consist of a spectrum of events of aberrant arousal arising from non-REM sleep stages 3 and 4 (deep) sleep, ranging from confusional arousals to sleepwalking to night terrors. There is often a family history of similar spells in parents or siblings, supporting a genetic predisposition. Precipitants include sleep deprivation, emotional stress, medical illness, and other conditions that contribute to disruption of normal sleeping patterns (Mahowald and Bornemann 2005).

In *REM sleep behavior disorder*, individuals "act out their dreams" due to an interruption of physiological muscle atonia during REM sleep. This disorder has been reported in one case series of children with ASD reported to have disrupted sleep who were studied with polysomnography (Thirumalai et al. 2002). REM sleep behavior disorder is usually associated with older age and has been related to degeneration of dopaminergic neurons in the substantia nigra, a subcortical region involved in motor control (see Chapter 15). REM sleep behavior disorder can also occur in association with psychotropic medications that affect REM sleep, such as the selective serotonin reuptake inhibitors (Mahowald and Schenck 2005). Related abnormalities, such as increased phasic muscle activity in REM sleep in mentally retarded individuals with autism (Diomedi et al. 1999), raise the possibility that neurostructural or neurochemical abnormalities involving the brainstem or subcortical regions may be associated with autism. If borne out in future investigations, the presence of REM sleep behavior in autism may provide valuable clues to the etiology of ASD.

Rhythmic movement disorder is characterized by repetitive motion of the head (including head banging), trunk or limbs, usually during the transition from wakefulness to sleep (Hoban 2003). It may also arise during sustained sleep. Although the condition most often affects infants and toddlers in a transient and self-limited fashion, it may persist in children with autism and other developmental disabilities.

IMPACT ON DAYTIME BEHAVIOR

In autism, short sleep duration has been associated with stereotypic behavior, as well as inflated overall autism scores and social skills deficits (Schreck et al. 2004). As association between sleep problems and repetitive behaviors (stereotyped, self-injurious, compulsive, ritualistic, restricted) and craving for sameness was reported in a cohort of children with autism (Gabriels et al. 2005), although this association may have been moderated by their

TABLE 12.2
Strategies for improving sleep in children with autism

Take a sleep history to identify treatable sleep disorders and consider polysomnography when appropriate

Behavioral treatments
• Sleep hygiene, e.g. avoidance of caffeine, engaging in regular exercise, having a bedtime routine
• Sleep restriction
• Extinction (training children to fall asleep on their own)

Pharmacologic treatments
• Antiepileptic drugs
• Antidepressants
• Other medications (e.g. clonidine)
• Melatonin

Light therapy

level of cognitive ability. Behavioral treatment of sleep problems in children with intellectual disabilities and challenging daytime behavior reduces parental stress, increases parents' satisfaction with their own and their child's sleep, and heightens their sense of control and ability to cope with their child's sleep (Wiggs and Stores 2004).

Treatment of a sleep disorder may improve daytime behavior. Associations between disordered breathing in sleep and aberrant daytime behaviors such as hyperactivity and aggressiveness are well documented in typically developing children (Chervin et al. 2002, Gottlieb et al. 2003), with improvement in problem behaviors after adenotonsillectomy (Goldstein et al. 2002). We evaluated a girl with ASD and obstructive sleep apnea whose sleep apnea was treated with adenotonsillectomy (Malow et al. 2006). Although she still retained her autism diagnosis on the Autism Diagnostic Observation Schedule (ADOS; Lord et al. 2000), her performance on this test and the Child Behavior Checklist (Achenbach and Rescorla 2001) documented improvement in a variety of domains, including social interaction and ability to focus.

EVALUATION AND TREATMENT OF SLEEP DISORDERS IN AUTISM

Defining the cause of the sleep disturbance is critical to appropriate intervention. For example, insomnia due to poor sleep hygiene may be responsive to behavioral interventions; insomnia due to impaired circadian control of sleep may be responsive to treatment with supplemental melatonin or other therapies that target the circadian cycle; daytime sleepiness due to obstructive sleep apnea should respond to treatment with adenotonsillectomy or other therapies; and nocturnal events due to epileptic seizures should respond to antiepileptic drugs. Table 12.2 outlines effective strategies in treating children with autism who have sleep disorders.

First, one should take a sleep history and refer for polysomnography or actigraphy as indicated. The sleep history should include the bed time, waking time, and any waking during the night, with estimated durations and associated behaviors. Daytime functioning should be assessed, including hyperactivity as well as sleepiness and daytime naps. Parents should be encouraged to keep a sleep diary to assess sleep latency, total sleep time, night wakings, and response to treatment. A sleep questionnaire such as the Children's Sleep Habits Questionnaire (Owens et al. 2000a) is a useful adjunctive tool to assess multiple domains of sleep problems including sleep-related breathing disorders, sleep anxiety, bedtime resistance and daytime sleepiness. A behavioral rating scale such as the Child Behavior Checklist (Achenbach and Rescorla 2001) will screen other behavioral domains including mood, anxiety, aggression and hyperactivity, which may impact sleep. When appropriate, a psychiatric evaluation to assess for bipolar disorder, depression or anxiety disorder should be obtained, as all of these conditions can affect sleep.

Treatable conditions such as sleep-related breathing disorders, restless legs syndrome, seizures or narcolepsy should be sought. Ask parents about the presence of snoring, apnea, snorting or gasping, sweating, screaming, or excessive leg movements or activity. Refer for *polysomnography* (PSG) if there is a concern for sleep-related breathing disorder or sleep-related seizures. A multiple sleep latency test may be performed the morning after polysomnography to assess objectively daytime sleepiness and symptoms of narcolepsy. In children diagnosed with obstructive sleep apnea, tonsillectomy and adenoidectomy is the first line of therapy. If symptoms persist or surgery is not an option, the child may be a candidate for continuous positive airway pressure (CPAP), which overcomes the upper airway obstruction with pressurized air delivered through a mask. Desensitization of patients to CPAP is required and can be achieved, often in conjunction with a respiratory therapist.

Actigraphy represents an alternative to PSG for documenting sleep disturbances in children with autism. In actigraphy, the child wears an activity meter on the wrist that quantifies movement and rest, which serve as surrogates of activity and sleep. Actigraphy is more convenient and less intrusive and expensive than PSG, and data can be collected for multiple nights (Ancoli-Israel et al. 2003). Although characterized as an objective measure of the rest (sleep)–activity (wake) cycle, actigraphy has its limitations in that periods of quiet wakefulness may be interpreted by the device as sleep, and periods of restless sleep may be interpreted by the device as wakefulness. Therefore, data from actigraphy is best interpreted in the context of sleep diaries (Sadeh and Acebo 2002). Simultaneous measurement of actigraphy and in-home or in-laboratory PSG can provide additional validation within an individual by assisting in the interpretation of periods of quiet wakefulness or restless sleep, and thereby improve the interpretation of multiple nights of actigraphy not accompanied by PSG.

Evaluate for behavioral causes of insomnia and educate parents on behavioral strategies to promote sleep. Sleep hygiene (habit) problems should be identified, and parents educated to pay attention to basic principles of sleep hygiene, including daytime exercise, a regular and consistent bedtime, a consistent bed that is not used for other activities (e.g. TV viewing or time-out), a structured calming bedtime routine, and dim evening lights. Caffeine (e.g. cola drinks) and stimulating activities should be avoided in the hour before bedtime. Discourage the use of sleep aids such as falling asleep with the TV on or with parents in physical contact. These sleep aids may promote sleep at bedtime but also contribute to night wakings – when the television or parent is not present, a brief arousal from sleep may become a prolonged night waking. The challenges of being a parent of a child with ASD may interfere with having the time and energy to teach a child to fall asleep on his or her own, and return to sleep with minimal assistance once awakened.

Teach parents how to teach their children to fall asleep on their own by helping the child settle into a relaxed state and by providing no stimulation or reinforcement for re-sisting sleep. Limiting daytime naps may also be effective in promoting more consolidated sleep at night. Visual supports showing what is expected of the child are a critical part of this approach in autism. A visual schedule for the bedtime routine and visual "back to bed" reminders on the door will communicate to the child the parental expectations. The child should be trained to follow the visual schedule after a cue from parents. This may be accomplished using physical prompts. Morning reinforcers (e.g. wrapped presents) for successfully meeting expectations may be incorporated into the routine. If the child has anxiety about falling asleep alone, parents may temporarily set up a bed or rocking chair next to the child's bed. No physical contact or eye contact should be made during this phase of treatment. The rocking chair can be gradually moved closer to the door on successive nights until it is through the door. Difficulty initiating sleep may also result from hypersensitivity to environmental stimuli, including noises in the bedroom or elsewhere in the home, or tactile hypersensitivity to bedclothes or blankets. Weighted blankets may sometimes be helpful in children with tactile sensitivities.

Pharmacologic Treatment

When behavioral therapies are ineffective, pharmacologic treatment can be considered, although this is not always necessary. There is a wide range of options for pharmacologic treatment, best used in conjunction with the behavioral techniques just described, and tailored to the cause of the individual child's sleep problem. With all medications, it is important to start with low doses and increase gradually, monitoring carefully for adverse effects as children with autism may be sensitive to certain classes of medications and unable to communicate side-effects.

Behavioral or Circadian Rhythm Sleep Disorders

If the sleep problem is primarily behavioral involving sleep initiation, or is circadian involving phase shift problems, a combination of sleep hygiene and melatonin may be useful. Synthetic melatonin, available as a dietary supplement, has a gentle sleep-pro-moting effect when used in combination with sleep hygiene and evening light dimming. Melatonin has been effective in open-label trials of sleep promotion in Asperger syn-drome, with a dose of 3 mg at bedtime decreasing sleep latency as measured by actigraphy

(Paavonen et al. 2003). Although melatonin's half life is less than an hour, in a subset of patients the onset of effect may be delayed for up to 1–2 hours. Therefore, it is recommended that melatonin initially be given 30 minutes before the desired bedtime, and moved to an earlier time depending on the onset of effect. Doses as low as 300 µg are physiologic and may be effective at promoting sleep, although doses of 1–3 mg are more sedating and more commonly used. Dosage may be started at 300 µg and rapidly titrated up to 3 mg if needed. Rarely, doses of up to 6 mg are needed. Oral melatonin is rapidly metabolized, and extended release melatonin, also available over the counter, may be necessary for the child with sleep maintenance difficulties. Once a sleep cycle is established for 6 weeks or more, the melatonin may be discontinued, although long term use is occasionally necessary to maintain the sleep cycle. Although melatonin is a dietary supplement, is not approved by the US Food and Drug Administration, and has not been rigorously tested for safety, efficacy or purity of preparation, no serious long term adverse effects have been seen in this widely used supplement. Clonidine is also useful for sleep initiation problems in the child who is mildly anxious or overaroused at night. Diphenhydramine and the benzodiazepines are other options.

PSYCHIATRIC OR NEUROLOGIC DISORDERS IMPACTING SLEEP

A helpful principle for prescribing sleep medications in children with coexisting neurologic or psychiatric disorders is to consider the overlapping neurological systems that are affected. Wherever possible, prescribe a medication for the coexisting condition that also assists with sleep, while avoiding those that cause insomnia. In children with coexisting epilepsy or bipolar disorder, mood stabilizing antiepileptics with sedating properties can be used. The antiepileptic regimen can be adjusted to administer a bedtime dose of medication that provides sedation and promotes sleep. Options include carbamazepine, levatiracetam, gabapentin or topiramate, which are usually dosed two or three times a day but can be adjusted to give the higher dose at bedtime. Valproic acid comes in an extended release form that can be given once a day, at bedtime. Lamotrigine tends to be more stimulating and may interfere with sleep, but may be an excellent choice in children with daytime sleepiness.

Children with comorbid bipolar disorder, extreme mood irritability, aggression or self-injurious behavior may benefit from treatment with the sedating atypical neuroleptics such as risperidone, olanzapine or quetiapine. The dosages of these medications can be adjusted to give the higher dose at bedtime.

In the anxious or depressed child, specific antidepressants that promote sleep may be considered. These include the highly sedating drugs mirtazapine, trazadone (should be avoided in males who cannot communicate reliably because of the risk of priapism), the mildly sedating selective serotonin reuptake inhibitor (SSRI) citralopram, and the tricyclic antidepressants (such as clomipramine, imipramine and nortryptilline). The sedating SSRIs or tricyclic antidepressants may also be useful for children with obsessional thoughts that interfere with sleep onset. Bupropion, venlafaxine, fluoxetine and sertraline are relatively stimulating and should be avoided in those with insomnia and reserved for those with daytime sleepiness without insomnia.

LIGHT THERAPY

Light therapy may be useful for children with circadian rhythm abnormalities in combination with chronotherapy, where the sleep–wake cycle is delayed over the course of several days until the desired bedtime is reached. Bright light administered in the morning "resets" the circadian clock and facilitates an earlier bedtime (Chesson et al. 1999). Although no definitive studies have been performed in autism, light of 2500 lux administered for 1–2 hours in the morning is recommended and is safe, based on experience from the pediatric seasonal affective disorder literature (Swedo et al. 1997). Dosage may be increased by 1000 lux every three days to a maximum of 10,000 lux. Lower dosages may require the longer treatment times. Cautions include the small risk of precipitating a manic episode in coexisting or unrecognized bipolar disorder (Schwitzer et al. 1990) and the risk of a photosensitivity reaction (usually precipitated by UV light exposure) (Bickers 2001). If a child has a photosensitizing condition or is taking photo-sensitizing medications (such as tetracyclines, sulfonamides, nonsteroidal anti-inflam-matory agents, and phenothiazines), the risk–benefit should be carefully weighed and a non-UV emitting light source should be used. There are several commercial light boxes available. An alternative to purchasing a commercial light box is for the patient to get exposed to bright light each morning. Adherence to sleep hygiene measures including a strict bedtime and wake time routine is necessary to prevent the return of a delayed bedtime. Close follow-up is recommended in children receiving light therapy to prevent relapse.

CONCLUSIONS

Sleep concerns are common in children with autism, with a variety of behavioral, phar-macological and other options for therapy. The cornerstone of treatment is to establish the etiology of the sleep concern, which is often multifactorial. Identifying and treating sleep disorders may result not only in more consolidated sleep, more rapid time to fall asleep, and avoidance of night wakings, but also impact favorably on daytime behavior.

ACKNOWLEDGMENTS

This work was funded by a Vanderbilt University Interdisciplinary Discovery Grant and by the Vanderbilt General Clinical Research Center (M01 RR-00095 from the National Center for Research Resources, National Institutes of Health).

REFERENCES

Achenbach TM, Rescorla LA (2001) *Manual for the ASEBA Preschool Forms and Profiles.* Burlington, VT: University of Vermont, Research Center for Children, Youth, and Families.
Ancoli-Israel S, Cole R, Alessi C, Chambers M, Moorcroft W, Pollak CP (2003) The role of actigraphy in the study of sleep and circadian rhythms. *Sleep* 26: 342–92.

Bickers DR (2001) Photosensitivity and other reactions to light. In: Braunwald E, Fauci AS, Kasper DL, Hauser SL, Longo DL, Jameson JL, eds. *Harrison's Principles of Internal Medicine, 15th edn.* New York: McGraw-Hill, pp. 345–7.

Chervin RD, Archbold KH, Dillon JE, Panahi P, Pituch KJ, Dahl RE, Guilleminault C (2002) Inattention, hyperactivity, and symptoms of sleep-disordered breathing. *Pediatrics* 109: 449–56.

Chesson AL, Littner M, Davila D, Anderson WM, Grigg-Damberger M, Harlse K, Johnson S, Wise M (1999) Practice parameters for the use of light therapy in the treatment of sleep disorders. *Sleep* 22: 641–60.

Christodulu KV, Durand VM (2004) Reducing bedtime disturbance and night waking using positive bedtime routines and sleep restriction. *Focus Autism Dev Disabil* 19: 130–9.

Chugani DC (2004) Serotonin in autism and pediatric epilepsies. *Ment Retard Dev Disabil Res Rev* 10: 112–6.

Diomedi M, Curatolo P, Scalise A, Placidi F, Caretto F, Gigli GL (1999) Sleep abnormalities in mentally retarded autistic subjects: Down's syndrome with mental retardation and normal subjects. *Brain Dev* 21: 548–53.

Gabriels RL, Cuccaro ML, Hill DE, Ivers BJ, Goldson E (2005) Repetitive behaviors in autism: relationships with associated clinical features. *Res Dev Disabil* 26: 169–81.

Goldstein NA, Fatima M, Campbell TF, Rosenfeld RM (2002) Child behavior and quality of life before and after tonsillectomy and adenoidectomy. *Arch Otolaryngol Head Neck Surg* 131: 52–7.

Gooley JJ, Saper CB (2005) Anatomy of the mammalian circadian system. In: Kryger MH, Roth T, Dement WC, eds. *Principles and Practice of Sleep Medicine.* Philadelphia: Elsevier/Saunders, pp. 335–50.

Gottlieb DJ, Vezina RM, Chase C (2003) Symptoms of sleep-disordered breathing in 5-year-old children are associated with sleepiness and problem behaviors. *Pediatrics* 112: 870–7.

Hering E, Epstein R, Elroy S, Iancu DR, Zelnik N (1999) Sleep patterns in autistic children. *J Autism Dev Disord* 29: 143–7.

Hoban T (2003) Rhythmic movement disorder in children. *CNS Spectr* 8: 135–8.

Honomichl RD, Goodlin-Jones BL, Burnham M, Gaylor E, Anders TF (2002) Sleep patterns of children with pervasive developmental disorders. *J Autism Dev Disord* 32: 553–61.

Hoshino Y, Watanabe H, Yashima Y, Kaneko M, Kumashiro H (1984) An investigation on sleep disturbance of autistic children. *Folia Psychiatr Neurol Jpn* 38: 45–51.

Jones B (2005) Basic mechanisms of sleep-wake states. In: Kryger MH, Roth T, Dement WC, eds. *Principles and Practice of Sleep Medicine.* Philadelphia: Elsevier/Saunders, pp. 136–53.

Levitt P, Eagleson KL, Powell EM (2004) Regulation of neocortical interneuron development and the implications for neurodevelopmental disorders. *Trends Neurosci* 27: 400–6.

Lord C, Risi S, Lambrecht L, Cook EH, Leventhal BL, DiLavore PC, Pickles A, Rutter M (2000) The Autism Diagnostic Observation Schedule–Generic: a standard measure of social and communication deficits associated with the spectrum of autism. *J Autism Dev Disord* 30: 205–23.

Mahowald MW, Bornemann MAC (2005) NREM sleep–arousal parasomnias. In: Kryger MH, Roth T, Dement WC, eds. *Principles and Practice of Sleep Medicine.* Philadelphia: Elsevier/Saunders, pp. 889–96.

Mahowald M, Schenck C (2005) REM sleep parasomnias. In: Kryger MH, Roth T, Dement WC, eds. *Principles and Practice of Sleep Medicine.* Philadelphia: Elsevier/Saunders, pp. 897–916.

Malow BA (2004) Sleep disorders, epilepsy, and autism. *Ment Retard Dev Disabil Res Rev* 10: 122–5.

Malow BA, McGrew SG, Harvey M, Henderson LM, Stone WL (2006) Impact of treating sleep apnea in a child with autism spectrum disorder. *Pediatr Neurol* 34: 325–8.

McCauley JL, Olson M, Delahanty R, Amin T, Nurmi EL, Organ EL, Jacobs MM, Folstein SE, Haines JL, Sutcliffe JS (2004) A linkage disequilibrium map of the 1-Mb 15q12 GABAA receptor subunit cluster and association to autism. *Am J Med Genet* 131: 51–9.

Nir I, Meir D, Zilber N, Knobler H, Hadjez J, Lerner Y (1995) Brief report: circadian melatonin, thyroid-stimulating hormone, prolactin, and cortisol levels in serum of young adults with autism. *J Autism Dev Disord* 25: 641–4.

Owens J, Opipari L, Nobile C, Spirito A (1998) Sleep and daytime behavior in children with obstructive sleep apnea and behavioral sleep disorders. *Pediatrics* 102: 1178–84.

Owens JA, Spirito A, McGuinn M (2000a) The Children's Sleep Habits Questionnaire (CSHQ): psychometric properties of a survey instrument for school-aged children. *Sleep* 23: 1043–51.

Owens JA, Spirito A, McGuinn M, Nobile C (2000b) Sleep habits and sleep disturbance in elementary school-aged children. *J Dev Behav Pediatr* 21: 27–36.

Paavonen EJ, von Wendt T, Vanhala NR, Aronen ET, von Wendt L (2003) Effectiveness of melatonin in the treatment of sleep disturbances in children with Asperger disorder. *J Child Adolesc Psychopharmacol* 13: 83–95.

Patzold LM, Richdale AL, Tonge BJ (1998) An investigation into sleep characteristics of children with autism and Asperger's disorder. *J Paediatr Child Health* 34: 528–33.

Richdale AL (1999) Sleep problems in autism: prevalence, cause, and intervention. *Dev Med Child Neurol* 41: 60–6.

Richdale AL, Prior MR (1995) The sleep/wake rhythm in children with autism. *Eur Child Adolesc Psychiatry* 4: 175–86.

Sadeh A, Acebo C (2002) The role of actigraphy in sleep medicine. *Sleep Med Rev* 6: 113–24.

Saper CB, Chou T, Scammell TE (2001) The sleep switch: hypothalamic control of sleep and wakefulness. *Trends Neurosci* 24: 726–31.

Schreck KA, Mulick JA, Smith AF (2004) Sleep problems as possible predictors of intensified symptoms of autism. *Res Dev Disabil* 25: 57–66.

Schwietzer PK (2005) Drugs that disturb sleep and wakefulness. In: Kryger MH, Roth T, Dement WC, eds. *Principles and Practice of Sleep Medicine.* Philadelphia: Elsevier/Saunders, pp. 499–518.

Schwitzer J, Neudorfer C, Blecha HG Fleischhacker WW (1990) Mania as a side effect of phototherapy. *Biol Psychiatry* 29: 532–4.

Segawa M, Katoh M, Katoh J, Nomura Y (1992) Early modulation of sleep parameters and its importance in later behavior. *Brain Dysfunct* 5: 211–23.

Stein MA, Mendelsohn J, Obermeyer WH, Amromin J, Benca R (2001) Sleep and behavior problems in school-aged children. *Pediatrics* 107: E60.

Stores G, Wiggs L (1998) Abnormal sleep patterns associated with autism: a brief review of research findings, assessment methods and treatment strategies. *Autism* 2: 157–69.

Swedo SE, Allen AJ, Glod CA, Clark CH, Teicher MH, Richter D, Hoffman C, Hamburger S, Dow S, Brown C, Rosenthal NE (1997) A controlled trial of light therapy for the treatment of pediatric seasonal affective disorder. *J Am Acad Child Adolesc Psychiatry* 36: 816–21.

Takase M, Taira M, Sasaki H (1998) Sleep–wake rhythm of autistic children. *Psychiatry Clin Neurosci* 52: 181–2.

Thirumalai SS, Shubin RA, Robinson R (2002) Rapid eye movement sleep behavior disorder in children with autism. *J Child Neurol* 17: 173–8.

Tordjman S, Anderson GM, Pichard N, Charbuy H, Touitou Y (2005) Nocturnal excretion of 6-sulphatoxymelatonin in children and adolescents with autistic disorder. *Biol Psychiatry* 57: 134–8.

Tuchman R, Rapin I (2002) Epilepsy in autism. *Lancet Neurol* 1: 352–8.

Wiggs L, Stores G (2004) Sleep patterns and sleep disorders in children with autistic spectrum disorders: insights using parent report and actigraphy. *Dev Med Child Neurol* 46: 372–80.

Williams PG, Sears LL, Allard A (2004) Sleep problems in children with autism. *J Sleep Res* 13: 265–8.

13
ATYPICAL SENSORY/PERCEPTUAL RESPONSIVENESS

Isabelle Rapin

A prominent, ubiquitous, and poorly understood symptom of autism, reported since the earliest days of its study (Kanner 1943, Frith 1991), is atypical responsiveness to stimuli in any or all sensory modalities. The same child may be oblivious of some stimuli in a modality and over-react to others in the same modality. Children differ greatly not only in the severity of this problem but also in which modality or modalities are affected. That atypical sensory behaviors involve more than one modality speaks against a dominant problem at the level of peripheral sensory receptors or conduction from receptors to cortex; rather it implicates perception, selective attention, short term memory and cognitive resource allocation. All these aspects of sensory processing require coordinated activity in widely distributed cortical/subcortical networks, which does not refute the possibility of peripheral/subcortical deficits in some children, or the coexistence of both. Much of current research on sensory function in autism is focused on the reciprocal role in the brain of bottom-up versus top-down deficits that may explain the association of defective and superior skills in the same individual. Yet impairment at the level of the sensory receptors cannot be dismissed as entirely irrelevant.

SENSORY DEPRIVATION AND AUTISM
The prevalence of autism is higher in blind than in sighted children (Brown et al. 1997, Hobson et al. 1999, Hobson and Bishop 2003); it is also higher in deaf than in hearing children (Rosenhall et al. 1999), although the evidence for the latter is not as strong as in the case of blindness and, especially, deaf-blindness. The much higher prevalence of "primary" autism – autism without other evidence of brain pathology – in blind individuals than in sighted peers suggests that the deprivation of visual experience itself, in particular inadequate ability to see facial expression and gestures, might play a direct causal role in the autism (Hobson and Bishop 2003). The autistic behaviors observed in some infants raised in the relative isolation of hospitals or orphanages (Spitz 1945, Rutter and O'Connor 2004), and also in infant monkeys reared on surrogate wire mothers (Harlow and Harlow 1962), argue for sensory deprivation as a potential cause of – or at least contributing factor to – autism. Although many of these behaviors regress rather rapidly when some of the deprived infants are placed in more nurturing environments

(Beckett et al. 2002), they do not in others. This reinforces the likelihood that in autism innate genetic susceptibility modulates the deleterious consequences of lack of stimulation for the developing brain.

Deafness or blindness may occasionally be coincidental in a child genetically predisposed to "primary" autism. The increased prevalence of autism in deaf or blind children is probably largely attributable to the condition responsible for the sensory impairment also affecting the critical brain circuits responsible for the autism. Such is the case with extremely preterm birth (Chase 1972), congenital rubella and cytomegalovirus infection (Chess et al. 1971, Yamashita et al. 2003), but also of certain genetic disorders associated with both gross brain malformations and retinal pathology, for example the variant of Joubert syndrome associated with severe visual impairment (Raynes et al. 1999) or an occasional case of septo-optic dysplasia with optic atrophy (Polizzi et al. 2005).

TYPES OF SENSORY PROBLEMS AND BEHAVIORAL SOURCES OF INFORMATION

Clinical observations and parental reports are the main sources of behavioral information on aberrant sensory function in autism, but with few exceptions this information is anecdotal and poorly documented. The assumption of aberrant sensory function is largely based on indirect motor evidence, for example averted or overly prolonged gaze suggesting impaired vision. Lack of response to sound and failure to speak are regularly the presenting symptoms that alert parents of toddlers on the autism spectrum that something is amiss. By far the most distressing sensory symptom is self-injury without apparent distress. Decreased sensitivity to pain seems to provide a more plausible explanation for self-injury than an extreme form of manipulative bad habit akin to motor stereotypy for which the same explanation is often given. Temple Grandin, an exceptionally insightful professional woman with autism, states that she cannot abide the sensation of the seams of underwear against her skin, but writes that she has a craving for the deep bodily sensation of being squeezed in a press (Grandin 1995). In a rare study that compared subjective sensory experience with detailed psychophysical evaluation of vision in 9 on average 12-year-old verbal children with high functioning autism (HFA) and matched controls, all the autistic children reported atypical sensory experiences in at least one modality, and 4 of them reported hypersensitivy in all five modalities (auditory most often, followed by vision, touch, olfaction, and taste) (Davis et al. 2006).

My search of the literature did not uncover empirical behavioral, electrophysiologic or imaging data on aberrant responses to temperature, touch, vibration, position, olfaction or taste in autism. Many parents report that not only do their children smell foods before tasting them, but they are also extremely selective in what they are willing to eat. Whether this is because of taste, smell or texture is difficult to say, but it can create a difficult challenge for parents (Gillberg and Coleman 2000). Many children on the autism spectrum react extremely negatively to certain smells and tastes; or they may sniff people, lick their hands, objects or furniture, or chew on their clothes, a particular toy or inedible objects, which brings up the possibility of enhanced sensitivity to taste and smell. According to Gillberg (1990), atypical responses to "sensory stimuli" were the strongest discriminators between autism and mental retardation in children below age 3 years. Parents of some children with autism report that they have a low threshold for motion sickness, whereas other children twirl for many minutes without seemingly getting dizzy (Ritvo et al. 1969). There is a small body of early research exploring vestibular function, but little in more recent reports. Rogers and Ozonoff (2005) call for at least two modalities to be tested in any one study and for the inclusion of smell, taste, vestibular function and other somatosensory modalities besides pain and its exclusive focus on self-injury.

Rogers et al. (2003) compared parental answers to items on the Autistic Diagnostic Interview-Revised (ADI-R) (Lord et al. 1994) regarding aberrant sensory reactions (and stereotypies, not discussed here) in 22 typically developing toddlers matched for mental age to the answers in three groups of developmentally disabled preschoolers: 26 with autism, 20 with fragile-X syndrome (fra-X) – 7 of whom were autistic – and 32 with nonautistic mental retardation. The parents of children in the autism and fra-X groups reported more aberrant sensitivity to touch, taste and smell, visual and auditory stimuli, and auditory filtering than those of children in the other two groups. Abnormal responses to taste and smell were more numerous in the autistic group than in the other three groups. The investigators concluded that, even though it was related to impaired adaptive behavior, abnormal sensory reactivity correlated with neither overall developmental level nor IQ in the autistic and mentally retarded groups. They also observed that in the autistic group the total sensory score correlated with restricted activities observed on the Autistic Diagnostic Observation Schedule–Generic (ADOS-G) (Lord et al. 1999).

Rogers and Ozonoff (2005) reviewed all (48) empirical controlled laboratory studies of sensory dysfunction in autism published between 1960 and 2005 and highlighted the problems of many early studies and their scarcity, especially in recent years. Studies often involved small groups of severely autistic children with broad ranges of IQs and ages. Diagnosis was not always rigorously documented and studies did not routinely exclude neurologically diagnosable disorders. Most controls were typically developing children, not nonautistic developmentally impaired children matched on both chronological age and mental age. The tentative conclusion of the review was that sensory hyporeactivity seemed to be the most consistent characteristic of autism.

Many older studies reporting deficient sensory function in autism enrolled younger, less rigorously selected, more severely autistic children; they did not have access to the anatomic and physiologic correlates of sensory function today's advanced technology provides. Contemporary research differs by the need to enroll older, tightly selected, attentive, motivated, non-retarded subjects capable of participating in the often tedious and demanding tasks required by current behavioral, electrophysiologic and imaging paradigms; it tends to emphasize superior rather than deficient sensory function in autism (Dakin and Frith 2005, Mottron et al. 2006). Its strict criteria have the drawback of limiting the generalizability of conclusions to this HFA subgroup of the autism spectrum. Broader studies are sorely needed if we hope to resolve the discrepancies between empirical observational studies and the flood of parental and clinical reports too numerous to be discounted despite their acknowledged biases and flaws.

COMPLEXITIES AND LIMITATIONS OF TESTING SENSORY FUNCTION IN CHILDREN ON THE AUTISTIC SPECTRUM

SUBJECT COMPLEXITIES

Inherent in all studies of children with disabilities is the matter of chronological age and maturation of the nervous system. A limitation of the field, and notably in autism, is that most studies are cross-sectional and many involve a wide range of ages. A dilemma is whether to match affected children on chronological age or mental age/IQ, as well as gender and social variables. Matching on both, which is now considered de rigueur, limits inclusion to HFA children and adults with "idiopathic" autism and excludes those with more severe deficits that might have stronger biologic correlates. The matter of symptomatic vs idiopathic autism and of where to cut within the autism spectrum in order to have tightly defined homogeneous subgroups was discussed in Chapter 1. Problems with unrepresentative small groups are exacerbated by the demands of ever more sophisticated measures.

STIMULUS AND TASK COMPLEXITIES

Much current research uses clever paradigms in which autistic subjects and controls listen to or view passively a standard repetitive stimulus, or two types of stimuli that differ in some stimulus parameter or type, or are to pay attention or respond actively in some way to rare deviants (oddballs) among the frequent standards that differ from the standards along a particular dimension of interest, or even by their absence, or they may be presented with an even rarer totally unexpected novel stimulus in the same or another modality. In electrophysiology, these different stimuli are presented in long runs and responses to each type of stimulus averaged off-line. For imaging, stimuli and tasks of varying complexity are presented in runs, and runs that make successively lesser processing demands are subtracted from those at the next higher level of complexity. In both types of measure, responses are averaged over many presentations on the assumption that performance will be stable during data collection. Comparisons are between group means of subjects and controls.

BEHAVIORAL MEASURES

Behavioral measures of stimulus discrimination include verbal reports or motor responses, such as reaction times and number of selective responses, omissions and false alarms to selected stimuli. Group means of subjects and controls are compared. Behavioral measures are optimally informative because they not only provide direct evidence on the arrival of stimulation to the brain but also show that it was processed in order to generate the response. Their major limitation is their inapplicability to the untestable or unreliable part of the autistic population.

PHYSIOLOGIC MEASURES

These measures are discussed in greater detail in Chapter 10 and in an excellent review (Steinschneider and Dunn 2002). A strength of electrophysiologic measures and magnetoencephalography (MEG) is their temporal resolution, which ranges from a fraction of a millisecond in the case of brainstem auditory evoked responses (BAERs) to hundreds of milliseconds in cortical event-related potentials (ERPs) and event-related magnetic fields (ERMFs). Their spatial resolution is limited because most are composites of electrophysiologic activity with varying latencies generated in a number of distinct brain regions. The locations at which they are recorded with maximum amplitude is a function of the orientation of their generators relative to the recording electrodes and does not necessarily indicate that their source is on the cortical surface in close proximity to the electrode. High amplitude does not necessarily signal a strong response as there are cases where it may indicate failure to allocate cognitive capacity appropriately between sensory channels. Identifying successive components from composite waves and extracting the location of their generators calls for complex mathematical formulas and assumptions. Evoked responses are exceedingly small and therefore require averaging over a large number of stimulus presentations. Comparisons are made across group averages. Data analysis is performed off line and is very time-consuming.

Brainstem auditory evoked responses

BAERs are averaged auditory responses measured in fractions of milliseconds during the first 10 ms following stimulation with extremely rapid trains of 1000 or more clicks or rarely more frequency-specific stimuli (Stapells and Oates 1997). They are the one electrophysiologic measure with clinical application to assessing hearing in individual children with autism because they can be tested even in sedated sleep. They provide a measure of conduction velocity between the cochlea and the pons (waves I–III) and between the pons and the lower midbrain (waves III–V), which decreases with maturation. BAERs are an extremely important tool for testing peripheral hearing in young and uncooperative children with autism because of the significant prevalence of autism associated with hearing loss (Jure et al. 1991, Rosenhall et al. 2003, Roper et al. 2003).

Early cortical "exogenous", "automatic", or "pre-attentional" event-related responses

P1 (P50) is generated partly in primary auditory cortex (A1 – Heschl's gyrus) (Steinschneider and Dunn 2002). It is followed by the N1 (N100) complex, which has multiple generators that include the planum temporale posterior to A1 and lateral superior temporal gyrus (auditory association cortex). P1 and N1 index the brain's automatic detection of the sensory volley. Their amplitude is sensitive to features such as the intensity of stimuli. The mismatch negativity (MMN) and corresponding mismatch field negativity, superposed on late N1 and early P2 (P200), are generated in response to the brain's pre-attentional detection of an unexpected change in an ongoing chain of stimuli, which implicates storage of the preceding stimulus in the short term prefrontal memory buffer.

Late cortical "endogeneous", "processing-contingent" event-related responses
Late ERPs are not modality specific; they index active evaluation of the relevance of perceived incoming stimuli. Auditory N2 (N200) peaks between 200 and 300 ms over lateral temporal and parietal cortices in response to target (attended) stimuli. It is lateralized to the left hemisphere in phonetic discrimination tasks, whereas later, more posterior components are associated with higher order tasks. P3 (P300) is a composite potential with a time course of several hundred milliseconds; it is recorded broadly over the vertex and has widespread generators. P3a, generated in prefrontal and limbic cortices, is a correlate of automatic switching of attention and orientation to rare or novel stimuli and habituates with repeated presentation. P3b has a number of generators, including a hippocampal one; its maximum amplitude is over parietal cortex and it coincides in time with the subject selecting the appropriate response to signal the active discrimination of a target. N4 (N400, Nc, or late frontal negativity) is also a prolonged composite with multiple generators. One of its generators is in posterior superior temporal cortex, with a left preponderance in response to semantically incongruous words in a sentence or to the detection of the mismatch between a word and picture.

Transcranial magnetic stimulation
This tool can be applied to stimulate or inhibit particular cortical areas transiently, making it possible to dissect out subcomponents of brain processes in electrophysiologic experiments. It is not discussed in this chapter.

IMAGING MEASURES
Morphometry
Brain morphometry provides a static tridimensional anatomic view of the brains of individuals and can be acquired in sleeping sedated children. The spatial resolution of MRI is in the millimeter range, and the time required to acquire the image of each slice is steadily decreasing from minutes to seconds. New techniques to image tracts increase its informational power. Images can be mathematically normalized to enable averaged inter-group comparisons, and parcellated to calculate the surfaces or volumes of particular brain structures. Computational techniques have even been devised to provide images of the opened cortical sulci. Correlating morphometric findings with behavioral variables for inter-group comparisons are performed off-line. All these analyses require sophisticated and powerful tools and are time-consuming.

Functional magnetic response imaging (fMRI)
fMRI documents increased oxygenated blood flow in regionally activated cortex or

subcortical areas, which can be mapped onto the subject's anatomic MRI or onto a normalized average brain map that exposes the entire cortical surface with opened sulci. Use of the subtraction technique mentioned earlier enables the detection of task-related changes in blood flow in brain regions or structures of interest. The spatial resolution is of the order of several millimeters and data acquision may be quite lengthy, of the order of many minutes, depending on how many different behavioral stimulus runs the experiment calls for. As in the case of morphometry, off-line analysis is often lengthy and complex.

Positron emission tomography (PET)

PET imagesthe metabolism of glucose and of some other ligands in activated brain areas. It suffers from the same temporal constraints as fMRI and its spatial resolution is even coarser. Its power is that it can provide data on the dynamic neurochemical events in specified systems of the brain. Its limitation is the requirement for radioactive ligands, which precludes its use in children under age 18 years unless it has a therapeutic medical indication.

To summarize, imaging studies and MEG require complex, expensive apparatus and expert personnel. Imaging and electrophysiologic approaches both call for powerful and labor-intensive computerized statistical analyses. They require different instrumentation and competencies. These limitations explain why most studies are carried out on small numbers of subjects (usually HFA children) and do not take advantage of the complementary time and spatial resolutions of electrophysiology and functional imaging in comprehensive studies using both technologies in the same subjects performing identical tasks.

AUDITORY SYSTEM
BEHAVIORAL EVIDENCE

Suspected hearing loss or failure of language development is probably the most frequent concern that brings parents of young children on the autism spectrum to their physician, unfortunately all too often to be reassured and told they are overanxious. This is particularly likely if they recount that the child is inconsistent, at times seeming deaf and at others screaming and covering his/her ears if someone turns on the vacuum cleaner. To reiterate what was said in Chapter 4, any doubt about hearing, especially if loss of words is reported, must be taken seriously and requires immediate referral for formal audiologic assessment, which often requires BAER testing. As stressed in Chapter 4, in some children with or without autism who are not deaf, inadequate or absent speech has to do with a selective deficiency in decoding acoustic language, usually at the level of the auditory cortex (Klein et al. 1995, 2000), occasionally due to pathology in subcortical auditory relays (Rapin and Gravel 2003).

Modern technology is making it possible not only to document impaired hearing in the laboratory but also to begin to understand the brain basis of extraordinary auditory talens in some individuals with autism (Kellerman et al. 2005). The fact that some children appear to experience discomfort to sounds that others can tolerate (Khalfa et al. 2004), or can hear some high pitched soft sounds not heard by the average person has long suggested better than average hearing threshold. An increased prevalence in autism of unusual musical ability and absolute pitch (ability to identify sound frequency out of context) is well documented (Bonnel et al. 2003). Many parents report that their non-verbal or poorly verbal preschooler can sing recognizable melodies on key and loves to listen to music. Musical savants are retarded autistic individuals with prodigious memories for music who can teach themselves an instrument and play without a score a piece of music they may have heard only once (Treffert 2005).

BAER ABNORMALITIES: EVIDENCE FOR SUBCORTICAL DYSFUNCTION IN AUTISM?

A recent well controlled study found no behavioral or physiologic difference in peripheral sensitivity between 40 autistic children and 40 matched nonautistic normal controls (Gravel et al. 2006). A number of early BAER studies did report abnormalities, but, as otoacoustic emissions and tests of middle ear function were not available in most, they must be interpreted cautiously as some no doubt included children with unsuspected middle ear effusions and perhaps neurologic conditions that might explain delayed or even absent BAERs (Klin 1993). A recent study of 73 autistic individuals from Canada disclosed prolonged wave I–III interpeak latencies in about half of the cases, suggesting dysfunction between neurons in the spiral ganglia and pontine cochlear nuclei; this same finding was also discovered in some nonautistic first degree relatives, raising the possibility of a genetic trait (Maziade et al. 2000). The same group (Thivierge et al. 1990) and others (e.g. Novick et al. 1980, Fein et al. 1981, Rosenhall et al. 2003) have reported prolonged III–V rather than I–III latencies in children or young adults with autism whose peripheral hearing was ostensibly normal. These observations underline the need for further rigorous studies of BAERs in larger numbers of subjects with defined selection criteria, in whom all potential confounding explanations for abnormal findings have been meticulously ruled out.

EARLY AUDITORY ERPs

In the aggregate, early studies of children with autism, with their previously mentioned limitations, showed few consistent differences from controls in latency or amplitude of N1, MMN or P2 in response to monaural vs binaural presentation, rate, intensity, or length of stimuli, clicks vs tones, pitch changes, and simple vs complex sounds or speech stimuli (see Chapter 10). If differences were found in autism they were almost all in the direction of smaller amplitudes or longer latencies (Novick et al. 1980, Courchesne et al. 1985, Buchwald et al. 1992).

Some more recent investigations evaluated early auditory ERP components to sound and speech as potential contributors to receptive–expressive language disorders in autism (Chapter 4). A MEG study of the impaired detection of rapid changes in tone frequency of oddballs in 11 low functioning autistic children and adults, compared to normal controls, suggested its relevance to their severely impaired language (Tecchio et al. 2003). Subjects in an earlier study were 6 young adults, 2 of them mildly autistic, diagnosed in childhood with verbal auditory agnosia (VAA), the most severe deficit in the decoding of the rapid speech sounds that characterize phonology (Klein et al. 1995). Maps of ERPs to tones and syllables revealed a 40 ms delay in the N1 component over lateral temporal cortex, but not over the vertex (A1), to tones and syllables. In 9 autistic children with adequate nonverbal intelligence, 4 of whom were essentially nonverbal, the MMN and P3a responses were absent to vowel changes. The deficit was interpreted as selective to speech discrimination because there was no difference from controls in responses to simple or complex tones or single vowel sounds (Ceponiene et al. 2003). Magnetic mismatch fields (MMFs) in 9 autistic adults did not differ from those of 19 normal controls in response to change in the duration of a tone, change of a tone to a vowel, and between 2 vowels, except that the latency in the MMF was delayed on the left in the cross phoneme change, suggesting a delay in automatic processing of changes in speech sounds in autism (Kasai et al. 2005). Recordings from single neurons in Heschl's gyrus in 2 patients being investigated for potential epileptic surgery while they were watching an English language film were shown to be highly correlated with location of activation on fMRI in normal subjects watching the same movie (Mukamel et al. 2005).

These studies and others support the view that auditory processing deficits at an early stage of decoding incoming speech are responsible for, or cannot be dismissed as contributors to the severely deficient language of a subset of individuals with autism. Severely deficient language associated with abnormality of early ERP components may represent an autistic endophenotype in which impaired sociability or cognitive impairment does not provide an adequate explanation for failure to acquire language at the expected age.

LATE AUDITORY ERPS

ERPs address the active processing of auditory stimuli (see Chapter 10). P300 was absent or smaller in each of 5 adolescents with autism compared to controls when they had to respond to the change in pitch of tones or to the absence of a stimulus in a train (Novick et al. 1980). In 8 verbal 8- to 10-year-old HFA children compared to normal peers, the N1c component to words was delayed over the left hemisphere, and the amplitude of the N4 component was not as expected smaller to target animal words to which they were to respond (Dunn et al. 1999) (decreased amplitude of P300 and N400 when a response is required is interpreted as evidence for failure to deploy processing capacity to the task at hand [Hoeksma et al. 2004]). The N4 findings were replicated in 10 8- and 9-year-olds and 8 11- and 12-year-olds, but delayed N1 latency over temporal derivations was limited to the younger group, a correlate of language processing maturation in the older children (Dunn and Bates 2005).

Because inadequate interpretation and production of prosody is so salient in autism (see Chapter 4), electrophysiologic correlates of its perception were sought in HFA adults and controls who were to respond selectively in an oddball paradigm to "Bob" spoken with the prosody of an assertion or a question, and to the prosody of happy or angry "Bob". There was no difference between the groups in behavioral responses, N1 or P2 waves to any of the stimuli, indicating normal processing of the auditory characteristics of the stimuli, and in both groups the amplitude of P3 was largest to emotional prosody. The groups did not differ in their behavioral responses to either the linguistic or the emotional prosody (Shriberg et al. 2001). There is such a dearth of formal studies of the perception of prosody in autism and, in particular, of its maturation, that this negative study cries for replication in children rather than adults.

IMAGING STUDIES

A number of *morphometric studies* have focused on brain areas relevant to auditory and language processing in autism. They are reviewed in depth in Chapter 8, together with functional imaging studies. The finding of atypical hemispheric asymmetry and reversed asymmetry of the volumes of regions concerned with language both in autistic children and in nonautistic children with developmental language disorders (DLDs) (Herbert et al. 2002; Herbert et al. 2005) was replicated in a new sample of autistic children with mixed receptive/expressive language disorders or DLD, but not in fluent autistic children (De Fosse et al. 2004). This morphometric study adds to the clinical and electrophysiologic evidence of heterogeneity of language disorders in autism. It is also consonant with a PET study that showed reversed dominance in 5 HFA men listening to speech and a tendency toward reduced activation of auditory cortex by sound (Muller et al. 1999).

A number of PET studies during speech activation revealed left or bitemporal hypo-metabolism in children with autism (Boddaert and Zilbovicius 2002, Boddaert et al. 2004a). The volume of gray matter in the upper lip of the posterior superior temporal sulcus, an area now known to be a node in networks concerned with the integration of multimodal sensory and limbic activities, including the processing of semantics, was found to be bilaterally smaller in 21 severely retarded children with autism compared to age-matched nonautistic retarded controls (Boddaert et al. 2004b). An fMRI study showed that listening passively to vocal stimuli failed to activate this region in 5 autistic men but did so in normal controls (Gervais et al. 2004).

Studies of auditory function in autism have produced mixed results. BAERs are mostly normal, while early obligatory ERPs to a variety of language and nonlanguage auditory stimuli are generally adequate or near adequate, even though they were delayed in a number of cases, perhaps a correlate of decreased perfusion in temporal cortex (Zilbovicius et al. 2000). Thus, subcortical factors do not seem to play a dominant role, with the caveat that what was found in individuals with HFA may not apply to the entire population, especially very young children. Automatic detection of change may be impaired in some autistic individuals, especially when the stimuli are speech sounds, in which case alterations may be lateralized. Morphometry and functional imaging show atypical lateralization of language-related cortex, perhaps only in individuals with autism and receptive–expressive language deficits. There is still lack of consensus on whether processing differences between language and non-language auditory stimuli are best explained by the complexity of the input (Bertone et al. 2005) or specific lateralized modules for language The most robust ERP deficits imply that they have more to do with auditory processing than with sensitivity or perception. Variability of findings among studies points to their limitations in terms of numbers of subjects, choice of controls and other confounding variables, but they also strongly point to the fact that autism is a heterogeneous syndrome so that a variety of auditory processing deficits are expected.

VISUAL SYSTEM
CLINICAL/BEHAVIORAL EVIDENCE
Clinicians generally assume that vision is not implicated in autism; in fact, they regularly regard vision as autistic persons' favored distance receptor channel. Yet atypical use of information in this modality is one of the most prominent symptoms of autism, with gaze avoidance, that is, an apparent repugnance to look at the face and eyes of others (Richer and Coss 1976, Klin et al. 2002), widely considered a signature of the disorder and assumed to index the social deficits of autism (Scharre and Creedon 1992). Parents report a variety of other unusual visual behaviors in their children, for example staring at spinning wheels or moving objects. Or children may gaze at their wriggling fingers with their heads tilted "out of the corner" of their deviated eyes (Mottron et al. 2006), perhaps signaling difficulty with foveation or peripheral vision, or atypical control of the extraocular muscles.

Standard ophthalmologic examination of 34 children with a wide range of severity and cognitive competence (Scharre and Creedon 1992) revealed refractive errors, strabismus, atypical optokinetic nystagmus and saccadic visual pursuit in a high proportion of children. Stereoscopy could be evaluated in only a minority of children. This high prevalence of abnormalities needs to be viewed cautiously because the subjects were unselected and some of the children may have had etiologies that affected both the eyes and the brain. Children on the spectrum without evidence of diagnosable brain pathologies, those with "primary" or "idiopathic" autism, can be presumed to have the same risk for visual deficits as their typically developing peers, but like all children they need to be screened by competent examiners to ascertain that there is indeed no overlooked peripheral visual pathology.

As was the case for audition, superior visual abilities are reported in a notable proportion of individuals with autism. These include extraordinary ability to analyze details of complex visual scenes, as depicted by Rain Man shown in the film to report the right number of sticks dropped on the floor without the need to count them. Superior pattern recognition, feature detection and short term visual memory have been documented repeatedly on neuropsychological testing. Visually gifted savants, like Steven Wiltshire who can study a complex of buildings and reproduce it with photographic exactitude, are awesome by any criteria (O'Connor and Hermelin 1987); they parallel musically gifted savants able to reproduce a complex piece of music heard but once, an ability that can occur in the face of significant cognitive deficiencies (Treffert 2005). A proposed explanation for visual savants' amazing skills is superior ability to process detail despite deficient ability for global perception (Frith and Happe 1994), and, in the visual modality, superiority of the parvocellular and inadequacy of the magnocellular systems.

EYE MOVEMENT CONTROL

Vision is a major player in the control of eye movements, together with other cortical and subcortical circuitry. There is still no consensus on the role played by the cerebellum and neocortex in oculomotor control and on their contributions to the atypical visual behaviors and gaze abnormalities of many individual with autism (Scharre and Creedon 1992, Mottron et al. 2006). Early investigators who focused on vestibular dysfunction attributed gaze abnormalities to dysfunction in that system (Slavik et al. 1984). This hypothesis seems to be refuted by the more recent demonstration of an intact vestibulo-ocular reflex, at least in a group of 13 HFA young teenagers, a group older and no doubt less severely affected than those studied by early investigators. Reports of saccadic fixation and dysmetric eye movements in visual pursuit may be a signature of disordered eye movement control by the dorsal cerebellar vermis–fastigial–pontine loop (Takarae et al. 2004a,b; Nowinski et al. 2005). Smallness in some individuals on the autism spectrum of lobules VI and VII of the dorsal vermis (Courchesne et al. 1988) seems a plausible correlate of disordered eye movement control (Kaufmann et al. 2003) as the disordered movements resemble those caused by dyscontrol of the brainstem oculomotor system seen in children following surgical removal of cerebellar neoplasms (Courchesne et al. 1994). On the other hand, study of visual pursuit, of the ability to maintain eccentric gaze, control visually guided saccades and suppress antisaccades (inhibition of looking at an unexpected target in the periphery of the visual field), supports the integrity of cerebellar–brainstem control of eye movements and suggests fronto-striatal or fronto-parietal dyscontrol (Minshew et al. 1999, Goldberg et al. 2002, Kemner et al. 2004, Nowinski et al. 2005).

Gaze aversion is widely attributed not to oculomotor dyscontrol but to social difficulties and the abnormal processing of faces, consisting for example of a preference for looking at the mouth rather than the eyes to gather information about another person's behavior (Richer et al. 1976, Klin et al. 2002). Other views are that aberrant gaze is the corollary of autistic rigidity, or of prolonged fixation on some small target because of the assumed inadequacy of the magnocellular visual system involved in processing movement and in wide scanning of scenes, discussed below. The inescapable conclusion is that even such a relatively well understood system as the control of the eye movements by vision is exceedingly complex and that there is probably no single explanation for its abnormalities in autism.

INPUT PATHWAYS FOR VISUAL STIMULI

Current research assumes that superiority in detection of fine visual detail in autism denotes dominance of the ventral visual system and inadequate attention to the "bigger picture" due to inadequacy of the dorsal system (Milne et al. 2002, Horton and Sincich 2004, Boeschoten et al. 2005, Dakin and Frith 2005). Large *magnocellular neurons* in the two ventral layers of the lateral geniculate nucleus receive their inputs mainly from the rods and large widely connected parasol ganglion cells of the retinal periphery. They project retinotopically onto more laterally placed neurons of the primary visual cortex (V1). These in turn form the *dorsal cortical visual stream*, which projects mainly to posterior parietal cortex and to the posterior superior temporal sulcus. This later maturing, more rapidly conducting system has low spatial, high temporal resolution, is exquisitely sensitive to motion, and is silent on color. It provides information about location in space and is therefore often referred to as the "where" pathway. Small *parvocellular neurons* in the four dorsal layers of the lateral geniculate nucleus receive their inputs mainly from the cones of the fovea and small tightly coupled sparsely connected ganglion cells of the central retina and project retinotopically onto more medial neurons in primary visual cortex (V1). These in turn form the *ventral cortical visual stream*, which, through successive relays, projects to inferotemporal cortex, including the fusiform gyrus, and also onto the posterior superior temporal sulcus (Dakin and Frith 2005). This earlier maturing, slower conducting "what" pathway has much finer spatial resolution, but lower temporal resolution, than the dorsal system. It is particularly suited to the processing of edges, form, texture and color required for the identification of static objects and pattern recognition. Detailed maps of the visual cortex produced by fMRI in a group of 8 HFA adults and controls were similar, suggesting equivalent retinal organization (Hadjikhani et al. 2004).

PROCESSING OF VISUAL STIMULI IN AUTISM

Research on visual function in autism, whether it relied on behavioral, ERP, or imaging measures, has not reached a consensus on whether the differences between the magno- and parvocellular systems provide an adequate explanation for the differing ways in which autistic people process visual information, or whether the differences are better ascribed to cognitive deficits, in particular in attention or the binding of stimulus characteristics that affect perception in other modalities as well as vision (weak central coherence theory) (Frith and Happe 1994, Plaisted et al. 2006). It is now widely accepted that even HFA individuals have suboptimal awareness of motion, for example of a stream of dots moving in one direction embedded in a background of randomly moving dots (Milne et al. 2002, Davis et al. 2006), contrasted with superior perception of rapid flicker, colors and shapes (Bertone et al. 2005). This combination may account for Ran Main's ability to count sticks at a glance and for many autistic persons' remarkable awareness of the details of a complex visual pattern, such as detecting a figure embedded in a noisy visual background which they ignore (Pellicano et al. 2005), and excelling at Block Design which calls for building a tri-dimensional design from a two-dimensional picture (Dakin and Frith

2005). Uncanny awareness of visual detail while showing apparent oblivion to the complex scene surrounding a visual target is widely ascribed to dominance of the ventral visual system stream and (or even because of) impairment of the dorsal visual system pathway.

A spectacular study of fra-X provides behavioral and pathological evidence for selective abnormality of the magnocellular/dorsal visual pathway in this overlapping condition (Kogan et al. 2004). The pattern of visual function in 9 fra-X men was similar to that in autism, with impaired detection of motion and preserved form perception. Pathologic examination of the lateral geniculate bodies of another fra-X male revealed that instead of the clear demarcation of the magno- and parvocellular layers in a control brain, the geniculates contained only small neurons. There was no immunohistochemical staining with an anti-FMRP antibody, whereas differential staining of the magno- and parvocellular layers was clear in the normal human and in 2 monkey brains.

Face recognition is uniquely important and starts to develop soon after birth as infants discriminate their caretakers from strangers long before their first birthday. Children with autism have well documented deficits in facial recognition, as shown in a study in which they were compared to children with developmental language disorders or mental retardation (Klin et al. 1999). Surprisingly, the scores of 24 more mildly affected boys with PDD-NOS were within expected norms, and scores were less strongly correlated to nonverbal IQ in the autistic boys than in the nonautistic comparison groups (Hauck et al. 1998). Typically developing controls had a better memory for faces than objects, whereas this was not the case for those with autism.

Specialization in face vs non-face perception has been documented in a number of ERP studies, which show differences between autistic and nonautistic controls at electrodes located over the posterior temporal regions of the scalp. For example, in 15 non-retarded adolescents and adults with autism spectrum disorders (ASDs) compared to matched normal controls, the latency of wave N170 was 18ms longer on average in the ASD group (McPartland et al. 2004). Whereas controls showed longer latencies to inverted than to upright faces, latencies were equal in the ASD group, suggesting lack of sensitivity to this configurational alteration (or superiority in processing a static object such as an inverted face, depending on one's hypothesis). The amplitude of N170 was greater to faces than to non-faces, and to inverted faces than to upright faces in both groups. The expected difference, with higher amplitude on the right, was borderline but less in the ASD group than in controls.

A number of fMRI studies indicate that faces, more than other visual stimuli, activate a region of the lateral aspect of the right fusiform gyrus in the ventral temporal lobe that receives its input from the parvocellular ventral visual pathway and has come to be considered "the" face processing area. This view has received a boost from a recent experiment that found a patch in the corresponding area of the monkey brain in which 97% of visually responsive neurons responded selectively to faces (Tsao et al. 2006). However, faces also activate other brain areas including the amygdala, temporal pole, medial frontal cortex and inferolateral frontal cortex (Schultz et al. 2003). Involvement of the dorsal visual stream may make it easier for people with autism to interpret static faces than the dynamic faces with moving facial features that express emotion. These facial movements activate a node in the posterior superior temporal sulcus on which networks that participate in visual, language and social processing converge. This area was reported to be smaller and underactivated in children with autism (Boddaert et al. 2004b, Gervais et al. 2004). Behavioral studies, ERPs and fMRI are starting to provide more realistic insights into how the brain proceeds in analyzing visual information.

SOMATOSENSORY SYSTEM AND SELF-INJURY
SOMATOSENSORY STIMULI
One of the hallmarks of autism is abnormal response to somatosensory stimulation, which, as in the case of audition and vision, consists of both heightened and blunted responses to touch and pain (other somatosensory modalities seem not to have been studied). Tactile defensiveness, reported by Temple Grandin and many parents of children with autism, is widely assumed to indicate lowering of the threshold for touch or pain. It was reported to be correlated with rigidity, verbal perseveration and visual stereotypies, but not to motor stereotypies or stereotyped object manipulation, in 28 children with developmental disabilities (Baranek et al. 1997), but I did not find a formal study of threshold to touch. Perhaps, as reported by Grandin (1995), sustained and widespread stimulation of low-threshold mechanosensors by squeezing is soothing to individuals averse to light touch (mechanical allodynia) because it generates a large field of surround inhibition that dampens the perception of temporally or spatially restricted mechanical stimuli, much in the way that scratching or rubbing quiets itch (Oaklander et al. 2002).

A single study that compared 10 severely retarded autistic children to retarded controls reported that those with autism responded more often to touch than sound (Kemner et al. 1994). This study has been widely interpreted as indicating preeminence in autism of proximal senses like touch, taste and smell over distal senses like vision and hearing. One experiment addressed directly the question of a selective deficit in processing of distal (visual) vs proximal (somatosensory) sensory modalities in four matched groups of 20 children each: HFA, attention deficit, dyslexia, and no deficit. In an oddball active/passive paradigm, ERPs to geometric patterns and to nonpainful electrical shocks to digits revealed no intergroup or intermodality difference specific to somatosensory function in the autistic group.

Ornitz (1974) hypothesized that paradoxical sensory responses of children with autism reflected inadequate integration and modulation of sensory inputs at the brainstem level, which he ascribed to dysfunctional vestibular connectivity (see below). He also speculated that motor stereotypies in autism might serve the purpose of increasing proprioceptive feedback, but this does not seem to have been followed up.

SENSITIVITY TO PAIN AND SELF-INJURIOUS BEHAVIORS
There is an extensive literature on self-injurious behaviors (SIBs) and the experience of

pain. Biting of the hand or wrist and head banging or hitting are the most common and persistent SIBs, but there are many others, including constant picking at scabs of sores that never have a chance to heal, in some cases resulting in permanent scarring. I have seen a 20 year old lose an eye to repeated poking, and head banging in a 16-month-old infant who slapped his head nonstop to the point of having two large temporal subgaleal fluid collections. No wonder SIBs are at the forefront of parental concerns in autism!

SIB is not limited to, but is highest in, the severely retarded severely autistic population. It is also prevalent in nonautistic seriously retarded individuals (Mace and Mace 1995, Schroeder et al. 1995, Breau et al. 2003) and, in muted form, in some HFA persons. A problem evaluating the reliability of the SIB literature is that the DSM/ICD classification systems limit the diagnosis of autism in retarded individuals to those whose autistic symptomatology is out of proportion to their IQ, making it likely that reports of SIB in severely retarded populations probably include many individuals who were also autistic. Even some normal people engage in mild SIBs like picking at scabs, biting the insides of their mouths, or occasionally hitting themselves in frustration, and some otherwise normal infants are head bangers (Sallustro and Atwell 1978). SIB is reported in some 30–70% of severely mentally retarded or autistic individuals, depending on the source of the population studied (Bartak and Rutter 1976, Schroeder et al. 1978, Sandman and Hetrick 1995). Although SIB tends to abate with age in outpatient populations, it creates huge management problems in some institutionalized adults because it responds poorly to standard psychotropic drugs.

There are many anecdotal reports by parents suggesting that their autistic children are remarkably tolerant of painful stimuli, and even unusually tolerant of the cold. It is logical, therefore, to assume that SIB denotes a raised threshold for pain. A study of the relationship of SIB to documented pain was performed in 101 severely retarded nonverbal children, 44 of whom had SIBs (Breau et al. 2003). Standardized questionnaires to caregivers regarding the location, variety and frequency of self-injury indicated that SIB in 31 children who did not have pain involved primarily the hand and head, whereas direct observations and reports on 13 children with acute or chronic pain showed that they localized their SIBs to the vicinity of the pain, perhaps to draw attention to it or alleviate it; they did not have an elevated threshold for pain and the time course of the SIB was related to the duration of the pain.

It is clear that most SIBs in autism are not responses to an actual pain, although the possibility of a real undiagnosed pain must of course be kept in mind. It is also clear that SIBs in autism (and in severe mental retardation) are largely environmentally influenced – or even driven – and that, whatever their underlying biologic pathophysiology, children use SIBs to manipulate their caregivers. Some consider SIBs a variant or extreme variant of motor stereotypies because both are seemingly purposeless rhythmic repetitive behaviors to some degree modulated by environmental contingencies (Bodfish et al. 2000).

The dominant view today is that SIB has an underlying biologic basis but is a highly idiosyncratic learned behavior (Symons 2005). Behaviorists point out that SIBs can have any one of three goals: getting attention, escaping an aversive situation, or obtaining some tangible object or reward (Carr and Smith 1995, Mace et al. 1995). In addition, there are some rare seemingly uncontrollable bouts of self-injury that may be very prolonged and do not have as clear antecedents or consequences as more ordinary SIBs; these are felt to be more directly biologically driven than those which clearly follow operant conditioning rules (Thompson et al. 1995, Kern et al. 2003).

Lesch–Nyhan syndrome may provide a model for extreme SIB, although these boys want to be restrained and often become extremely agitated when restraints are removed, suggesting that their experience of SIB is aversive. But even in this disease, where the evidence for a biologic cause of SIB is overwhelming, although not understood, environmental issues still play a modulatory role (Hall et al. 2001). Autopsies in 3 cases revealed that dopamine (DA) levels were only 10–30% of those found in controls in DA terminals in the striatum, whereas serotonin terminals were increased, indicating a profound alteration in the balance of the principal neurotransmitters (Lloyd et al. 1981). Thus far, SIB in Lesch–Nyhan syndrome has been resistant to pharmacologic medications.

The DA theory of SIB in autism posits that DA depletion in the nigrostriatal tract leads to D1 receptor supersensitivity. Poor response of SIB to DA receptor blockers like haloperidol is attributed to their unselective binding to both D1 and D2 receptors. Anecdotal reports of spectacular reduction of SIB in an occasional adult with intractable SIB following administration of olanzapine, which has better affinity for D1 receptors than the other neuroleptics, seems to support the DA theory in a subset of individuals with SIB (Schroeder et al. 1995); unfortunately, olanzapine's unfavorable safety profile severely limits its use.

The other biologic line of research on SIB focuses on endogenous opioids and has two facets (Thompson et al. 1995; Sandman et al. 1995, 2002). The analgesia hypothesis states that self-injury raises levels of enkephalins to compensate for dysregulation of the opioid system which is set too low in a subset of individuals with SIB; the addiction hypothesis posits that SIB, because it releases endorphins, is experienced as pleasureful, which helps perpetuate it by an addictive mechanism. The opioid theory is bolstered by the effectiveness of naltrexone, a *mu* opiate receptor blocker, in some half of individuals with intractable SIB (Sandman et al. 1995, Symons et al. 2004). Evidence that SIB raises beta-endorphins promptly and selectively supports the opioid theory (Sandman et al. 2000), although random plasma and CSF metabolite levels were inconsistent (Gillberg 1995, Sandman et al. 1995). Several trials of naltrexone to block opioid receptors were disappointingly negative in autism, perhaps because they focused on its core symptoms (sociability, language and stereotypy) rather than more narrowly on SIB. An interesting potential animal model is that male, and not female, neonatal rats treated with capsaicin, which poisons small afferent pain fibers and thus chronically blunts the experience of pain, have reduced brain weights and are hyperactive (Newson et al. 2005). There was increased neuronal density not only in several cortical areas but also in the caudate/putamen. Although the investigators viewed it as a model of schizophrenia, it might also be relevant to autism and mental retardation with SIB. The DA and opioid theories may pertain only to distinct subgroups of individuals with SIB; the two may in fact have some common ground inasmuch as DA plays a key role in addiction and reward systems.

The therapeutic consequences to draw from the research on SIBs are that this complex behavioral trait arises, in most individuals, from learned context-dependent contingencies in predisposed individuals with an as yet poorly understood complex biologic vulnerability. A few cases may reflect largely endogeneous factors unrelated to environmental triggers, and others may be entirely learned. A review of drug trials indicates that it is important to characterize the circumstances in which SIB arises for two reasons: first, behavioral approaches to control require an understanding of the message the child is attempting to convey by the behavior so as not to reinforce it and second, identifying the antecedents and consequences is required in order to manipulate them selectively. Any drug trial must also attempt to define the category of SIB as each calls for a different pharmacologic approach (Mace and Mace 1995). It is clear that even this differentiated approach is far from universally successful in doing away with this distressing symptom. In addition to targeted investigations of their biology, progress calls for much more careful and sophisticated description and quantitation of SIBs (Brasic et al. 1997) and their circumstances than heretofore available.

VESTIBULAR SYSTEM AND POSTURAL CONTROL

Some children on the autism spectrum spin without apparent vertigo, rock, or crave to be tossed up or held upside down, whereas others easily get car sick and have postural instability, again suggesting both blunted and increased sensitivity in this sensory system. Maintaining a stable erect posture even when the head or body are out of alignment calls for the coordination of three sensory systems: vision to inform about the horizon, proprioception about the location and angles of muscles and joints relative to one another, and the vestibular system to report on gravity and angular acceleration of the head. All three sensory systems project to the cerebellum which plays a key role in integrating their inputs with extraocular muscle control. The vestibulo-cerebellar system seems to be functional in autism (Goldberg et al. 2000); this system is involved in the stabilization of retinal images of stationary objects during transient head rotation or tilt (vestibulo-ocular reflex). Visual fixation suppresses nystagmus induced by the semicircular canals during and after induced rotation. Evidently dancers and skaters learn to use visual fixation to avoid losing their balance after rapid spins. Post-rotational nystagmus was stated to be shorter in children with autism than in controls when they were tested in a lighted room with their eyes open, whereas it did not differ in the dark (Ritvo et al. 1969). The authors also found that when the beds of sleeping children were rocked, it prolonged REM bursts in normal children but not in those with autism (Ornitz 1974). The investigators interpreted their findings, together with clinical evidence of sensorimotor hypo- and hyperfunction in autism, as evidence of inadequate brainstem modulation of sensory inputs and motor outputs by vestibulo-cerebellar and vestibulo-spinal influences, although this vestibular–brainstem hypothesis soon came under criticism on both experimental and theoretical grounds (Maurer and Damasio 1979).

Very little research seems to have been done on the vestibular system in autism following this spate of early work, yet occupational therapists use vestibular stimulation in some of the most popular therapies currently offered to children with autism (Ayres and Tickle 1980, Slavik et al. 1984). A recent but sobering review of sensory and motor interventions provided to these children points out that there is little empirical evidence for their efficacy or specificity (Baranek 2002).

There are some intriguing findings that suggest that further work on postural control in autism may be fruitful. Depending on the demands of the task, children with autism standing with their eyes occluded on a stabilometric platform had paradoxically decreased or increased ability to maintain the erect posture without swaying (Kohen-Raz et al. 1992). Children with autistic disorder, but not those with Asperger syndrome, were reported to be less sensitive to the effects of visually perceived environmental motion on posture than unaffected controls (Gepner et al. 1995, Gepner and Mestre 2002). These findings were discussed in the context of the blunted visual perception of motion by the magnocellular dorsal visual system mentioned earlier, or of increased postural rigidity reflecting aberrant visuocerebellar processing in a subset of children with autism. These fragmentary data can only provide food for armchair speculation until more rigorous research on proprioception and vestibular function in autism is performed.

POTENTIAL UNDERLYING CAUSES OF MULTIMODAL ABERRANT SENSORY FUNCTION IN AUTISM

This review of the confusing field of sensory functioning in children with autism leads to several conclusions. First, clinical observation and now research data indicate that there is indeed a mixture of hyper- and hypofunction in this disorder. Second, it emphasizes what is stated again and again in this book: autism, even "idiopathic" autism in cognitively competent individuals without a diagnosable underlying etiology, is not a "disease". Therefore nothing or very little one can say about autism applies to the entire population on the spectrum. This means that studies of small groups of affected individuals are unlikely to be representative of the entire population of persons with autistic symptomatology. It is particularly likely that findings in HFA may not apply to those who are more severely affected. Third, whether or not there are subtle dysfunctions at subcortical levels is an open question that needs further study. Fourth, the explanatory power of cognitive theories regarding the influence of neuropsychologic factors on sensory function in autism is attractive but will remain inadequate until its brain basis is better understood.

HYPER- AND HYPOSENSITIVITY TO SENSORY STIMULI

As pointed out several times, the accumulated testimonies of parents and clinicians are simply too numerous to be denied. Autistic savants with truly extraordinary talents are the best examples of this paradox (Treffert 2005). Although true savants are exceptionally rare, the many more numerous individuals on the autism spectrum can be shown with appropriate tools to have both talents and deficiencies, often in the same modality. There is now experimental demonstration of superior and decreased function in the same individual, the best examples being in the visual modality (Bertone et al. 2005) in which there is at least a plausible anatomic explanation. Most of the research in other modalities has focused on deficiencies; it is time to look for both, and in particular in thus far neglected modalities like taste, smell, proprioception, temperature and vestibular function.

EVIDENCE FOR SUBCORTICAL OR EARLY CORTICAL SENSORY/PERCEPTUAL (BOTTOM-UP) DEFICITS

Full processing of sensory inputs requires that they be received by the peripheral sensory transducers and transmitters, and undergo preliminary processing at each relay of largely segregated input channels, mainly by subcortical loops, as they are transmitted to subcortical and early cortical receptors to be perceived, attended to, and stored in a short term memory buffer while their features are extracted. There is now irrefutable evidence of bottom-up deficits in three sensory modalities. The strongest evidence for both deficits and strengths in early processing in autism comes from the behavioral, electrophysiologic, imaging and, now, pathologic (if one accepts the fra-X findings of Kogan et al. (2004) as relevant to autism) studies of the visual system. In the auditory modality, there is some evidence for subtle deficits in frequency tuning of the cochlea or subcortical relays (Plaisted et al. 2003, Alcantara et al. 2004) and for conduction abnormalities in the BAERs in a relatively genetically homogeneous sample (Thivierge et al. 1990; Maziade et al. 2000). Inconsistencies of latencies of the preattentive peaks of auditory ERPs, with delays or even absent responses in some studies (Ceponiene et al. 2003, Tecchio et al. 2003, Kasai et al. 2005), support early processing deficits but also inhomogeneity of samples. Contradictory findings in studies of the vestibular–oculomotor systems lead to the same conclusion, as findings implicate involvement of both cerebellar–brainstem and cortical control mechanisms (Minshew et al. 1999, Takarae et al. 2004). This bottom-up evidence cannot be discarded when considering potential later mechanisms to explain aberrant responses of persons with autism to sensory stimuli.

EVIDENCE FOR COGNITIVE (TOP-DOWN) INFLUENCES ON SENSORY PERCEPTION

Electrophysiology has shown the complexities of early largely automatic cortical steps required before incoming stimuli can be consciously evaluated in the light of previously stored relevant inputs, ongoing organismic needs and priorities are evaluated, and a decision is reached on whether and how the sensory input is to be acted upon. Activation of the widespread networks gives rise to the late activity-contigent composite ERPs on the scalp and is referred to behaviorally as top-down processing. Inadequacy in coordinating the binding activities of these widespread endogeneous cortical/subcortical networks influences all inputs to the cortex and its outputs as well.

This overarching cognitively based new view of autism is characterized by a higher order top-down processing disorder that affects the integration of sensory inputs and grew out of the "theory of mind" proposed by Frith, Leslie, Happe and their British collaborators some 20 years ago (Baron-Cohen et al. 1985, Leslie and Frith 1988, Frith 1989, Happe and Frith 1999), which showed that children with autism were concrete and did not take full advantage of what was in full view to interpret what was happening around them. It has progressed way beyond its narrow early focus on reading other people's intentions to propose that what is wrong in autism is a focus on details because of failure to integrate sensory inputs into a coherent whole (Happe and Frith 1999). This top-down deficiency, referred to as "weak central coherence", is now widely embraced because of its attractive explanatory powers for many autistic behaviors. To reiterate, bottom-up and top-down deficits both exist and neither accounts for all aspects of atypical sensory processing in autism.

The weak central coherence hypothesis of the British psychologists has highlighted the superiorities (and associated deficiencies) of HFA individuals and savants (Dakin and Frith 2005, Mottron et al. 2006). Most elaborated in the visual domain, it is also supported by some auditory evidence (Heaton et al. 2001; Bonnel et al. 2003; Bertone et al. 2003, 2005; Heaton 2003; Kellerman et al. 2005). In the visual domain, superiority in local processing tied to the parvosystem, and weakness in global processing tied to the magnosystem provides a neat coherent anatomo-physiologic explanation for bottom-up differences. Superior awareness of minute details and behavioral rigidity could explain, at least in part, some expert knowledge because of willingness to devote hundreds of hours to some narrow field of interest like timetables or the butterflies of Madagascar. Lack of attention to global aspects of environments, and difficulty looking at and interpreting facial expression could explain deficiencies in the multichannel processing required for sophisticated decision making, executive skills, and gauging social contingencies.

Such broad behavioral deficits must reflect some type of underlying general brain dysfunction. A speculative one relates to the speed of neuronal activity. Sensory processing is generally slower in autism (and developmental language disorder) than in normal individuals (Oram Cardy et al. 2005) and, as is well known, considerably faster in older children and adults than in infants. This speeding up with maturation might contribute to improvement in language processing in autistic and nonautistic children with impaired language comprehension, as this skill is dependent on fast neural activity. Impaired rapid neuronal processing transcending dysfunction in the magnocellular system and affecting other sensory systems besides vision might contribute to problems interpreting rapidly received stimuli such as speech. Might the smallness of neurons in cortical minicolumns (Buxhoeveden and Casanova 2002, Casanova et al. 2002) and subcortical relays in the limbic system and cerebellum (Bauman and Kemper 1985, Bauman and Kemper 2005) play a part in difficulties that clearly go beyond a single sensory system?

Another biologic factor that may bear on the weak central coherence hypothesis are high frequency gamma EEG oscillations that involve the thalamus and cortex and play an important role in binding and synchronizing incoming sensory stimuli and neural activity (see Chapter 10). Gamma oscillations over parietal cortex in 6 HFA adolescents differed from those of controls during a visual discrimination task that they performed as well as their control peers (Brown et al. 2005). Synchronized gamma oscillations are also involved in the processing of rapid stimuli like tone frequency and speech in human auditory cortex (Brown et al. 2005, Mukamel et al. 2005). An oscillating circuit that involves the climbing fibers of the inferior olive on cerebellar Purkinje cells is required for the maintenance of EEG gamma oscillations (Welsh et al. 2005). Abnormalities in the inferior olive, as well as in the cerebellum (Bauman et al. 1997), might thus contribute to inefficient sensory processing in autism.

Finally, processing of local details is known to engage left hemisphere activity more strongly than right and was clearly demonstrated in children with early lateralized brain lesions (Nass 2002). The opposite is the case for gauging social expression, prosody, taking in complex situations at a glance, and other skills that require attention to the global scene. There is now a large neuropsychological, electrophysiological and imaging literature that explores the local/global dichotomy in autism and its consequences for attention, memory, reasoning and cognitive style (Dakin and Frith 2005, Mottron et al. 2006). The interhemispheric dichotomy of better left than right processing in autism may have some truth but is clearly too simplistic. For example, a counter example that springs to mind is inadequate language in those children with poor receptive-expressive skills. What is a much more attractive view than an all-or-none theory is to think of graded difference in competence for complex skills, most of which engage both hemispheres, albeit plausibly to different degrees, and do so to varying degrees in different individuals, especially those with atypical brains.

CONCLUSION

If this whirlwind review has had the virtue of bringing out how much more there is to learn about the complexities of sensory processing in autism and its neurologic basis, that simplistic views that consider only deficits and ignore superior skills are grossly inadequate, and how many research questions remain to be answered, it will have had a useful role. It has also stressed repeatedly, because it is so often ignored by researchers what clinicians know well: autism is heterogeneous, even in well matched samples, because it is not a single disease and the expectation that deficits (or superiorities) represent universal traits is fallacious. Investigators need to heed the recommendations of Rogers and Ozonoff (2005) regarding research design and sample choices and to be aware of pitfalls in the interpretation of limited results. Finally, until deficits in thus far neglected sensory modalities are tackled, devising rational and effective therapies will continue to elude us, and precious time and large sums of money will continue to be spent on treatments lacking an empirical basis or demonstrated effectiveness.

ACKNOWLEDGMENTS
Many thanks to Drs S Moshé, M Steinschneider and RF Tuchman for their constructive suggestions.

REFERENCES

Alcantara JI, Weisblatt EJ, Moore BC, Bolton PF (2004) Speech-in-noise perception in high-functioning individuals with autism or Asperger's syndrome. *J Child Psychol Psychiatry* 45: 1107–14.

Ayres AJ, Tickle LS (1980) Hyper-responsivity to touch and vestibular stimuli as a predictor of positive response to sensory integration procedures by autistic children. *Am J Occup Ther* 34: 375–81.

Baranek GT (2002) Efficacy of sensory and motor interventions for children with autism. *J Autism Dev Disord* 32: 397–422.

Baranek GT, Foster LG, Berkson G (1997) Tactile defensiveness and stereotyped behaviors. *Am J Occup Ther* 51: 91–5.

Baron-Cohen S, Leslie AM, Frith U (1985) Does the autistic child have a "theory of mind"? *Cognition* 21: 37–46.

Bartak L, Rutter M (1976) Differences between mentally retarded and normally intelligent autistic children. *J Autism Child Schizophr* 6: 109–20.

Bauman ML, Kemper TL (1985) Histoanatomic observations of the brain in early infantile autism. *Neurology* 35: 866–74.

Bauman ML, Kemper TL (2005) Neuroanatomic observations of the brain in autism: a review and future directions. *Int J Dev Neurosci* 23: 183–7.

Bauman ML, Filipek PA, Kemper TL (1997) Early infantile autism. *Int Rev Neurobiol* 41: 367–86.

Beckett C, Bredenkamp D, Castle J, Groothues C, O'Connor TG, Rutter M (2002) Behavior patterns associated with institutional deprivation: a study of children adopted from Romania. *J Dev Behav Pediatr* 23: 297–303.

Bertone A, Mottron L, Jelenic P, Faubert J (2003) Motion perception in autism: a "complex" issue. *J Cogn Neurosci* 15: 218–25.

Bertone A, Mottron L, Jelenic P, Faubert J (2005) Enhanced and diminished visuo-spatial information processing in autism depends on stimulus complexity. *Brain* 128: 2430–41.

Boddaert N, Zilbovicius M (2002) Functional neuroimaging and childhood autism. *Pediatr Radiol* 32: 1–7.

Boddaert N, Chabane N, Belin P, Bourgeois M, Royer V, Barthelemy C, Mouren-Simeoni MC, Philippe A, Brunelle F, Samson Y, Zilbovicius M (2004a) Perception of complex sounds in autism: abnormal auditory cortical processing in children. *Am J Psychiatry* 161: 2117–20.

Boddaert N, Chabane N, Gervais H, Good CD, Bourgeois M, Plumet MH, Barthelemy C, Mouren MC, Artiges E, Samson Y, Brunelle F, Frackowiak RS, Zilbovicius M (2004b) Superior temporal sulcus anatomical abnormalities in childhood autism: a voxel-based morphometry MRI study. *Neuroimage* 23: 364–9.

Bodfish JW, Symons FJ, Parker DE, Lewis MH (2000) Varieties of repetitive behavior in autism: comparisons to mental retardation. *J Autism Dev Disord* 30: 237–43.

Boeschoten MA, Kemner C, Kenemans JL, Engeland H (2005) The relationship between local and global processing and the processing of high and low spatial frequencies studied by event-related potentials and source modeling. *Brain Res Cogn Brain Res* 24: 228–36.

Bonnel A, Mottron L, Peretz I, Trudel M, Gallun E, Bonnel AM (2003) Enhanced pitch sensitivity in individuals with autism: a signal detection analysis. *J Cogn Neurosci* 15: 226–35.

Brasic JR, Barnett JY, Ahn SC, Nadrich RH, Will MV, Clair A (1997) Clinical assessment of self-injurious behavior. *Psychol Rep* 80: 155–60.

Breau LM, Camfield CS, Symons FJ, Bodfish JW, Mackay A, Finley GA, McGrath PJ (2003) Relation between pain and self-injurious behavior in nonverbal children with severe cognitive impairments. *J Pediatr* 142: 498–503.

Brown C, Gruber T, Boucher J, Rippon G, Brock J (2005) Gamma abnormalities during perception of illusory figures in autism. *Cortex* 41: 364–76.

Brown R, Hobson RP, Lee A, Stevenson J (1997) Are there "autistic-like" features in congenitally blind children? *J Child Psychol Psychiatry* 38: 693–703.

Buchwald JS, Erwin R, Van Lancker D, Guthrie D, Schwafel J, Tanguay P (1992) Midlatency auditory evoked responses: P1 abnormalities in adult autistic subjects. *Electroencephalogr Clin Neurophysiol* 84: 164–71.

Buxhoeveden DP, Casanova MF (2002) The minicolumn hypothesis in neuroscience. *Brain* 125: 935–51.

Carr EG, Smith CE (1995) Biological setting events for self-injury. *Ment Retard Dev Disabil Res Rev* 1: 94–8.

Casanova MF, Buxhoeveden DP, Switala AE, Roy E (2002) Minicolumnar pathology in autism. *Neurology* 58: 428–32.

Ceponiene R, Lepisto T, Shestakova A, Vanhala R, Alku P, Naatanen R, Yaguchi K (2003) Speech-sound-selective auditory impairment in children with autism: they can perceive but do not attend. *Proc Natl Acad Sci USA* 100: 5567–72.

Chase JB (1972) *Retrolental Fibroplasia and Autistic Symptomatology.* New York: American Foundation for the Blind.

Chess S, Korn SJ, Fernandez PB (1971) *Psychiatric Disorders of Children with Congenital Rubella.* New York: Brunner/Mazel.

Courchesne E, Courchesne RY, Hicks G, Lincoln AJ (1985) Functioning of the brain-stem auditory pathway in non-retarded autistic individuals. *Electroencephalogr Clin Neurophysiol* 61: 491–501.

Courchesne E, Yeung-Courchesne R, Press GA, Hesselink JR, Jernigan TL (1988) Hypoplasia of cerebellar vermal lobules VI and VII in autism. *N Engl J Med* 318: 1349–54.

Courchesne E, Townsend J, Akshoomoff NA, Saitoh O, Yeung-Courchesne R, Lincoln AJ, James HE, Haas RH, Schreibman L, Lau L (1994) Impairment in shifting attention in autistic and cerebellar patients. *Behav Neurosci* 108: 848–65.

Dakin S, Frith U (2005) Vagaries of visual perception in autism. *Neuron* 48: 497–507.

Davis RA, Bockbrader MA, Murphy RR, Hetrick WP, O'Donnell BF (2006) Subjective perceptual distortions and visual dysfunction in children with autism. J Autism Dev Disord (in press).

De Fosse L, Hodge SM, Makris N, Kennedy DN, Caviness VS, McGrath L, Steele S, Ziegler DA, Herbert MR, Frazier JA, Tager-Flusberg H, Harris GJ (2004) Language-association cortex asymmetry in autism and specific language impairment. *Ann Neurol* 56: 757–66.

Dunn MA, Bates JC (2005) Developmental change in neural processing of words by children with autism. *J Autism Dev Dis* 35: 361–76.

Dunn M, Vaughan HG, Kreutzer J, Kurtzberg D (1999) Electrophysiologic correlates of semantic classification in autistic and normal children. Dev Neuropsychol 16: 75-99.

Fein D, Skoff B, Mirsky AF (1981) Clinical correlates of brainstem dysfunction in autistic children. J Autism Dev Disord 11: 303-315.

Frith U (1989) *Autism: Explaining the Enigma.* Oxford: Basil Blackwell.

Frith U (1991) *Autism and Asperger Syndrome.* Cambridge: Cambridge University Press.

Frith U, Happe F (1994) Autism: beyond "theory of mind". *Cognition* 50: 115–32.

Gepner B, Mestre DR (2002) Brief report: postural reactivity to fast visual motion differentiates autistic from children with Asperger syndrome. *J Autism Dev Disord* 32: 231–8.

Gepner B, Mestre D, Masson G, de Schonen S (1995) Postural effects of motion vision in young autistic children. *Neuroreport* 6: 1211–4.

Gervais H, Belin P, Boddaert N, Leboyer M, Coez A, Sfaello I, Barthelemy C, Brunelle F, Samson Y, Zilbovicius M (2004) Abnormal cortical voice processing in autism. *Nat Neurosci* 7: 801–2.

Gillberg C (1990) Autism and pervasive developmental disorders. *J Child Psychol Psychiatry* 310: 91–119.

Gillberg C (1995) Endogeneous opioids and opiate antagonists in autism: brief review of empirical findings and implications for clinicians. *Dev Med Child Neurol* 37: 239–45.

Gillberg C, Coleman M (2000) *The Biology of the Autistic Syndromes, 3rd edn. Clinics in Developmental Medicine No. 153/154.* London: Mac Keith Press.

Goldberg MC, Landa R, Lasker A, Cooper L, Zee DS (2000) Evidence of normal cerebellar control of the vestibulo-ocular reflex (VOR) in children with high-functioning autism. *J Autism Dev Disord* 30: 519–24.

Goldberg MC, Lasker AG, Zee DS, Garth E, Tien A, Landa RJ (2002) Deficits in the initiation of eye movements in the absence of a visual target in adolescents with high functioning autism. *Neuropsychologia* 40: 2039–49.

Grandin T (1995) *Thinking in Pictures and Other Reports from my Life with Autism.* New York: Doubleday.

Gravel JS, Dunn M, Lee WW, Ellis MA (2006) Peripheral audition of children on the autistic spectrum. *Ear Hear* 27: 299–312.

Hadjikhani N, Chabris CF, Joseph RM, Clark J, McGrath L, Aharon I, Feczko E, Tager-Flusberg H, Harris GJ (2004) Early visual cortex organization in autism: an fMRI study. *Neuroreport* 15: 267–70.

Hall S, Oliver C, Murphy G (2001) Self-injurious behaviour in young children with Lesch–Nyhan syndrome. *Dev Med Child Neurol* 43: 745–9.

Happe F, Frith U (1999) How the mind reads the mind. *Neurosci News* 2: 16–25.

Harlow HF, Harlow M (1962) Social deprivation in monkeys. *Sci Am* 207: 136–46.

Hauck M, Fein D, Maltby N, Waterhouse L, Feinstein C (1998) Memory for faces in children with autism. *Child Neuropsychol* 4: 187–98.

Heaton P (2003) Pitch memory, labelling and disembedding in autism. *J Child Psychol Psychiatry* 44: 543–51.

Heaton P, Pring L, Hermelin B (2001) Musical processing in high functioning children with autism. *Ann NY Acad Sci* 930: 443–4.

Herbert MR, Harris GJ, Adrien KT, Ziegler DA, Makris N, Kennedy DN, Lange NT, Chabris CF, Bakardjiev A, Hodgson J, Takeoka M, Tager-Flusberg H, Caviness VS (2002) Abnormal asymmetry in language association cortex in autism. *Ann Neurology* 52: 588–96.

Herbert MR, Ziegler DA, Deutsch CK, O'Brien LM, Kennedy DN, Filipek PA, Bakardjiev AI, Hodgson J, Takeoka M, Makris N, Caviness VS (2005) Brain asymmetries in autism and developmental language disorder: a nested whole-brain analysis. *Brain* 128: 213–26.

Hobson RP, Bishop M (2003) The pathogenesis of autism: insights from congenital blindness. *Philos Trans R Soc Lond B Biol Sci* 358: 335–44.

Hobson RP, Lee A, Brown R (1999) Autism and congenital blindness. *J Autism Dev Disord* 29: 45–56.

Hoeksma MR, Kemner C, Verbaten MN, van Engeland H (2004) Processing capacity in children and adolescents with pervasive developmental disorders. *J Autism Dev Disord* 34: 341–54.

Horton JC, Sincich LC (2004) A new foundation for the visual cortical hierarchy. In: Gazzaniga MS, ed. *The Cognitive Neurosciences, 3rd edn.* Cambridge MA: Massachussetts Institute of Technology, pp. 233–43.

Jure R, Rapin I, Tuchman RF (1991) Hearing-impaired autistic children. *Dev Med Child Neurol* 33: 1062–72.

Kanner L (1943) Autistic disturbances of affective contact. *Nerv Child* 2: 217–50.

Kasai K, Hashimoto O, Kawakubo Y, Yumoto M, Kamio S, Itoh K, Koshida I, Iwanami A, Nakagome K, Fukuda M, Yamasue H, Yamada H, Abe O, Aoki S, Kato N (2005) Delayed automatic detection of change in speech sounds in adults with autism: a magnetoencephalographic study. *Clin Neurophysiol* 116: 1655–64.

Kaufmann WE, Cooper KL, Mostofsky SH, Capone GT, Kates WR, Newschaffer CJ, Bukelis I, Stump MH, Jann AE, Lanham DC (2003) Specificity of cerebellar vermian abnormalities in autism: a quantitative magnetic resonance imaging study. *J Child Neurol* 18: 463–70.

Kellerman GR, Fan J, Gorman JM (2005) Auditory abnormalities in autism: toward functional distinctions among findings. *CNS Spectr* 10: 748–56.

Kemner C, Verbaten MN, Cuperus JM, Camfferman G, van Engeland H (1994) Visual and somatosensory event-related brain potentials in autistic children and three different control groups. *Electroencephalogr Clin Neurophysiol* 92: 225–37.

Kemner C, van der Geest JN, Verbaten MN, van Engeland H (2004) In search of neurophysiological markers of pervasive developmental disorders: smooth pursuit eye movements? *J Neural Transm* 111: 1617–26.

Kern L, Bailin D, Mauk JE (2003) Effects of a topical anesthetic on non-socially maintained self-injurious behavior. *Dev Med Child Neurol* 45, 769–71.

Khalfa S, Bruneau N, Roge B, Georgieff N, Veuillet E, Adrien JL, Barthelemy C, Collet L (2004) Increased perception of loudness in autism. *Hear Res* 198: 87–92.

Klein SK, Kurtzberg D, Brattson A, Kreutzer JA, Stapells DR, Dunn MA, Rapin I, Vaughan HG (1995) Electrophysiologic manifestations of impaired temporal lobe auditory processing in verbal auditory agnosia. *Brain Lang* 51: 383–405.

Klein SK, Tuchman RF, Rapin I (2000) The influence of premorbid language skills and behavior on language recovery in children with verbal auditory agnosia. *J Child Neurol* 15: 36–43.

Klin A (1993) Auditory brain stem responses in autism: Brain stem dysfunction or peripheral hearing loss? *J Autism Dev Dis* 23: 15–35.

Klin A, Sparrow SS, de Bildt A, Cicchetti DV, Cohen DJ, Volkmar FR (1999) A normed study of face recognition in autism and related disorders. *J Autism Dev Disord* 29: 499–508.

Klin A, Jones W, Schultz R, Volkmar F, Cohen D (2002) Visual fixation patterns during viewing of naturalistic social situations as predictors of social competence in individuals with autism. *Arch Gen Psychiatry* 59: 809–16.

Kogan CS, Boutet I, Cornish K, Zangenehpour S, Mullen KT, Holden JJ, Der Kaloustian VM, Andermann E, Chaudhuri A (2004) Differential impact of the FMR1 gene on visual processing in fragile X syndrome. *Brain* 127: 591–601.

Kohen-Raz R, Volkmar FR, Cohen DJ (1992) Postural control in children with autism. *J Autism Dev Disord* 22: 419–32.

Leslie AM, Frith U (1988) Autistic children's understanding of seeing, knowing and believing. *Br J Clin Psychol* 6: 315–24.

Lloyd KG, Hornykiewicz O, Davidson L, Shannak K, Farley I, Goldstein M, Shibuya M, Kelley WN, Fox IH (1981) Biochemical evidence of dysfunction of brain neurotransmitters in the Lesch–Nyhan syndrome. *N Engl J Med* 305: 1106–11.

Lord C, Rutter M, Le Couteur A (1994) Autism Diagnostic Interview–Revised: A revised version of a diagnostic interview for caregivers of individuals with possible pervasive developmental disorders. *J Autism Dev Dis* 24: 659–85.

Lord C, Rutter M, DiLavore P, Rial S (1999) *Autism Diagnostic Observation Schedule – WPS Edition.* Los Angeles: Western Psychological Services.

Mace FC, Mace JE (1995) Bio-behavioral diagnosis and treatment of self-injury. *Ment Retard Dev Disabil Res Rev* 1: 104–10.

Maurer RG, Damasio AR (1979) Vestibular dysfunction in autistic children. *Dev Med Child Neurol* 21: 656–9.

Maziade M, Merette C, Cayer M, Roy MA, Szatmari P, Cote R, Thivierge J (2000) Prolongation of brainstem auditory-evoked responses in autistic probands and their unaffected relatives. *Arch Gen Psychiatry* 57: 1077–83.

McPartland J, Dawson G, Webb SJ, Panagiotides H, Carver LJ (2004) Event-related brain potentials reveal anomalies in temporal processing of faces in autism spectrum disorder. *J Child Psychol Psychiatry* 45: 1235–45.

Milne E, Swettenham J, Hansen P, Campbell R, Jeffries H, Plaisted K (2002) High motion coherence thresholds in children with autism. *J Child Psychol Psychiatry* 43: 255–63.

Minshew NJ, Luna B, Sweeney JA (1999) Oculomotor evidence for neocortical systems but not cerebellar dysfunction in autism. *Neurology* 52: 917–22.

Mottron L, Dawson M, Soulieres I, Hubert B, Burack J (2006) Enhanced perceptual functioning in autism: an update, and eight principles of autistic perception. *J Autism Dev Dis* 36: 27–43.

Mukamel R, Gelbard H, Arieli A, Hasson U, Fried I, Malach R (2005) Coupling between neuronal firing, field potentials, and FMRI in human auditory cortex. *Science* 309: 951–4.

Muller R-A, Behen ME, Rothermel RD, Chugani DC, Muzik O, Mangner TJ, Chugani HT (1999) Brain mapping of language and auditory perception in high-functioning autistic adults: a PET study. *J Autism Dev Dis* 29: 19–31.

Nass R (2002) Plasticity: mechanisms, extent and limits. In: Segalowitz SJ, Rapin I, eds. *Child Neuropsychology, 2nd edn.* Amsterdam: Elsevier Science, pp. 29–68.

Newson P, Lynch-Frame A, Roach R, Bennett S, Carr V, Chahl LA (2005) Intrinsic sensory deprivation induced by neonatal capsaicin treatment induces changes in rat brain and behaviour of possible relevance to schizophrenia. *Br J Pharmacol* 146: 408–18.

Novick B, Vaughan HG, Kurtzberg D, Simson R (1980) An electrophysiologic indication of auditory processing defects in autism. *Psychiatry Res* 3: 107–14.

Nowinski CV, Minshew NJ, Luna B, Takarae Y, Sweeney JA (2005) Oculomotor studies of cerebellar function in autism. *Psychiatry Res* 137: 11–9.

Oaklander AL, Cohen SP, Raju SV (2002) Intractable postherpetic itch and cutaneous deafferentation after facial shingles. *Pain* 96: 9–12.

O'Connor N, Hermelin B (1987) Visual and graphic abilities of the idiot savant artist. *Psychol Med* 17: 79–90.

Oram Cardy JE, Flagg EJ, Roberts W, Brian J, Roberts TP (2005) Magnetoencephalography identifies rapid temporal processing deficit in autism and language impairment. *Neuroreport* 16: 329–32.

Ornitz EM (1974) The modulation of sensory input and motor output in autistic children. *J Autism Child Schizophr* 4: 197–215.

Pellicano E, Gibson L, Maybery M, Durkin K, Badcock DR (2005) Abnormal global processing along the dorsal visual pathway in autism: a possible mechanism for weak visuospatial coherence? *Neuropsychologia* 43: 1044–53.

Plaisted K, Saksida L, Alcantara J, Weisblatt E (2003) Towards an understanding of the mechanisms of weak central coherence effects: experiments in visual configural learning and auditory perception. *Philos Trans R Soc Lond B Biol Sci* 358: 375–86.

Plaisted K, Dobler V, Bell S, Davis G (2006) The microgenesis of global perception in autism. *J Autism Dev Disord* (in press).

Polizzi A, Pavone P, Iannetti P, Gambardella A, Ruggieri M (2005) CNS findings in three cases of septo-optic dysplasia, including one with semilobar holoprosencephaly. *Am J Med Genet A* 136: 357.

Rapin I, Gravel JS (2003) "Auditory neuropathy": physiologic and pathologic evidence calls for more diagnostic specificity. *Int J Pediatr Otorhinolaryngol* 67: 707–28.

Raynes HR, Shanske A, Goldberg S, Burde R, Rapin I (1999) Joubert syndrome: monozygotic twins with discordant phenotypes. *J Child Neurol* 14: 649–54.

Richer JM, Coss RG (1976) Gaze aversion in autistic and normal children. *Acta Psychiatr Scand* 53: 193–210.

Ritvo ER, Ornitz EM, Eviatar A, Markham CH, Brown MB, Mason A (1969) Decreased post-rotatory nystagmus in early infantile autism. *Neurology* 19: 653–8.

Rogers SJ, Ozonoff S (2005) Annotation: what do we know about sensory dysfunction in autism? A critical review of the empirical evidence. *J Child Psychol Psychiatry* 46: 1255–68.

Rogers SJ, Hepburn S, Wehner E (2003) Parent reports of sensory symptoms in toddlers with autism and those with other developmental disorders. *J Autism Dev Disord* 33: 631–42.

Roper L, Arnold P, Monteiro B (2003) Co-occurrence of autism and deafness: diagnostic considerations. *Autism* 7: 245–53.

Rosenhall U, Nordin V, Brantberg K, Gillberg C (2003) Autism and auditory brain stem responses. *Ear Hear* 24: 206–14.

Rosenhall U, Nordin V, Sandstrom M, Ahlsen G, Gillberg C (1999) Autism and hearing loss. *J Autism Dev Disord* 29: 349–57.

Rutter M, O'Connor TG (2004) Are there biological programming effects for psychological development? Findings from a study of Romanian adoptees. *Dev Psychol* 40: 81–94.

Sallustro F, Atwell CW (1978) Body rocking, head banging, and head rolling in normal children. *J Pediatr* 93: 704–8.

Sandman CA, Hetrick WP (1995) Opiate mechanisms in self-injury. *Ment Retard Dev Disabil Res Rev* 1: 130–7.

Sandman CA, Hetrick W, Talyor D, Marion S, Chicz-Demet A (2000) Uncoupling of proopio-melanocortin (POMC) fragments is related to self-injury. *Peptides* 21: 785–91.

Sandman CA, Touchette P, Marion S, Lenjavi M, Chicz-Demet A (2002) Disregulation of pro-opiomelanocortin and contagious maladaptive behavior. *Regul Pept* 108: 179–85.

Scharre JE, Creedon MP (1992) Assessment of visual function in autistic children. *Optom Vis Sci* 69: 433–9.

Schroeder S, Schroeder C, Smith D, Dalldorf J (1978) Prevalence of self-injurious behavior in a large state facility for the retarded. *J Autism Child Schizophr* 8: 261–9.

Schroeder SR, Hammock RG, Mulick JA, Rojahn J, Walson P, Fernald W, Meinhold P, Saphare G (1995) Clinical trials of D1 and D2 dopamine modulating drugs and self-injury in mental retardation and developmental disability. *Ment Retard Dev Disabil Res Rev* 1: 120–9.

Schultz RT, Grelotti DJ, Klin A, Kleinman J, Van der Gaag C, Marois R, Skudlarski P (2003) The role of the fusiform face area in social cognition: implications for the pathobiology of autism. *Philos Trans R Soc Lond B Biol Sci* 358: 415–27.

Shriberg LD, Paul R, McSweeny JL, Klin AM, Cohen DJ, Volkmar FR (2001) Speech and prosody characteristics of adolescents and adults with high-functioning autism and Asperger syndrome. *J Speech Lang Hear Res* 44: 1097–115.

Slavik BA, Kitsuwa-Lowe J, Danner PT, Green J, Ayres AJ (1984) Vestibular stimulation and eye contact in autistic children. *Neuropediatrics* 15: 33–6.

Spitz RA (1945) Hospitalism: an enquiry into the genesis of psychiatric conditions in early childhood. *Psychoanal Study Child* 1: 53–74.

Stapells DR, Oates P (1997) Estimation of the pure-tone audiogram by the auditory brainstem response: a review. *Audiol Neurootol* 2: 257–80.

Steinschneider M, Dunn M (2002) Electrophysiology in developmental neuropsychology. In: Segalowitz S, Rapin I, eds. *Handbook of Neuropsychology, vol. 8. Child Neuropsychology, 2nd edn.* Amsterdam: Elsevier Science, pp. 91–146.

Symons FJ (2005) Self-injurious behavior and sequential analysis: context matters. *Am J Ment Retard* 110: 323–6.

Symons FJ, Thompson A, Rodriguez MC (2004) Self-injurious behavior and the efficacy of naltrexone treatment: a quantitative synthesis. *Ment Retard Dev Disabil Res Rev* 10: 193–200.

Takarae Y, Minshew NJ, Luna B, Krisky CM, Sweeney JA (2004a) Pursuit eye movement deficits in autism. *Brain* 127: 2584–94.

Takarae Y, Minshew NJ, Luna B, Sweeney JA (2004b) Oculomotor abnormalities parallel cerebellar histopathology in autism. *J Neurol Neurosurg Psychiatry* 75: 1359–61.

Tecchio F, Benassi F, Zappasodi F, Gialloreti LE, Palermo M, Seri S, Rossini PM (2003) Auditory sensory processing in autism: a magnetoencephalographic study. *Biol Psychiatry* 54: 647–54.

Thivierge J, Bedard C, Cote R, Maziade M (1990) Brainstem auditory evoked response and subcortical abnormalities in autism. *Am J Psychiatry* 147: 1609–13.

Thompson T, Symons F, Delaney D, England C (1995) Self-injurious behavior as an endogeneous neurochemical self-administration. *Ment Retard Dev Disabil Res Rev* 1: 137–48.

Treffert DA (2005) The savant syndrome in autistic disorder. In: Casanova MF, ed. *Recent Developments in Autism Research.* New York: Nova Science, pp. 27–55.

Tsao DY, Freiwald WA, Tootell RBH, Livingstone MS (2006) A cortical region consisting entirely of face-selective cells. *Science* 311: 670–4.

Welsh JP, Ahn ES, Placantonakis DG (2005) Is autism due to brain desynchronization? *Int J Dev Neurosci* 23: 253–63.

Yamashita Y, Fujimoto C, Nakajima E, Isagai T, Matsuishi T (2003) Possible association between congenital cytomegalovirus infection and autistic disorder. *J Autism Dev Disord* 33: 455–9.

Zilbovicius M, Boddaert N, Belin P, Poline JB, Remy P, Mangin JF, Thivard L, Barthelemy C, Samson Y (2000) Temporal lobe dysfunction in childhood autism: A PET study. Positron emission tomography. *Am J Psychiatry* 157: 1988–93.

14
MOTOR DEFICITS IN AUTISM

Jennifer C Gidley Larson and Stewart H Mostofsky

HISTORICAL PERSPECTIVE

In 1943, Kanner presented 11 case studies of what he termed "early infantile autism". Among the other well-known deficits of sociability and communication, Kanner described stereotyped behaviors and commented that many of the children were clumsy in both gait and gross motor performance. In addition, many parents reported that as infants almost all of the children had a failure to assume the anticipatory posture for being picked up out of the crib; even after being picked up, the infants remained passive and would not adjust their body to the correct position for being held. In addition to confirming the lack of postural adjustment, Eveloff (1960) reported a single case of a child with autistic disorder (AD) who demonstrated poor body awareness and boundaries, as well as odd posturing and facial grimacing in the event of an overwhelming emotion. Shortly after Kanner's publication, Ritvo and Provence (1953, cited in Williams et al. 2004) reported evidence of deficient imitative learning in a 21-month-old boy with AD. The child's mother noted that her son could not play pat-a-cake simply by watching her, instead she had to move his hands through the appropriate actions of the game for him to learn the pattern of movements.

Evidence accumulated since those initial descriptions indicates that impairments in motor development are a common, if not consistent, finding in children with autism spectrum disorders (ASDs), equally present across high functioning and low functioning individuals. In one of the initial studies that examined basic motor functioning in autism, Ornitz et al. (1977) found that disturbances in motility (hand flaps, finger flicks, body posture, incorrect gesturing, toe walking, and darting or lunging movements) were present in approximately 70% of their ASD group. Additionally, they found that parents reported significant delays in motor development in children, later diagnosed with ASD, as young as 6–12 months. Similar findings of motor disturbance are found throughout the literature on autism (DeMyer et al. 1972, Vilensky et al. 1981, Jones and Prior 1985, Rapin 1991, Hallett et al. 1993, Haas et al. 1996, Rogers et al. 1996, Teitelbaum et al. 1998, Baranek 2002, Green et al. 2002, Noterdaeme et al. 2002). These include abnormalities in basic aspects of motor control, including gait, posture, coordination and tone, as well as difficulties with imitation and with pantomime of complex gestures (often referred to as dyspraxia); each of these motor abnormalities will be discussed in greater depth throughout the chapter. The chapter will also highlight how characterization of motor dysfunction can increase insight into the brain mechanisms underlying ASD; motor signs can serve as markers for deficits in parallel brain systems important for control of the social and communication skill impairments that characterize autism, and by using tests of motor function for which neurologic basis is well mapped out, it may be possible to gain understanding of the neural circuits impaired in autism.

BASIC MOTOR DEFICITS

Despite the historical findings and the abundant literature that suggests otherwise, motor impairments, including dystonia, unusual gait, posture, balance and coordination, and abnormal performance of complex motor movements, are not considered a core feature of autism. However, motor "mannerisms" such as repetitive and stereotyped behaviors, hand flapping, finger flicking, body rocking and unusual twisting of the hands are listed as a defining feature of autism in the DSM-IV classification system (APA 1994), all of which testify to dysfunction of the motor system.

Motor dysfunction in ASD appears to be evident during infancy (Kanner 1943; Eveloff 1960; Ornitz et al. 1977; Teitelbaum et al. 1998, 2004; Baranek 1999; Watson et al. 2003). Its presence at such an early age suggests that motor abnormalities may be a core deficit of ASD. In a retrospective video analysis of infants aged 9–12 months, Baranek (1999) found that a combination of sensory–motor behaviors, including anticipatory posturing, correctly discriminated children with autism from typically developing children and those with developmental disabilities. Teitelbaum et al. (1998), also by way of childhood videos, analyzed infantile movements using Eshkol–Wachman movement notation (Eshkol and Wachman 1958). In children later diagnosed with ASD, they detected deviations from expected motor development in lying, sitting and standing and found that the children experienced difficulties in sequencing movements appropriately when learning to roll, crawl and walk. Using the same movement notation, Teitelbaum et al. (2004) observed similar motor patterns in infants later diagnosed with Asperger syndrome (ASP). A weakness of the two Teitelbaum studies is the lack of a typically developing comparison group. Nevertheless, these studies suggest that abnormal motor signs may be observable from birth.

Beyond infancy, basic motor deficits have been found in gait, coordination, posture and tone in both children and adults with autism. Maurer and Damasio (1982) observed a variety of disturbances in action, posture and tone in children with autism, including asymmetrical and odd postures while standing and walking, as well as diminished arm swing and flexed elbows during walking, disturbances which, they suggested, resembled those seen in patients with basal ganglia dysfunction. Vilensky et al. (1981) used a motion analyzer to measure components of locomotion (upper-limb movements, orientation of elbows, posture, foot–ground contact, etc.) after filming children walking on a track. When compared to normal children, the ASD group was found to spend a greater amount of time in the stance phase (period between initial foot–ground contact and toe-off), to have shorter stride lengths, and to land more flat footed or on their toes (rather than heel to toe); upper-limb movement was reduced or uncoordinated, and the hands and fingers showed dystonic posture. These abnormalities were thought to be similar to those seen in Parkinsonism, and the authors suggested that the motor disturbances seen in ASD might be a result of an impaired basal ganglia function.

In a more recent study, Hallett et al. (1993) examined the locomotion of 5 adults with autism. Four of the subjects were mildly ataxic, 2 had unstable balance, and all 5 showed decreased range of motion at the ankle and abnormal upper-limb posturing; however, in contrast to the findings of Vilensky et al. (1981), these AD adults showed normal gait velocity and step length. In addition, 3 of the subjects presented with neurological soft signs suggestive of cerebellar dysfunction, and the authors posited a role of the cerebellum in the motor disturbances in autism. Furthermore, hypotonia, which is often observed in children with ASD (Maurer and Damasio 1982), can be associated with cerebellar abnormalities (Takanashi et al. 1999, Varan et al. 2001).

Standardized motor examinations have also been used to examine motor impairments in children with autism. Our own group (Jansiewicz et al. 2005) used the Physical and Neurological Examination for Subtle Signs (PANESS; Denckla 1985) to assesses gait (in particular stressed gait maneuvers, including tandem gait and walking on heels, toes and sides of the feet), balance, speed of repetitive and patterned movements, dysrhythmia and overflow movements. We found that children with ASD made significantly more errors than typically developing controls on almost all measures, showing greater difficulty with balance (both right and left feet, eyes open), and in performance of all stressed gait maneuvers; they also displayed significantly more overflow and dysrhythmia than did controls and were slower on timed repetitive movements of the hands and feet.

Beyond basic aspects of motor coordination, children with ASD have also been found to show deficits in motor response preparation and planning. In a task of motor reprogramming, using a reciprocating sequence on a four-button box with an occasional "oddball" movement that disturbed the sequence, causing the child to move in an unexpected direction, Rinehart et al. (2001) reported that children with high functioning autism (HFA) and ASP had normal ability to execute these movements, while their reaction time for movement preparation was abnormally slow. This finding is consistent with an earlier study that also observed a disruption in motor planning in children with autism; the investigator (Hughes 1996) postulated that this disruption might be due to a more widespread deficit in the ability to perform goal-directed sequenced movements.

Other findings suggest that deficits in intersensory processing of the visual, vestibular and proprioceptive inputs, important for guiding motor execution, may also contribute to the motor deficits of ASD. Some studies suggest over-reliance on visual feedback to maintain balance and stability, while others point to disruption of the vestibular or proprioceptive systems, in either case suggesting abnormalities of multimodal intersensory integration (Weimer et al. 2001, Minshew et al. 2004).

DEFICITS IN IMITATION

In addition to the more broadly defined basic motor dysfunctions just discussed, one of the most consistently reported motor findings in the autism literature is deficit in imitation (for detailed reviews, see Smith and Bryson 1994, Rogers et al. 1996, Williams et al. 2004). Children with ASD consistently imitate less and make specific errors when compared to both clinical and typically developing controls (Smith and Bryson 1994, Williams et al. 2001, Rogers et al. 2003). These deficits have been observed in both high and low functioning individuals with autism and across a wide age range (from early childhood through adulthood), suggesting that impaired imitation may be a fundamental deficit in autism.

Impairments in imitation were first reported by DeMyer et al. (1972), who found that children with autism performed poorly on body imitation, better in motor-object imitation, and best in spontaneous object use. Similarly, Jones and Prior (1985) found that children with AD exhibited significant deficits in imitation both for gesture, assessed by the Imitation of Gestures Test (Berges and Lezine 1965), and for dynamic movements (i.e. swinging movements of arms and legs, lateral and vertical extensions), assessed by the Test of Dynamic Body Movement (constructed for that study). Children with AD were matched on chronological age and mental age to typically developing children. The AD group was significantly impaired in both gesture and dynamic movements; in fact, the 6- to 10-year-old AD children were not yet performing at a preschool level when compared to the control groups. The investigators also observed that the children with AD had difficulties integrating their hands in bimanual coordination, and that the movements were awkward and "out of control". In more recent studies, children with autism have been found to show impairments in imitating simple body movements (Rogers and Pennington 1991), imitating both meaningful and non-meaningful sequential movements (Rogers et al. 1996), and imitating both orofacial movements and actions on objects (Rogers et al. 2003). Adults with HFA and ASP show significant impairments when imitating a simple movement sequence in a *mirror-image* fashion (i.e. movements by experimenter's left hand correspond to movements by subject's right hand) (Avikainen et al. 2003).

Several lines of evidence suggest the deficits seen in imitation are to a certain degree specific to ASDs and may be a differentiating factor between ASDs and other childhood disorders. Findings across a number of studies reveal that children with autism demonstrate specific weaknesses and errors in tasks of imitation when compared to children with ADHD (Ohta 1987), Down syndrome (Libby et al. 1997), nonspecific developmental delay (Charman et al. 1997, Stone et al. 1997), mental retardation, hearing impairment, language impairment (Stone et al. 1990), and fragile-X syndrome (Rogers et al. 2003) (for a comprehensive review, see Williams et al. 2004).

While imitative deficits are widely reported in ASD, the precise underpinnings of these deficits are still unknown. Possible mechanisms have been explored to explain this deficit in imitation, including memory and symbolic content (Smith and Bryson 1994,

Rogers et al. 1996), executive function (Rogers et al. 1996, Dawson et al. 2001), motor function (Damasio and Maurer 1978, Smith and Bryson 1998), motor planning and sequencing (Hughes 1996, Rogers et al. 1996 Minshew et al. 1997), and praxis (DeMyer et al. 1981, Rogers et al. 1996, Mostofsky et al. 2006).

PERFORMANCE OF SKILLED MOTOR GESTURES

One prominent hypothesis suggests that deficits in imitation reflect a more global impairment in praxis. While impairments in imitation of gestures have been the most often reported, several investigators have also documented impairments in pantomime of skilled motor gestures in response to verbal command or during actual tool use (DeMyer et al. 1972, 1981; Hammes and Langdell 1981; Jones and Prior 1985; Ohta 1987; Hertzig et al. 1989; Rogers et al. 1996). Imitation and pantomime tasks are used to assess limb praxis in neurologically impaired adults (Gonzales Rothi et al. 1997, Heilman and Gonzalez Rothi 2003), and it was the findings of impairments in both imitation and pantomime that led DeMyer et al. (1972) to first suggest that imitation problems in autism may be associated with "dyspraxia"; subsequently, these impairments have prompted several investigators to also suggest that a dyspraxic deficit may be associated with autism (DeMyer et al. 1981, Jones and Prior 1985, Ohta 1987, Rogers et al. 1996).

DeMyer and colleagues posited that, to imitate actions properly, one must have an intact visual memory and an appropriate concept of body movement and image, and that the consequence of a defective or disturbed body image is dyspraxia. In agreement with DeMyer, Jones and Prior (1985) postulated that the abnormal and impaired imitation and errors of orientation and coordination seen in children with AD during performance of skilled motor tasks might be characterized as dyspraxia. A similar pattern of deficits has been described in ASD (DeMyer et al. 1972, Jones and Prior 1985, Smith and Bryson 1994, Rogers et al. 1996, Williams et al. 2004, Mostofsky et al. 2006).

After finding impairments reflecting widespread deficits in imitation and pantomime in high-functioning adolescents with ASD, Rogers et al. (1996) suggested that there might be a "generalized dyspraxia" in autism. In a subsequent study of toddlers with ASD, the same group (Rogers et al. 2003) failed to find differences between typically developing children and those with autism on tests of "praxis". However, the praxis battery used in the toddlers was limited to performing novel actions with actual objects (e.g. removing a ball from a fish bowl or climbing out of a cardboard box) and did not incorporate more classic tests of praxis, such as pantomimed use of imagined tools, which are difficult to administer to toddlers. Accordingly, the findings may exclude difficulty only with motor planning/execution and not with abilities to acquire (learn), store, recall or transcode spatio-temporal representations of complex movements, which are critical to praxis (Heilman and Gonzalez Rothi 2003).

Consistent with earlier findings, our own group has found that high functioning children with ASD show significantly more errors than do typically developing controls in performing gestures not only to imitation, but also to command (i.e. pantomime) and with actual tool use (Mostofsky et al. 2006). Analysis of error types revealed that the ASD group made significantly more spatial, content/concretization and body-part-for-tool errors. Spatial errors were the most prevalent type in both children with ASD and controls, accounting for a majority of errors in both groups. The findings suggest that deficits in performance of skilled motor tasks may be secondary to impaired acquisition of spatial representations of movement and/or the motor sequence programs necessary to execute them. The findings from our analysis of praxis error types in children with autism reveal a pattern of deficits consistent with that observed in adults with acquired ideomotor apraxia. Despite the similar characterization, the neurologic basis of developmental dyspraxia, in which there may be impaired acquisition of motor and sensory representations of skilled gestures, likely differs from that of adult-onset apraxia/dyspraxia in which there is loss of previously acquired representations. It is possible that developmental dyspraxia can result from a deficit in gestural representation or execution similar to that seen in adults (Cermak 1985). Alternatively, impairments in mechanisms involved in procedural learning, important for acquisition of motor skills, may contribute to developmental dyspraxia observed in children with ASD, in contrast to adult apraxia involving loss of previously learned skills (Mostofsky et al. 2000).

MOTOR LEARNING

In the context of the developmental disorder of autism, these "dyspraxic" deficits could be secondary to a fundamental problem with acquiring motor skills, i.e. motor skill learning. Indeed, in a review of "imitation and action in autism", Smith and Bryson (1994) cited Wing (1969), noting that, "Clumsy children with autism reportedly have particular difficulty learning organized patterns of movements (e.g., skipping and dancing . . .)". Furthermore, there is evidence that procedural learning occurs as early as 3 months of age in humans (Haith et al. 1993, Nelson 1995). It follows that a developmental impairment in motor skill learning would be expected to affect the ability to perform skilled movements beginning in infancy. This would be consistent with findings in children with autism of qualitative abnormalities in early motor milestones such as sitting, crawling and walking (Losche 1990, Teitelbaum et al. 1998).

In most neuropsychological models, motor skill learning is included in a broader construct of procedural learning, which refers to the process by which skills and actions are acquired implicitly (without conscious recall) through repeated exposure to, and practice of, a task (Squire 1986); this is in contrast to declarative learning, which refers to acquisition of facts that can be recalled explicitly (with conscious recall). Mostofsky et al. (2000) found children with ASD to be impaired in a task of motor sequence learning (Serial Reaction Time Task, SRTT). When compared to typically developing children, the ASD group demonstrated an impaired ability to learn implicitly a visual-motor sequence. These findings are supported by preliminary data collected in our laboratory using a rotary pursuit (RP) task (personal data, unpublished). Motor skill (procedural) learning was measured by time-on-target across blocks and trials of the task; we observed that the ASD group demonstrated significantly less learning of this novel motor task than did the control group. Because both tasks (SRTT and RP) are visually guided, inadequacy suggests a deficit in visual–motor sequence learning in ASD.

In contrast to impaired motor sequence learning, we found that children with HFA demonstrate normal motor adaptation during a catching task in which adaptation was primarily dependent on somatosensory/proprioceptive feedback (Mostofsky et al. 2004). One interpretation from this pattern of findings is that motor sequence learning is impaired in autism, with spared adaptation. Another distinction is that for both the SRTT and RP task, motor learning is visually guided; this is in contrast to catch adaptation, in which changes in upward arm movement are produced in response to a force perturbation conveyed through somatosensory/proprioceptive feedback. It follows that in autism there may be impaired ability to use visual feedback to guide motor skill learning. This would be consistent with deficits in motor imitation that depend on visual feedback to guide the acquisition and developmental of complex imitative gestures. Consistent with these observations, Ricks and Wing (1975) commented, "Often the only way to teach motor skills to a young autistic child is to move his limbs through the action which is required", suggesting difficulty with visuomotor learning compared with motor learning dependent on somatosensory/proprioceptive feedback. Further, Asperger (see Miyahara et al. 1997) commented that autistic children have movement problems because they do not learn by watching other people in daily life. A deficit in motor learning may help explain the variety of complex motor impairments reported in the literature, and might point to the underlying neural mechanisms that underlie failure to perform complex gestures such as waving goodbye or blowing a kiss that are critical for communication and social interaction.

MOTOR DEFICITS IN AUTISTIC DISORDER VERSUS ASPERGER SYNDROME

Clumsiness has been traditionally ascribed to ASP and not AD (Szatmari et al. 1989, Klin et al. 1995, Green et al. 2002; for a review, see Macintosh and Dissanayake 2004), despite empirical studies that consistently report an equal prevalence of motor impairments in both (Ghaziuddin et al. 1994, Manjiviona and Prior 1995, Macintosh and Dissanayake 2004, Jansiewicz et al. 2006). Perhaps it was the relative lack of impairment in communication that made early investigators of ASP emphasize motor clumsiness they may have considered incongruous. Contemporary research, however, shows that motor deficits are present across the entire autism spectrum, suggesting that some motor dysfunction may be a fundamental component of the ASDs. Ghaziuddin et al. (1994) used the Bruiniks–Oseretsky test of motor proficiency (Bruininks 1978) to assess clumsiness and found no differences between ASP and AD. In a follow-up study of motor coordination, Ghaziuddin and Butler (1998) found that children with AD were clumsier than those with PDD-NOS, who in turn were clumsier than those with ASP. Manjiviona and Prior (1995) concluded that motor clumsiness is not a differentiating characteristic between

AD and ASP after they found similar impairments on all three domains of the Test of Motor Impairment – Henderson Revision (manual dexterity, ball skills, and balance). As noted earlier, children with HFA and ASP demonstrate similar degrees of impairment as assessed by the PANESS (Jansiewicz et al. 2006). We have also found that children with HFA and ASP perform equally poorly on imitation and pantomime of skilled motor gestures (Mostofsky et al. 2006).

NEUROLOGICAL BASIS OF MOTOR DEFICITS IN AUTISM AND RELATION TO SOCIAL/COMMUNICATIVE IMPAIRMENTS

Investigations of motor dysfunction provide a window into some of the neural circuits impaired in autism (see Chapter 15). Neurologic, neuropsychologic, post-mortem, neurophysiologic and neuroimaging studies have long suggested that motor impairments observed in autism may stem from dysfunction in frontal and subcortical structures and circuits. Impaired balance, distal and proximal limb coordination (Jansiewicz et al. 2006), visual pursuit (Takarae et al. 2004), motor planning (Hughes 1996) and procedural learning (Mostofsky et al. 2000) are all suggestive of disturbed frontal–subcortical function.

Findings of hypotonia and gait abnormalities reported by Hallet et al. (1993) suggest cerebellar dysfunction in ASD. Consistent with this, cerebellar pathology is one of the more regular findings on post-mortem examination (Williams et al. 1980, Ritvo et al. 1986, Bauman and Kemper 1994, Bailey et al. 1998, Fatemi et al. 2002). Additionally, structural imaging studies have revealed abnormalities in the size of the cerebellar vermis (Courchesne et al. 1988, 1994; Hashimoto et al. 1995; Kates et al. 1998) and hemispheric volume (Gaffney et al. 1987, Murakami et al. 1989, Piven et al. 1997, Hardan et al. 2001, Sparks et al. 2002), although the findings are discrepant (e.g. increased or decreased hemisphere volume) (see Chapter 8).

Other clinical reports discussed earlier, such as those of Damasio and Maurer (1978) and Vilensky et al. (1981), suggest that autism may be associated with a disturbance of basal ganglia function. However, post-mortem and imaging studies have thus far failed to reveal consistent abnormalities in either frontal or basal ganglia regions (Gaffney et al. 1987, Piven et al. 1996, Kates et al. 1998, Abell et al. 1999, Sears et al. 1999, Carper and Courchesne 2000, Carper et al. 2002, McAlonan et al. 2002, Hardan et al. 2003). More recently, functional neuroimaging studies have revealed differences in frontal-subcortical circuits. Using positron emission tomography (PET), Chugani et al. (1999) observed that levels of serotonin synthesis in the frontal cortex, thalamus and contralateral dentate nucleus were much lower in children with AD than in age-matched controls; they suggested that abnormalities in a "dento-thalamo-cortical" circuit may underlie the disorder (see also Muller et al. 1998). Using functional magnetic resonance imaging (fMRI), several groups of investigators have reported differences in frontal-subcortical activation, including that associated with performance of simple motor tasks (Allen et al. 2004; see also Allen and Courchesne 2003). Others hypothesize impaired cerebral–cerebellar connections to be the neuropathological basis of autism (Carper and Courchesne 2000, Muller et al. 2001, Skoyles 2002).

Dysfunction within cortical–subcortical connection circuits may contribute to impaired development of motor coordination/execution as well as of ability to perform skilled motor gestures thought to reflect developmental dyspraxia. In traditional adult models the terms apraxia and dyspraxia are reserved for individuals who demonstrate impaired ability to perform skilled motor tasks *despite normal motor dexterity*. In contra-distinction, children with autism have been found to show deficits in basic aspects of motor execution (Jansiewicz et al. 2006). Given that autism is a developmental disorder, it may be that common neural mechanisms underlie impairments in basic aspects of motor coordination and in performance of skilled motor tasks. One possibility is that impaired motor coordination results in poor performance on examination for praxis. Alternatively, rather than a direct cause-and-effect relationship, it may be that these find-ings are epiphenomena, with both motor coordination and skilled performance resulting from abnormal development within shared frontal–subcortical regions/circuits important for motor execution/coordination and learning of skilled motor acts (for review, see Doyon et al. 2003). Differing from adult acquired ideomotor apraxia, developmental dys-praxia, including that observed in autism, may be due to a neurologic anomaly that affects the acquisition (i.e. *learning*) of motor skills. Frontal and parietal regions important for storage and implementation of spatial representations of complex motor gestures have been shown to be important for procedural motor learning (Grafton et al. 1998, Ghilardi et al. 2000, Muller et al. 2002, Daselaar et al. 2003, Doyon et al. 2003, Schendan et al. 2003). Also critical for motor learning are subcortical regions, including the striatum and cerebellum, which are thought to be associated with the encoding of motor sequence programs and the retrieval of learned movement sequences; additionally the cerebellum is associated with early learning phases of sequential movement (for review, see Doyon et al. 2003). It may be that the subcortical structures in circuit with the cortical structures are critical for motor skill learning, so that dysfunction within this circuit is contributing to impaired acquisition of motor skills in children with ASD. Abnormalities in cortical systems underlying motor imitation have been hypothesized to contribute to the impaired development of motor, as well as social and communicative, skills observed in autism (Williams et al. 2001), and cerebellar/basal ganglia connectivity to these regions may be critical to understanding impaired learning of motor and social/communicative skills acquired through imitation.

Motor imitation in humans appears to depend on a neural network that includes the inferior frontal operculum (Broca's area 44), superior parietal, and superior temporal sulcus (STS) regions. Findings from fMRI suggest that area 44 is the human analogue of monkey area F5, which contains "mirror neurons" (MNs) necessary for motor imitation (Gallese et al. 1996, Iacoboni et al. 2001, Rizzolatti et al. 2001, Rizzolatti et al. 2002). Strong evidence from both monkey and human research suggests that there is a broader MN system that includes not only Broca's area, but also more posterior areas that are critical to motor imitation including the rostral superior parietal region and the STS. These regions are involved in the encoding of visual/spatial representations of observed movements; the STS is particularly important for sensory processing and storing sensory representations of the kinesthetic traces of an observed movement (remote effects) (Iacoboni et al. 2001; Rizzolatti et al. 2001, 2002); additionally, the superior temporal regions are thought to contribute to visual-motor learning (Heilman and Gonzalez Rothi 1993, Haaland et al. 2000, Johnson et al. 2002). An fMRI study suggests the STS also participates in active motor feedback, in which observed actions and the reafferent motor related copies of the actions made by the imitator are monitored in the STS to help the imitator recognize whether the action made was the same as the action observed (Iacoboni et al. 2001). Recent imaging findings yield evidence of a dysfunctional MN system in individuals with ASD (Nishitani et al. 2004, Oberman et al. 2005, Theoret et al. 2005), and investigators have postulated that this dysfunction may contribute to the social and communicative deficits fundamental to autism.

Development of social and communicative gestures (e.g. waving, blowing a kiss) involves learning complex patterns of movements, many of which may be acquired through motor imitation. Furthermore, there is strong evidence that neural systems involved in motor imitation are also critical for understanding others' actions, which requires mapping the visual representation of the observed action onto one's own motor representation of the same action (Rizzolatti and Arbib 1998, Rizzolatti et al. 2001). Infants as young as newborns engage in imitation of facial expression and manual gestures (Meltzoff and Moore 1977, 1983; Field and Walden 1982), and neural systems involved in imitation may therefore also be important for development of socio-communicative skills such as empathy, self/other recognition, shared attention, and a sense of "other minds", or what is called Theory of Mind (ToM) (Meltzoff and Gopnik 1993, Gallese et al. 1996, Rizzolatti and Arbib 1998, Frith and Frith 1999, Blakemore and Decety, 2001). A contribution of the mirror system in the pathophysiology of autism has been hypothesized (Williams et al. 2001), although it does not entirely account for how, from a developmental perspective, abnormalities in this mirror system alone would result in impaired *acquisition/learning* of complex motor skills and gestures.

Rizzolatti et al. (2001) proposed that the mechanisms necessary for imitating *complex* motor actions and gestures likely require integration of the cortical system of MNs with neural systems important for motor learning, hypothesizing that the MN system provides the basis for recognizing and segmenting complex motor actions into "strings of discrete elements", with frontal–subcortical motor learning systems being important for assembling these discrete elements in order to construct a new motor action. As noted earlier, several groups, including our own, have observed deficits in motor imitation in autism, and our group has observed abnormalities in visuomotor sequencing learning in children with autism (Mostofsky et al. 2000, 2001).

It follows that cerebellar/basal ganglia connectivity to cortical mirror regions may be critical to understanding impaired acquisition of complex motor skills and gestures in autism. The cerebellum, which is consistently reported as abnormal in post-mortem studies of autism, appears to be particularly important for combining simpler elements of movement into more complex coordinated synergies (Thach et al. 1992), and abnormalities in cerebellar–cerebral connections, observed on PET by Chugani et al. (1999), may play a prominent role in impaired development of imitation and complex gestures in autism.

SUMMARY

Abnormalities on motor examination have often afforded valuable insights into developmental disorders of the brain. Motor abnormalities, including those involving basic aspects of motor execution such as gait, posture, coordination, and tone, as well as impaired imitation and pantomime of skilled motor gestures, are well documented in children and adults with ASD. These motor abnormalities are present across the autism spectrum, even in those with HFA or ASP. As autism is a developmental disorder, it may be that the motor deficits are due to impaired ability to learn specific skills.

There is evidence from clinical, post-mortem and imaging studies for the existence of autism-related abnormalities in frontal-subcortical circuits as well as parietal regions important for motor execution, imitation and learning. Neural systems important for motor imitation and motor/procedural learning may be important not only for the development of motor skills but also for socialization and communication, and thus dysfunction within these neural systems may contribute to a number of the deficits associated with autism. Further investigation into the neural basis of motor deficits in autism may thereby help illuminate the neurologic basis of this disorder.

REFERENCES

Abell F, Krams M, Ashburner J, Passingham R, Friston K, Frackowiak R, Happe F, Frith C, Frith U (1999) The neuroanatomy of autism: a voxel-based whole brain analysis of structural scans. *Neuroreport* 10: 1647–51.

Allen G, Courchesne E (2003) Differential effects of developmental cerebellar abnormality on cognitive and motor functions in the cerebellum: an fMRI study of autism. *Am J Psychiatry* 160: 262–73.

Allen G, Muller RA, Courchesne E (2004) Cerebellar function in autism: functional magnetic resonance image activation during a simple motor task. *Biol Psychiatry* 56: 269–78.

APA (1994) *Diagnostic and Statistical Manual of Mental Disorders, 4th edn (DSM-IV).* Washington, DC: American Psychiatric Association.

Avikainen S, Wohlschlager A, Liuhanen S, Hanninen R, Hari R (2003) Impaired mirror-image imitation in Asperger and high-functioning autistic subjects. *Curr Biol* 13: 339–41.

Bailey A, Luthert P, Dean A, Harding B, Janota I, Montgomery M, Rutter M, Lantos P (1998) A clinicopathological study of autism. *Brain* 121: 889–905.

Baranek GT (1999) Autism during infancy: a retrospective video analysis of sensory-motor and social behaviors at 9–12 months of age. *J Autism Dev Disord* 29: 213–24.

Baranek GT (2002) Efficacy of sensory and motor interventions for children with autism. *J Autism Dev Disord* 32: 397–422.

Bauman ML, Kemper TL (1994) *Neuroanatomic Observations of the Brain in Autism.* Baltimore: Johns Hopkins University Press.

Berges J, Lezine I (1965) *The Imitation of Gestures. Clinics in Developmental Medicine No. 18.* London: Spastics International Medical Publications.

Blakemore SJ, Decety J (2001) From the perception of action to the understanding of intention. *Nat Rev Neurosci* 2: 561–7.

Bruininks RH (1978) *Bruininks–Oseretsky Test of Motor Proficiency: Examiner's Manual.* Circle Pines, MN: American Guidance Service.

Carper RA, Courchesne E (2000) Inverse correlation between frontal lobe and cerebellum sizes in children with autism. *Brain* 123: 836–44.

Carper RA, Moses P, Tigue ZD, Courchesne E (2002) Cerebral lobes in autism: early hyperplasia and abnormal age effects. *Neuroimage* 16: 1038–51.

Cermak S (1985) Development dyspraxia. In: Roy EA, ed. *Neuropsychological Studies of Apraxia and Related Disorders. Advances in Psychology, vol. 23.* Amsterdam: North-Holland, pp. 225–48.

Charman T, Swettenham J, Baron-Cohen S, Cox A, Baird G, Drew A (1997) Infants with autism: an investigation of empathy, pretend play, joint attention, and imitation. *Dev Psychol* 33: 781–9.

Chugani DC, Muzik O, Behen M, Rothermel R, Janisse JJ, Lee J, Chugani HT (1999) Developmental changes in brain serotonin synthesis capacity in autistic and nonautistic children. *Ann Neurol* 45: 287–95.

Courchesne E, Yeung-Courchesne R, Press GA, Hesselink JR, Jernigan TL (1988) Hypoplasia of cerebellar vermal lobules VI and VII in autism. *N Engl J Med* 318: 1349–54.

Courchesne E, Townsend J, Saitoh O (1994) The brain in infantile autism: posterior fossa structures are abnormal. *Neurology* 44: 214–23.

Damasio AR, Maurer RG (1978) A neurological model for childhood autism. *Arch Neurol* 35: 777–86.

Daselaar SM, Rombouts SA, Veltman DJ, Raaijmakers JG, Jonker C (2003) Similar network activated by young and old adults during the acquisition of a motor sequence. *Neurobiol Aging* 24: 1013–9.

Dawson G, Osterling J, Rinaldi J, Carver L, McPartland J (2001) Brief report: Recognition memory and stimulus-reward associations: indirect support for the role of ventromedial prefrontal dysfunction in autism. *J Autism Dev Disord* 31: 337–41.

DeMyer MK, Alpern GD, Barton S, DeMyer WE, Churchill DW, Hingtgen JN, Bryson CQ, Pontius W, Kimberlin C (1972) Imitation in autistic, early schizophrenic, and non-psychotic subnormal children. *J Autism Child Schizophr* 2: 264–87.

DeMyer MK, Hingtgen JN, Jackson RK (1981) Infantile autism reviewed: a decade of research. *Schizophr Bull* 7: 388–451.

Denckla MB (1985) Revised Neurological Examination for Subtle Signs (1985). *Psychopharmacol Bull* 21: 773–800.

Doyon J, Penhune V, Ungerleider LG (2003) Distinct contribution of the cortico-striatal and cortico-cerebellar systems to motor skill learning. *Neuropsychologia* 41: 252–62.

Eshkol N, Wachman A (1958) *Movement Notation.* London: Weidenfeld & Nicolson.

Eveloff HH (1960) The autistic child. *Arch Gen Psychiatry* 3: 66–81.

Fatemi SH, Halt AR, Realmuto G, Earle J, Kist DA, Thuras P, Merz A (2002) Purkinje cell size is reduced in cerebellum of patients with autism. *Cell Mol Neurobiol* 22: 171–5.

Field TM, Walden TA (1982) Production and discrimination of facial expressions by preschool children. *Child Dev* 53: 1299–311.

Frith CD, Frith U (1999) Interacting minds – a biological basis. *Science* 286: 1692–5.

Gaffney G, Tsai L, Kuperman S, Minchin S (1987) Cerebellar structure in autism. *Am J Dis Child* 141: 1330–2.

Gallese V, Fadiga L, Fogassi L, Rizzolatti G (1996) Action recognition in the premotor cortex. *Brain* 119: 593–609.

Ghaziuddin M, Butler E (1998) Clumsiness in autism and Asperger syndrome: a further report. *J Intellect Disabil Res* 42: 43–8.

Ghaziuddin M, Butler E, Tsai L, Ghaziuddin N (1994) Is clumsiness a marker for Asperger syndrome? *J Intellect Disabil Res* 38: 519–27.

Ghilardi M, Ghez C, Dhawan V, Moeller J, Mentis M, Nakamura T, Antonini A, Eidelberg D (2000) Patterns of regional brain activation associated with different forms of motor learning. *Brain Res* 871: 127–45.

Gonzales Rothi LJ, Raymer AM, Heilman KM (1997) Limb praxis assessment. In: Gonzales Rothi LJ, Heilman KM, eds. *Apraxia: the Neuropsychology of Action.* Hove, Sussex: Psychology Press, pp. 61–74.

Grafton ST, Hazeltine E, Ivry RB (1998) Abstract and effector-specific representations of motor sequences identified with PET. *J Neurosci* 18: 9420–8.

Green D, Baird G, Barnett AL, Henderson L, Huber J, Henderson SE (2002) The severity and nature of motor impairment in Asperger's syndrome: a comparison with specific developmental disorder of motor function. *J Child Psychol Psychiatry* 43: 655–68.

Haaland KY, Harrington DL, Knight RT (2000) Neural representations of skilled movement. *Brain* 123: 2306–13.

Haas RH, Townsend J, Courchesne E, Lincoln AJ, Schriebman L, Yeung-Courchesne R (1996) Neurologic abnormalities in infantile autism. *J Child Neurol* 11: 84–92.

Haith MM, Wentworth N, Canfield RL (1993) The formation of expectations in early infancy. In: Rovee-Collier C, Lipsitt LP, eds. *Advances in Infancy Research, vol. 8.* Norwood, NJ: Ablex, pp. 217–49.

Hallett M, Lebiedowska MK, Thomas SL, Stanhope SJ, Denckla MB, Rumsey J (1993) Locomotion of autistic adults. *Arch Neurol* 50: 1304–8.

Hammes JG, Langdell T (1981) Precursors of symbol formation and childhood autism. *J Autism Dev Disord* 11: 331–46.

Hardan AY, Minshew NJ, Harenski K, Keshavan MS (2001) Posterior fossa magnetic resonance imaging in autism. *J Am Acad Child Adolesc Psychiatry* 40: 666–72.

Hardan AY, Kilpatrick M, Keshavan MS, Minshew NJ (2003) Motor performance and anatomic magnetic resonance imaging (MRI) of the basal ganglia in autism. *J Child Neurol* 18: 317–24.

Hashimoto T, Tayama M, Murakawa K, Yoshimoto T, Miyazaki M, Harada M, Kurdora Y (1995) Development of the brainstem and cerebellum in autistic patients. *J Autism Dev Disord* 25: 1–18.

Heilman KM, Gonzalez Rothi L (1993) Apraxia. In: Heilman KM, Valenstein E, eds. *Clinical Neuropsychology 3rd edn.* New York: Oxford University Press, pp. 141–63.

Heilman KM, Gonzalez Rothi L (2003) Apraxia. In: Heilman KM, Valenstein E, eds. *Clinical Neuropsychology 4th edn.* New York: Oxford University Press, pp. 215–35.

Hertzig ME, Snow ME, Sherman M (1989) Affect and cognition in autism. *J Am Acad Child Adolesc Psychiatry* 28: 195–9.

Hughes C (1996) Brief report: planning problems in autism at the level of motor control. *J Autism Dev Disord* 26: 99–107.

Iacoboni M, Koski LM, Brass M, Bekkering H, Woods RP, Dubeau MC, Mazziotta JC, Rizzolatti G (2001) Reafferent copies of imitated actions in the right superior temporal cortex. *Proc Natl Acad Sci USA* 98: 13995–9.

Jansiewicz E, Goldberg MC, Newschaffer CJ, Denckla MB, Landa RJ, Mostofsky SH (2006) Motor signs distinguish children with high functioning autism and Asperger's syndrome from controls. *J Autism Dev Disord* (in press).

Johnson SH, Rotte M, Grafton ST, Kanowski M, Gazzaniga MS, Heinze J (2002) Beyond the dorsal stream: a distributed left hemisphere system for the representation of skilled action. Paper presented at the 9th Annual Meeting of the Cognitive Neuroscience Society, April 14–16, San Francisco, CA.

Jones V, Prior M (1985) Motor imitation abilities and neurological signs in autistic children. *J Autism Dev Disord* 15: 37–46.

Kanner L (1943) Autistic disturbances of affective contact. *Nerv Child* 2: 217–50.

Kates WR, Mostofsky SH, Zimmerman AW, Mazzocco MM, Landa R, Warsofsky IS, Kaufmann WE, Reiss AL (1998) Neuroanatomical and neurocognitive differences in a pair of monozygous twins discordant for strictly defined autism. *Ann Neurol* 43: 782–91.

Klin A, Volkmar FR, Sparrow SS, Cicchetti DV, Rourke BP (1995) Validity and neuropsychological characterization of Asperger syndrome: convergence with nonverbal learning disabilities syndrome. *J Child Psychol Psychiatry* 36: 1127–40.

Libby S, Powell S, Messer D, Jordan R (1997) Imitation of pretend play acts by children with autism and Down syndrome. *J Autism Dev Disord* 27: 365–83.

Losche G (1990) Sensorimotor and action development in autistic children from infancy to early childhood. *J Child Psychol Psychiatry* 31: 749–61.

Macintosh K, Dissanayake C (2004) Annotation: The similarities and differences between autistic disorder and Asperger's disorder: a review of the empirical evidence. *J Child Psychol Psychiatry* 45: 421–34.

Manjiviona J, Prior M (1995) Comparison of Asperger syndrome and high-functioning autistic children on a test of motor impairment. *J Autism Dev Disord* 25: 23–39.

Maurer RG, Damasio AR (1982) Childhood autism from the point of view of behavioral neurology. *J Autism Dev Disord* 12: 195–205.

McAlonan GM, Daly E, Kumari V, Critchley HD, van Amelsvoort T, Suckling J, Simmons A, Sigmundsson T, Greenwood K, Russell A, Schmitz N, Happe F, Howlin P, Murphy DG (2002) Brain anatomy and sensorimotor gating in Asperger's syndrome. *Brain* 125: 1594–606.

Meltzoff A, Gopnik A (1993) The role of imitation in understanding persons and developing a theory of mind. In: Baron-Cohen S, Tager-Flusberg H, Cohen DJ, eds. *Understanding Other Minds: Perspectives from Autism.* Oxford University Press, New York, pp. 335–66.

Meltzoff AN, Moore MK (1977) Imitation of facial and manual gestures by human neonates. *Science* 198: 74–8.

Meltzoff AN, Moore MK (1983) Newborn infants imitate adult facial gestures. *Child Dev* 54: 702–9.

Minshew NJ, Goldstein G, Siegel DJ (1997) Neuropsychologic functioning in autism: profile of a complex information processing disorder. *J Int Neuropsychol Soc* 3: 303–16.

Minshew NJ, Sung K, Jones BL, Furman JM (2004) Underdevelopment of the postural control system in autism. *Neurology* 63: 2056–61.

Miyahara M, Tsujii M, Hori M, Nakanishi K, Kageyama H, Sugiyama T (1997) Brief report: motor incoordination in children with Asperger syndrome and learning disabilities. *J Autism Dev Disord* 27: 595–603.

Mostofsky SH, Goldberg MC, Landa RJ, Denckla MB (2000) Evidence for a deficit in procedural learning in children and adolescents with autism: implications for cerebellar contribution. *J Int Neuropsychol Soc* 6: 752–9.

Mostofsky SH, Goldberg MC, Cutting LE, Denckla MB (2001) Impaired procedural learning of rotary pursuit in children with autism. Paper presented at the International Meeting for Autism Research, November 9–10, San Diego, CA.

Mostofsky SH, Bunoski R, Morton SM, Goldberg MC, Bastian AJ (2004) Children with autism adapt normally during a catching task requiring the cerebellum. *Neurocase* 10: 60–4.

Mostofsky SH, Dubey P, Jerath VK, Jansiewicz EM, Goldberg MC, Denckla MB (2006) Developmental dyspraxia is not limited to imitation in children with autism spectrum disorders. *J Int Neuropsychol Soc* (in press).

Muller RA, Chugani DC, Behen ME, Rothermel RD, Muzik O, Chakraborty PK, Chugani HT (1998) Impairment of dentato-thalamo-cortical pathway in autistic men: language activation data from positron emission tomography. *Neurosci Lett* 245: 1–4.

Muller RA, Pierce K, Ambrose JB, Allen G, Courchesne E (2001) Atypical patterns of cerebral motor activation in autism: a functional magnetic resonance study. *Biol Psychiatry* 49: 665–76.

Muller RA, Kleinhans N, Pierce K, Kemmotsu N, Courchesne E (2002) Functional MRI of motor sequence acquisition: effects of learning stage and performance. *Brain Res Cogn Brain Res* 14: 277–93.

Murakami JW, Courchesne E, Press GA, Yeung-Courchesne R, Hesselink JR (1989) Reduced cerebellar hemisphere size and its relationship to vermal hypoplasia in autism. Arch Neurol 46: 689–94.

Nelson CA (1995) The ontogeny of human memory: a cognitive neuroscience perspective. *Dev Psychol* 31: 723–38.

Nishitani N, Avikainen S, Hari R (2004) Abnormal imitation-related cortical activation sequences in Asperger's syndrome. *Ann Neurol* 55: 558–62.

Noterdaeme M, Mildenberger K, Minow F, Amorosa H (2002) Evaluation of neuromotor deficits in children with autism and children with a specific speech and language disorder. *Eur Child Adolesc Psyhciatry* 11: 219–25.

Oberman LM, Hubbard EM, McCleery JP, Altschuler EL, Ramachandran VS, Pineda JA (2005) EEG evidence for mirror neuron dysfunction in autism spectrum disorders. *Brain Res Cogn Brain Res* 24: 190–8.

Ohta M (1987) Cognitive disorders of infantile autism: a study employing the WISC, spatial relationship conceptualization, and gesture imitations. *J Autism Dev Disord* 17: 45–62.

Ornitz EM, Guthrie D, Farley AH (1977) The early development of autistic children. *J Autism Child Schizophr* 7: 207–29.

Piven J, Arndt S, Bailey J, Andreasen N (1996) Regional brain enlargement in autism: a magnetic resonance imaging study. *J Am Acad Child Adolesc Psychiatry* 35: 530–6.

Piven J, Saliba K, Bailey J, Arndt S (1997) An MRI study of autism: the cerebellum revisited. *Neurology* 49: 546–51.

Rapin I (1991) Autistic children: diagnosis and clinical features. *Pediatrics* 87: 751–60.

Ricks DM, Wing L (1975) Language, communication and the use of symbols in normal and autistic children. *J Autism Child Schizophr* 5: 191–221.

Rinehart NJ, Bradshaw JL, Brereton AV, Tonge BJ (2001) Movement preparation in high-functioning autism and Asperger disorder: a serial choice reaction time task involving motor reprogramming. *J Autism Dev Disord* 31: 79–88.

Ritvo A, Provence S (1953) Form perception and imitation in some autistic children. *Psychoanal Study Child* 8: 155–61.

Ritvo ER, Freeman BJ, Scheibel AB, Duong T, Robinson H, Guthrie D, Ritvo A (1986) Lower Purkinje cell counts in the cerebella of four autistic subjects: initial findings of the UCLA-NSAC Autopsy Research Report. *Am J Psychiatry* 143: 862–6.

Rizzolatti G, Arbib MA (1998) Language within our grasp. *Trends Neurosci* 21: 188–94.

Rizzolatti G, Fogassi L, Gallese V (2001) Neurophysiological mechanisms underlying the understanding and imitation of action. *Nat Rev Neurosci* 2: 661–70.

Rizzolatti G, Fogassi L, Gallese V (2002) Motor and cognitive functions of the ventral premotor cortex. *Curr Opin Neurobiol* 12: 149–54.

Rogers S, Bennetto L, McEvoy R, Pennington BF (1996) Imitation and pantomime in high-functioning adolescents with autism spectrum disorders. *Child Dev* 67: 2060–73.

Rogers SJ, Pennington BF (1991) A theoretical approach to the deficits in infantile autism. *Dev Psychopathol* 3: 137–62.

Rogers SJ, Hepburn SL, Stackhouse T, Wehner E (2003) Imitation performance in toddlers with autism and those with other developmental disorders. *J Child Psychol Psychiatry* 44: 763–81.

Schendan HE, Searl MM, Melrose RJ, Stern CE (2003) An FMRI study of the role of the medial temporal lobe in implicit and explicit sequence learning. *Neuron* 37: 1013–25.

Sears LL, Vest C, Mohamed S, Bailey J, Ranson BJ, Piven J (1999) An MRI study of the basal ganglia in autism. *Prog Neuropsychopharmacol Biol Psychiatry* 23: 613–24.

Skoyles JR (2002) Is autism due to cerebral–cerebellum disconnection? *Med Hypotheses* 58: 332–6.

Smith IM, Bryson SE (1994) Imitation and action in autism: a critical review. *Psychol Bull* 116: 259–73.

Smith IM, Bryson SE (1998) Gesture imitation in autism. 1: Nonsymbolic postures and sequences. *Cogn Neuropsychol* 15: 747–70.

Sparks BF, Friedman SD, Shaw DW, Aylward EH, Echelard D, Artru AA, Maravilla KR, Giedd JN, Munson J, Dawson G, Dager SR (2002) Brain structural abnormalities in young children with autism spectrum disorder. *Neurology* 59: 184–92.

Squire LR (1986) Mechanisms of memory. *Science* 232: 1612–9.

Stone WL, Lawmanek KL, Fishel PT, Fernandez MC, Altemeier WA (1990) Play and imitation skills in the diagnosis of autism in young children. *Pediatrics* 86: 267–72.

Stone WL, Ousley OY, Littleford CD (1997) Motor imitation in young children with autism: what's the object? *J Abnorm Child Psychol* 25: 475–85.

Szatmari P, Bartolucci G, Bremner R (1989) Asperger's syndrome and autism: comparison of early history and outcome. *Dev Med Child Neurol* 31: 709–20.

Takanashi J, Sugita K. Barkovich AJ, Takano H, Kohno Y (1999) Partial midline fusion of the cerebellar hemispheres with vertical folia: a new cerebellar malformation? *AJNR Am J Neuroradiol* 20: 1151–3.

Takarae Y, Minshew NJ, Luna B, Krisky CM, Sweeney JA (2004) Pursuit eye movement deficits in autism. *Brain* 127: 2584–94.

Teitelbaum O, Benton T, Shah PK, Prince A, Kelly JL, Teitelbaum P (2004) Eshkol–Wachman movement notation in diagnosis: the early detection of Asperger's syndrome. *Proc Natl Acad Sci USA* 101: 11909–14.

Teitelbaum P, Teitelbaum O, Nye J, Fryman J, Maurer RG (1998) Movement analysis in infancy may be useful for early diagnosis of autism. *Proc Natl Acad Sci USA* 95: 13982–7.

Thach WT, Goodkin HP, Keating JG (1992) The cerebellum and the adaptive coordination of movement. *Annu Rev Neurosci* 15: 403–42.

Theoret H, Halligen E, Kobayashi M, Fregni F, Tager-Flusberg H, Pascual-Leone A (2005) Impaired motor facilitation during action observation in individuals with autism spectrum disorder. *Curr Biol* 8: R84–5.

Varan B, Akman A, Coskun M, Sagduyu A, Aydin P (2001) Joubert syndrome: a rare cause of hypotonia and developmental delay in infancy and childhood. *Eur J Med* 6: 58–60.

Vilensky JA, Damasio AR, Maurer RG (1981) Gait disturbances in patients with autistic behavior: a preliminary study. *Arch Neurol* 38: 646–9.

Watson LR, Baranek GT, DiLavore PC (2003) Toddlers with autism: developmental perspectives. Infants *Young Child* 16: 201–14.

Weimer AK, Schatz AM, Lincoln A, Ballantyne AO, Trauner DA (2001) "Motor" impairment in Asperger syndrome: evidence for a deficit in proprioception. *J Dev Behav Pediatr* 22: 92–101.

Williams JH, Whiten A, Singh T (2004) A systematic review of action imitation in autistic spectrum disorder. *J Autism Dev Disord* 34: 285–99.

Williams JH, Whiten A, Suddendorf T, Perrett DI (2001) Imitation, mirror neurons and autism. *Neurosci Biobehav Rev* 25: 287–95.

Williams RS, Hauser SL, Purpura DP, DeLong GR, Swisher CN (1980) Autism and mental retardation: neuropathologic studies performed in four retarded persons with autistic behavior. *Arch Neurol* 37: 749–53.

15

PATHOPHYSIOLOGY OF AUTISM: EVALUATION OF SLEEP AND LOCOMOTION

Masaya Segawa and Yoshiko Nomura

The pathophysiology of autism remains incompletely understood, and there are still controversies about the neurons/neuronal systems whose dysfunction underlies this disorder. There is now quite good agreement about the clinical features and course of the autism spectrum disorders (ASDs). The age-dependent unfolding of its characteristic symptoms, which become apparent in infancy and full-blown by age 3 years, is followed by an essentially non-progressive course. This course is that of a maturational disorder. The neuronal systems implicated in its pathophysiology attain a critical level of maturation in early infancy. They modulate by parallel projecting axons the maturation of hierarchically organized neuronal systems as they develop from lower to higher levels of the central nervous system (CNS). Some neuronal dysfunctions may thus not become clinically manifest until the affected neurons attain a critical level of maturation. Consequently, the symptoms caused by dysfunction of neurons at lower, earlier maturing levels of the hierarchy become clinically manifest earlier than those due to dysfunction of neurons at higher later maturing levels. The functional activity of these neuronal systems is influenced by environmental factors to which males are more vulnerable than females.

These features suggest that brainstem aminergic neurons may be primary contributors to the pathogenesis of autism because their widely distributed axons throughout the brain modulate its function from lower to higher levels (Role and Kelly 1991). Among them, serotonergic (5HT) neurons are considered the favored candidates inasmuch as they fulfill all of the characteristics just outlined (see Chapters 6 and 9). Sleep and locomotion are modulated independently by distinct brainstem aminergic neurons that also modulate movements in sleep. Both sleep and locomotion develop from infancy to childhood according to highly regulated developmental programs, each at their particular critical ages. The sleep–wake (S-W) cycle is modulated by environmental factors; in particular it is entrained to the 24 hour diurnal light/dark cycle and other time cues. Cues for awakening activate the ascending aminergic neurons of the brainstem, that is, the 5HT and the noradrenergic (NA) neurons, and peptides of the mesencephalon (Pace-Schott and Hobson 2002). Consequently, either abnormalities of these environmental factors influencing the neural pathways or primary disorders of the neural systems themselves may be responsible for disorders of sleep and locomotion.

We suggest that evaluation of characteristics of disordered sleep and locomotion may provide particularly insightful information on underlying disorders of monoamine systems and their role in the pathogenesis of autism. This view prompts us to summarize our studies and review those of others concerned with disordered sleep and locomotion in children of various ages with autistic symptomatology (Segawa 1982, 1985, 1999a).

SLEEP DISORDERS IN AUTISM

Sleep disorders are both common and prominent in autism; their clinical features are reviewed in Chapter 12. They are often very troublesome (Segawa 1982, Inamura 1984, Hoshino et al. 1984, Segawa 1985, Clements et al. 1986, Quine 1991, Taira et al. 1998, Patzold et al. 1998, Hering et al. 1999, Gail Williams et al. 2004, Wiggs and Stores 2004, Limoges et al. 2005), although their prevalence varies a great deal (Hoshino et al. 1984, Clements et al. 1986, Richdale and Prior 1995, Wiggs and Stores 1996, Patzold et al. 1998). Many parents complain spontaneously that disordered sleep creates a major problem for their families, yet, perhaps surprisingly, it may be necessary to ask other parents specifically about sleep to bring its disorders to light.

SLEEP–WAKE CYCLE ABNORMALITIES

One focus of our research is the evaluation of S-W cycles by asking parents to keep diaries of their children's sleep and wake times using the day-by-day plot method. The amount of data collected ranged from months to years in individual children. Plots on 63 children with autism aged 1 to 12 years revealed abnormalities in their circadian S-W cycles (Segawa 1982) (Fig. 15.1). Some exhibited a free running pattern that conformed to the endogenous 25 hour cycle oscillation (see below) (Segawa 1985) (Fig. 15.2). We subsequently restudied 85 patients, 70 male and 15 female, at ages ranging from 1 year 10 months to 24 years 8 months (mean 8.3 ± 4.5 years), whose S-W cycles we had been able to assess in early infancy. Only 27 (32%) of them had developed the expected normal circadian S-W cycle by 5 months; it was delayed in 45 (54%), and the other 12 (14%) continued to have frequent night-time awakenings and lacked any definite circadian rhythm (Segawa et al. 1992a). These abnormalities of the S-W cycle were ameliorated by providing environmental stimulation that enforced daytime wakefulness (Figs. 15.1, 15. 3) and were further improved by the administration of 5-hydroxytryptophan (5HTP) (Segawa 1982) (Fig. 15.3). In contrast to the disordered S-W cycle, body movements and/or rolling over during sleep occurred regularly and clock-dependently. We concluded that these movements were probably independent from the normality or disorder of the S-W cycle (Segawa 1982) (Fig. 15.3).

Normally, the circadian S-W cycle entrained to the 24 hour day–night cycle has developed by 4 months of age (Parmelee et al. 1964). Prior to that, a free running rhythm, which reflects a biological rhythm with a 25 hour cycle organized by the suprachiasmatic

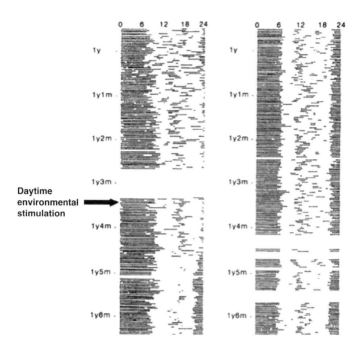

Fig. 15.1. Sleep–wake cycles of a child with autism (left) and a normal subject (right) aged 12–18 months. Each horizontal bar represents time spent in sleep and successive lines successive days. The numbers plotted at the top are 24 hour clock times. The arrow shows the date at which intensification of daytime environmental stimulation to foster wakefulness was started in this autistic child. Note the better consolidation (fewer awakenings) of night-time sleep and, after about a month, earlier falling asleep coincident with a decrease in daytime naps. Note also that the normal infant had already well consolidated night-time sleep and fell asleep earlier than the child with autism but took rather irregular daytime naps during the observation period.

nuclei, appears around 1–2 months of age. Within the next month or two the child's brain begins to entrain to the day–night, light–dark diurnal cycle (Segawa 1999b). The sleep pattern will be further modified as children mature. Young children consolidate their daytime sleep to twice a day, then to once a day (Ma et al. 1993), and eventually they give up the requirement for naps (Webb 1971). The biphasic S-W cycle is finally established by 5 years of age.

Our observations of sleep in autism suggest that there may be a failure in the development of the circadian S-W cycle owing to failure to entrain to the day–night cycle dating back to early infancy. This failure implicates involvement of the 5HT neurons among the ascending brainstem aminergic neurons that modulate development of the circadian S-W cycle in early infancy despite normal development of the neuronal systems responsible for the 25 hour biological rhythm. Rolling over during sleep tends to occur before entering into rapid eye movement (REM) sleep (Segawa et al. 1987). The REM–non-REM

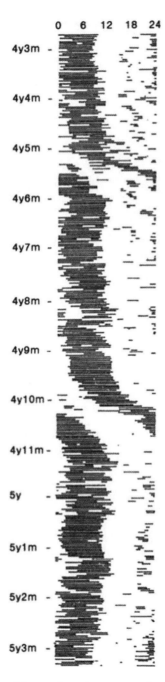

Fig. 15.2. Free running pattern of sleep–wake cycles over a year in a child with autism. Each horizontal bar indicates time asleep. Successive horizontal lines depict consecutive days. The numbers at the top indicate clock time.

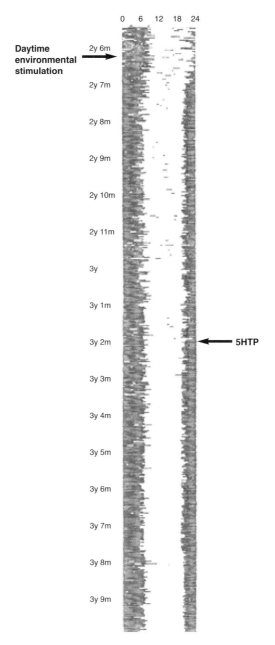

Fig. 15.3. Sleep–wake cycles and body movements in a child with autism. Each horizontal bar indicates time asleep. Each short vertical bar signals the time of rolling over. The first arrow shows the date when intensification of daytime stimulation to foster wakefulness was instigated. The second arrow shows the date when 5HTP was started. Note that the onset of daytime-enhanced stimulation quite promptly resulted in earlier falling asleep in the evening and decreased night-time awakenings.

(NREM) cycle in adults has a 90 minute periodicity, which means that REM sleep occurs clock-dependently. Although the cycle is shorter in children, after early infancy REM sleep occurs periodically, nearly clock-dependently. Because rolling over occurs periodically, this suggests that it is a "REM-on" gross movement and, therefore, that the periodic occurrence of REM sleep or REM–NREM cycle, is preserved in autism. The preservation of the REM-NREM rhythm in autism was also confirmed by polysomnograms (PSGs) (Ornitz 1972, Hashimoto and Tayama 1985).

ABNORMALITIES OF SLEEP COMPONENTS IN AUTISM

Polysomnography (PSG) refers to the continuous recording of biological phenomena throughout night-time sleep. "Sleep components" are state-dependent biologic features of sleep that are under the control of specific neurons or neural systems. PSGs in our clinic include recordings of the electroencephalogram (EEG), electro-oculogram, electromyograms (EMGs) of various muscles, as well a record of respiration and an electrocardiogram. The EMG is recorded by surface electrodes on the muscles of the chin, upper and lower limbs, sternocleidomastoideus and rectus abdominalis. PSGs measure components of sleep that reflect the ongoing functional states of the neuronal systems responsible for these biological components of sleep. These follow characteristic patterns of developmental change. Thus PSG in infants and children opens a window onto brain function, and it is therefore a useful tool for investigating physiological or pathological conditions, as well as for determining the maturity of specific neuronal systems.

PSG provides the opportunity to scrutinize the components of sleep continuously and noninvasively, and it contributes to the understanding of the pathophysiology of infantile autism. The parameters of REM sleep that develop during the fetal period, which include phasic movements, rapid eye movements (REMs) and atonia of the musculus mentalis, are preserved in autism. Their preservation points to normal development of the dopaminergic (DA) and cholinergic neurons that control the execution of these motor parameters during the fetal period. However, abnormalities in the maturation of the appearance of the bursts of REMs in REM sleep, which is normally complete by 2-24 weeks of postnatal age, have been found in autism (Ornitz 1972, 1983; Hashimoto and Tayama 1985; Elia et al. 1991). Furthermore, PSGs document leakage of the components of REM sleep, namely REMs and atonia, into NREM sleep (Hashimoto and Tayama 1985). The neural system (or systems) that executes REMs is normal but the one that modulates rapid eye movement bursts is affected. The former system develops early in the fetal period, whereas the latter develops later, in early infancy.

PSGs in children with autism reveal preservation of the normal REM–NREM cycle (Ornitz 1972, 1983; Tanguay et al. 1976; Hashimoto and Tayama 1985), as well as of the sleep structure and ratio of sleep stages (Hashimoto and Tayama 1985). Two types of movements during sleep have been analyzed across sleep stages: gross movements (GMs), defined as generalized movements lasting more than 2 seconds that involve the trunk muscles, and twitch movements (TMs), which are short muscle contractions lasting less than 0.5s and are restricted to one muscle. The frequency of these movements is assessed per unit time in each sleep stage. No difference was found in 11 children with autism (ages 1 year 10 months to 8 years 9 months) compared to age-matched normal children (Hashimoto and Tayama 1985). In contrast, the number of GMs was lower and that of TMs was higher in REM stage in a cohort of older children with autism compared to normal controls.

A recent study of adults with ASDs, compared to controls, showed a longer sleep latency, more frequent nocturnal awakenings, lower sleep efficiency, increased stage 1 sleep, decreased NREM sleep and slow wave sleep, fewer EEG spindles in stage 2 sleep, and a smaller number of REM s during REM sleep (Limoges et al. 2005). These abnormalities may be attributable to impairment of daytime wakefulness, with resulting prolongation of sleep latency and decrease of the efficacy of sleep-onset slow wave sleep; this latter abnormality in turn disturbs REM sleep by increasing TMs during REM sleep (Segawa 2002). Increase of the TMs of REM sleep causes a decrease in the number of rapid eye movements (Segawa et al. 1988). In another study of the PSGs of autistic individuals in whom disrupted sleep and nocturnal awakenings revealed a REM sleep behavior disorder, clonazepam helped to consolidate sleep and improve daytime performance (Thirumalai et al. 2002).

SLEEP COMPONENT ABNORMALITIES AS INDICATORS OF THE PATHOPHYSIOLOGY OF AUTISM

The components of REM sleep develop during fetal life (Segawa 1999c). Most of these components are in place by 40 weeks of gestation, with the notable exception of the atonia of postural muscle, which is not limited to REM sleep until about 3–4 months of postnatal life (Parmelee and Stern 1972). Irruption of the components of REM sleep into NREM sleep is prevented by the NA and 5HT neurons of the brainstem that inhibit the activity of the cholinergic neurons which execute REM sleep (Hobson et al. 1975, Sakai 1985). As is the case with the abnormalities in circadian S-W cycle, leakage of the atonia of REM into NREM sleep implies abnormalities of the 5HT neurons that modulate the development of sleep parameters during the first 4 months of postnatal life.

The patterns of GMs and TMs across sleep stages in autism just discussed are similar to those observed in a patient with DA receptor supersensitivity (Tanaka et al. 1989). The TMs of REM sleep reflect activity of the nigrostriatal DA neurons (Segawa et al. 1988). Thus, these age-related changes of TMs in autism suggest that DA activity decreases with age but that its transmission increases with age in late childhood, probably due to the occurrence of receptor supersensitivity.

ABNORMALITIES OF LOCOMOTION IN AUTISM

Evaluation of crawling in 97 individuals with autism, 78 male and 19 female, whose ages ranged from 1 year 10 months to 24 years 8 months, revealed that about a quarter of them did not crawl in infancy (Segawa and Nomura 1991). Among the 72 who did, we were

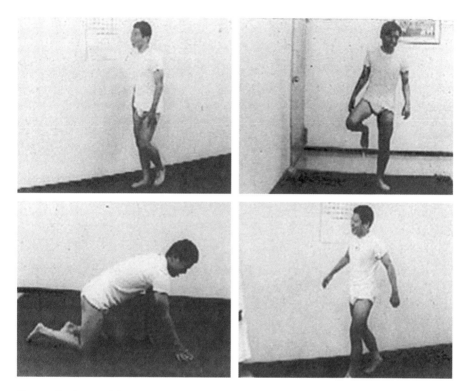

Fig. 15.4. Abnormal locomotion of autism. *Top left:* lack of associated arm movement while walking. *Top right:* stepping with spontaneous back-kicking of the leg and lack of arm swing. *Bottom left:* when asked to crawl the individual does so with flexed fingers and toes. *Bottom right:* being asked to walk on his toes brings back normal associated arm swing.

able to assess how they crawled in 39 of them. Of those, only 5 did it in the expected way, that is palm on the floor with fingers outstretched and dorsal surface of the foot or toes on the floor. Although most of the children began to walk by 2 years of age, less than 10% of them walked with a normal arm swing before age 5 years (Segawa 1982, Segawa et al. 1992a). Toe-walking without spasticity is not rare among children with autism, although we do not have an exact proportion of those who do (Segawa et al. 1992a). We also lack photographs or video recordings of the children. However, we consider that crawling in a flexed posture is an important and reliable sign of abnormality of locomotion in autism.

We recorded surface EMGs during locomotion in 17 autistic children aged 3–17 years. Fourteen of them lacked coordination of the upper and lower limbs, and in 11 the physiological flexors predominated in crawling and walking, in contrast with the dominance of extensor muscles in normal controls (Segawa and Nomura 1991). The abnormality of interlimb coordination in locomotion improved when the children were asked to walk on their toes (Fig. 15.4).

IMPLICATIONS OF LOCOMOTOR ABNORMALITIES FOR THE PATHOPHYSIOLOGY OF AUTISM

Locomotion is controlled by an intraspinal circuit that connects the two stepping generators, located in the cervical and lumbosacral segments of the spinal cord. The spinal generators are triggered by tonic innervations from the brainstem aminergic neurons that project onto them (Miller and van der Burg 1973). In the absence of this brainstem innervation, tonic proprioceptive inflow from the muscle spindles of the upper or lower limbs to the spinal generators can trigger these circuits and induce locomotion (Miller and van der Burg 1973). Improvement of locomotion in autistic subjects with toe-walking suggests normal function of the propriospinal locomotor circuitry and that the cause of the locomotor abnormalities just described might be dysfunction or hypofunction of the brainstem aminergic projectons to the spinal cord stepping generators. This suggestion is supported by the disappearance of atonic NREM (leakage of the atonia of REM sleep into NREM sleep) following locomotor training (Segawa 1999a). This implies that activity of the aminergic neurons is improved, in particular the 5HT neurons which modulate the antigravity muscles.

It is noteworthy that the neurons responsible for the axial atonia of the REM stage are similar in both location and biochemical character to those of the pedunculo-pontine nucleus and to neurons in the putative mesencephalic locomotor region (Mori and Takakusaki 1988, Mori et al. 1988). These systems are activated by cholinergic agonists and inhibited by NA and 5HT agonists (Mori et al. 1988). Activation of the cholinergic inputs results in postural atonia and cessation of locomotion, and activation of the NA and 5HT inputs restores posture and facilitates locomotion (Mori et al. 1992).

Animal experiments show that decreased tonic innervation, mostly due to a decrease of the monoaminergic influence on the spinal stepping generator, causes cessation or disturbance of locomotion, and is dose dependent (Bradley and Smith 1988). Decreased monoaminergic innervation results in increased and prolonged activation of the flexor muscles of the limbs (Bradley and Smith 1988). These features are similar to those observed in surface EMG in autism.

INTERVENTIONS
SLEEP DISORDERS

The relevance of abnormalities of the S-W cycle and of locomotion to the pathophysiology of autism is suggested by the alleviation of the symptoms of autism following improvement of these abnormalities. Interventions to improve sleep patterns in 27 children under age 4 years consisted of enforcing daytime wakefulness and regular night-time sleep (Segawa et al. 1992b). Consistent times that varied by no more than 30 minutes were set for evening bedtime and getting up in the morning. Parents were instructed to avoid daytime naps by strengthening cues for wakefulness and to avoid environmental factors that might disturb night-time sleep and daytime wakefulness. No medication was administered. Parents' day-by-day plots of 24 hour sleep/wake diaries were checked once a

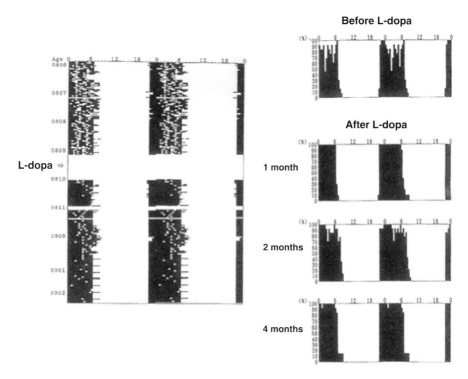

Fig. 15.5. Effect of small doses of L-dopa on night-time awakenings in a child with autism (see text). *Left:* "Sleep–wake rhythm" shown by "double track method"; x-axis indicates clock time; horizontal black bars denote times asleep, and white parts indicate times awake. *Right:* "Sleep-rate" shown by "double track method" in the same child before and after L-dopa; x-axis indicates clock time; y-axis indicates percentage of each 30 minute unit of time spent in sleeping during one month.

month to reinforce treatment parameters. Based on these diaries, the intervention resulted in improvements in sleep that were discernible within 1–2 months. Improvement of the circadian S-W cycle was observed in all of the children by age 45.5 ± 9.8 months. Improvement in sleep efficiency was associated with improved social relatedness and accommodation to novel environments in 19 of the 27 children. However, alleviation of insistence on sameness, hyperkinesis, aggressiveness, and panic states was observed in 13 children. Interestingly, the age at which the circadian S-W cycle improved coincided with the emergence of hand dominance in 25 of the children and with the utterance of one or a few meaningful words in 19 of them.

There are children who benefit from medication to improve sleep (see also Chapter 12). As shown in Figure 15.5, clock-dependent awakenings, that is, the awakenings during REM sleep mentioned earlier, persisted in some children with autism in whom the circadian S-W cycle had normalized. These undesirable awakenings were improved by small doses of L-dopa (0.5 mg/kg/day of plain L-dopa). Such small doses of L-dopa alleviate supersensitized DA receptors and improve DA transmission in the basal ganglia (Tanaka et al. 1989). Consequently, we postulate that these awakenings are due to abnormal increases in DA transmission that result from DA receptor supersensitivity. This therapy improved not only the clock-dependent awakenings during night sleep, but also aggressiveness, panic states and hyperkinesis (Segawa 1998). However, improvement of the S-W cycle did not improve the children's IQ levels.

Abnormality of melatonin regulation may also play a role in the sleep disorders of autism (Chamberlain and Herman 1990, Rapin and Katzman 1998, Patzold et al. 1998). Melatonin improves S-W cycle disorders (Jan and O'Donnell 1996). It is also reported to be effective in autism with mental retardation by prolonging nocturnal sleep and regulating the S-W cycle when given at 11 p.m. (Hayashi 2000). Abnormality of melatonin secretion is not necessarily causative as it might be a secondary consequence of the abnormal circadian S-W cycle that is not synchronized to the day–night light–dark cycle.

LOCOMOTOR DISORDERS

As to the disorders of locomotion, we instructed the parents to encourage their children to walk or run on roads or fields with mild up and down slopes, and also to climb stairs. Pedaling a tricycle was recommended for younger children. Improvement of locomotion was evaluated by normalization of the stepping pattern, that is, stepping with coordinated upper limb movements and without backward kicking of the legs. The result of these exercises was the lifting forward of the leg associated with spontaneous coordinated arm movement. Within one to several months, most children were able to walk with normal inter-limb coordination.

Improvement in the IQ paralleled the improvement of locomotion provided it was attained in early childhood, before age 5 years (Segawa 1998, 1999a). Improvement in certain neurological signs of autism in tandem with improvement of the IQ and locomotion provides clues to their underlying mechanisms. Children with infantile autism have difficulty closing their eyes and mouth on command or in imitation, and tend to flap their arms when attempting to imitate pronation/supination movements (Segawa et al. 1992b). These abnormalities signal orofacial and limb kinetic apraxia caused by inadequate functional specialization of the cortex. Ages at improvement of locomotion were correlated with the ages at which children were able to close their eyes or mouth on command and to imitate pronation/supination movements. They were also correlated with the ages at which leakage of atonia into NREM sleep disappeared (Segawa 1999a), all of which implicate 5HT neuronal dysfunction.

DISCUSSION

Analysis of sleep and locomotion in autism suggest that 5HT dysfunction plays a fundamental role in its pathophysiology (see Chapters 6 and 9). In rodents, early lesions in the 5HT neurons cause a disturbance of social relatedness (Valzelli 1978) and failure to accommodate to novel environments (Takahashi et al. 1986). Thus, early dysfunction of the 5HT neurons that modulate development of the circadian S-W cycle may explain autistic behaviors, in particular impaired social relatedness and accommodation to novel environments. The 5HT neurons contribute to preventing leakage of the atonia of REM sleep into NREM sleep and are also involved in the control of locomotion, including the development of postural tone, normal bipedal stepping, and upright walking with co-ordinated arm movements. They also participate in the development of the functional specialization of the cortex. Thus we postulate that dysfunction of the 5HT neuronal system plays an important role in the abnormalities of sleep and locomotion, the bipedal stepping and upright walking posture in autism, as well as in its cognitive deficits.

The results of PSG suggest that early abnormalities of the NA and DA neurons also play a role in autism. Early lesions of the dorsal bundle of the locus coeruleus interfere with the extinction of episodic memory (Mason 1979, Tanaka et al. 1987). This deficit is relevant to the often outstanding rote memory and insistence on sameness of many individuals with autism. Hyperkinesis and aggressiveness implicate dysfunction of DA neurons. The age at which TMs increase in REM sleep in autism coincides with the age at which hyperkinesis, aggression and panic behaviors tend to appear. The observation that small doses of L-dopa have beneficial effects on the clock-dependent awakenings during sleep, but that higher doses aggravate these symptoms, suggests that they may be attributable to DA receptor supersensitivity (Segawa 1998).

Histochemical examination of the human brain revealed that the activity of tyrosine hydroxylase in the caudate nucleus is high in early childhood and decreases with age (McGeer and McGeer 1973). This indicates that the activity of the nigrostriatal DA neurons decreases with age. In autism, increase in DA transmission in later childhood does not reflect an increase of the activities of the DA neurons or of DA content; rather, it suggests the existence of DA receptor supersensitivity resulting from the decrease of DA activity in early life, as shown in the findings in PSG described earlier.

We had the opportunity to examine a girl with tuberous sclerosis with a subependy-mal nodule located in the thalamostriatal sulci of the left caudate nucleus who had had West syndrome responsive to ACTH as an infant (Tanaka et al. 1989). She later devel-oped rotatory seizures towards the right that were aggravated by administration of 3–4 mg/kg/day of L-dopa, but which improved when the dose was lowered to 0.5 mg/kg/day. The locus of the nodule suggested that it was causing a mechanical block in the nigro-striatal DA pathway. This patient resembles the animal model of Ungerstedt (1971) in that her PSG pointed to DA receptor supersensitivity, which was aggravated by large doses and alleviated by small doses of L-dopa (Tanaka et al. 1989). Thus different responses to small and large doses of L-dopa observed in autistic patients suggest that both these behavioral abnormalities, as well as the patients' clock-dependent awakenings, reflect exaggeration of DA transmission attributable to DA receptor supersensitivity.

Rats reared in isolation who had undergone early depletion of the 5HT and NA neurons, when placed in the same cage with mice kill them without any intent of eating them (muricide) (Valzelli and Garattini 1972). Rats with early pharmacological depletion of 5HT and NA given L-dopa are aggressive towards their mates rather than exhibiting the expected normal social behavior (Ueda et al. 2004). These observations suggest that increased DA transmission in the brain, coupled with hypofunctioning of the 5HT and NA neurons, is responsible for aggressive behavior.

In the rat, daily handling between birth and weaning plays a role in the development of functional lateralization of the cortex (Sherman et al. 1980). Delay beyond age 4 months in the development of the circadian S-W cycle may be analogous to the consequences of insufficient handling at early ages in the rat: both reflect inadequate sensitivity to daytime cues for wakefulness or nursing in autism. We suggest that this delay may contribute to delay in the development of the functional lateralization of the cortex, and also to the development of meaningful words (Segawa et al. 1992b). MRI studies reveal that postnatal growth of the corpus callosum spurts around the second month, starting at the genu, followed by a period of rapid growth of the splenium between 4 and 6 months of age (Barkovich and Kjos 1988). It is intriguing that the period for the development of the circadian S-W cycle coincides with the spurt in the development of the corpus callosum.

Abnormality of the 5HT neurons involved in postural tone and locomotion may induce developmental abnormalities in the functional specialization of the cortex, with, as a consequence, impaired development of intelligence.

Abnormalities in the development of locomotion are one of the characteristic symptoms of both Rett syndrome (RS) and Down syndrome. We have observed in these diseases that both the ability to utter meaningful words, and IQ/DQ levels, tend to be higher in those whose crawling or walking was less delayed (Segawa 1999a, 2001a). Neurohistochemical studies in RS suggest that failure of locomotion (crawling) caused by dysfunction of the brainstem aminergic neurons affects the nigrostriatal DA neurons through dysfunction of the pedunculo-pontine nucleus (PPN) (Segawa 2001b), as was observed in monkey experiments with excitotoxic unilateral lesions in the PPN (Kojima et al. 1997).

With normalization of locomotion, both orofacial and limb kinetic apraxia improved in autism (Segawa 1999a). A monkey experiment showed that attainment of the ability of bipedal upright walking with coordinated upper limb swing activates the supplementary motor area (SMA) through activation of the fastigial nucleus of the cerebellum (Shigemi Mori, personal communication 2003). The fastigial nucleus is one of the key nuclei that integrate the function of the higher and lower locomotor systems and send the signal to execute locomotion to the nucleus of the reticulospinal tract (Mori et al. 2000). The results of experiments in the monkey suggest that inciting bipedal upright walking activates the fastigial nucleus and, consequently, the SMA. Our clinical experience leads us to postulate that improvement of locomotion in autism improves the cortical function by activating the fastigial nucleus.

The neuropathological studies in autism indicate that, besides abnormalities that suggest maturational arrest, there are indications of ongoing changes (Kemper and Bauman

1998). That is, the fastigial, globoid and emboliform nuclei, which have no connection with the atrophic Purkinje cells, appear hypertrophic in young children but become atrophic with age in autistic adults. The age-related change in the fastigial nucleus observed at autopsy may be related to failure of normal upright walking. We propose that in late infancy the brainstem 5HT neurons involved in the development of postural tone induce crawling and modulate the function of the DA neuron through the PPN. In early childhood these 5HT neurons are implicated in bipedal upright locomotion and are also involved in the development of the functional specialization of the cortex via the deep cerebellar nuclei.

SUMMARY

Delay in the development of the circadian S-W cycle, sleep parameters and locomotion appear to be early biologic signs of autism. Each is caused by the dysfunction of the specific brainstem aminergic neurons responsible for particular neurobehavioral signs and symptoms of autism. Failure in locomotion may lead to dysfunction of the midbrain DA neuron through dysfunction of the PPN. Their dysfunction is responsible in turn for particular neuropsychological and behavioral symptoms that appear age-dependently after early childhood. It may be that in autism the dysfunction of these DA neurons may impact on the functional development of the frontal cortex. The 5HT neurons and their specific receptors have been shown to play a role in the development of specific functions of the brain at critical ages (Gaspar et al. 2003). In the rat, the axons of 5HT neurons involved in morphogenesis are pruned during the first 7 postnatal days (Koh et al. 1991). These observations provide a scientific basis for early detection of their abnormalities and for attempts to correct them by enhanced environmental stimulation and locomotor training. Assessment of developmental abnormalities of the S-W cycle and locomotion yield valuable insights into the involvements of specific aminergic neuronal circuits and provide a window into the pathophysiology of autism.

REFERENCES

Barkovich AJ, Kjos BO (1988) Normal postnatal development of the corpus callosum as demonstrated by MR imaging. *AJNR* 9: 487–91.

Bradley NS, Smith JL (1988) Neuromuscular patterns of stereotypic hindlimb behaviors in the first two postnatal months. II. Stepping in spinal kittens. *Brain Res Dev Brain Res* 38: 53–67.

Chamberlain RS, Herman BH (1990) A novel biochemical model linking dysfunctions in brain melatonin, proopiomelanocortin peptides, and serotonin in autism. *Biol Psychiatry* 28: 773–93.

Clements J, Wing L, Dunn G (1986) Sleep problems in handicapped children: a preliminary study. *J Child Psychol Psychiatry* 27: 399–407.

Elia M, Ferri R Musumeci SA, Bergonzi P (1991) Rapid eye movement modulation during night sleep in autistic subjects. *Brain Dysfunct* 4: 348–54.

Gail Williams P, Sears LL, Allard A (2004) Sleep problems in children with autism. *J Sleep Re*s 13: 265–8.

Gaspar P, Cases O, Maroteaux L (2003) The developmental role of serotonin: news from mouse molecular genetics. *Nat Rev Neurosci* 4: 1002–12.

Hayashi E (2000) Effect of melatonin on sleep–wake rhythm: the sleep diary of an autistic male. *Psychiatry Clin Neurosci* 54: 383–4.

Hering E, Epstein R, Elroy S, Iancu DR, Zelnik N (1999) Sleep patterns in autistic children. *J Autism Dev Disord* 29: 143–7.

Hashimoto T, Tayama M. (1985) Polysomnographic studies on autism: phasic events during sleep. In: Annual report of "Studies on the Prevention and Treatment of Early Infantile Autism from the Standpoint of Developmental Neurobiology."] Ministry of Health and Welfare of Japan, pp. 11–8 (Japanese).

Hobson JA, McCarley RW, Wyzinski PW (1975) Sleep cycle oscillation: reciprocal discharge by two brainstem neuronal groups. *Science* 189: 55–8.

Hoshino Y, Watanabe H, Yashima Y, Kaneko M, Kumashiro H (1984) An investigation on sleep disturbance of autistic children. *Folia Psychiatr Neurol Jpn* 38: 45–51.

Inamura K (1984) [Sleep–wake patterns in autistic children.] *Jpn J Child Adolesc Psychiatry* 25: 205–17 (Japanese).

Jan JE, O'Donnell ME (1996) Use of melatonin in the treatment of paediatric sleep disorders. *J Pineal Res* 21: 193–9.

Kemper TL, Bauman M (1998) Neuropathology of infantile autism. *J Neuropathol Exp Neurol* 57: 645–52.

Koh T, Nakazawa M, Kani K, Maeda T (1991) Investigations of origins of serotonergic projection to developing rat visual cortex: a combined retrograde tracing and immunohistochemical study. *Brain Res Bull* 27: 675–84.

Kojima J, Yamaji Y, Matsumura M, Nambu A, Inase M, Tokuno H, Takada M, Imai H (1997) Excitotoxic lesions of the pedunculopontine tegmental nucleus produce contralateral hemi-parkinsonism in the monkey. *Neurosci Lett* 226: 111–4.

Limoges E, Mottron L, Bolduc C, Berthiaume C, Godbout R (2005) Atypical sleep architecture and the autism phenotype. *Brain* 8: 1049–61.

Ma G, Segawa M, Nomura Y, Kondo Y, Yanagitani M, Higurashi M (1993) The development of sleep-wakefulness rhythm in normal infants and young children. *Tohoku J Exp Med* 171: 29–41.

Mason ST (1979) Noradrenaline and behaviour. *Trends Neurosci* 2: 82–4.

McGeer EG, McGeer PL. (1973) Some characteristics of brain tyrosine hydroxylase. In: Mandel J, ed. *New Concepts in Neurotransmitter Regulation.* New York, London: Plenum, pp. 53–68.

Miller S, van der Burg J (1973) The function of long propriospinal pathways in the co-ordination of quadrupedal stepping in the cat. In: Stein RB, Pearson KG, Smith RS, Redford JB, eds. *Control of Posture and Locomotion. Advances in Behavioral Biology, vol. 7.* New York, London: Plenum, pp. 561–77.

Mori S, Takakusaki K (1988) Integration of posture and locomotion. In: Amblard B, Berthoz A, Mori S, eds. *Posture and Gait Development, Adaptation and Modulation.* Amsterdam, New York, Oxford: Excerpta Medica, pp. 341–54.

Mori S, Takakusaki K, Shimoda N, Tanaka H (1988) [Suppression of the muscle tone and control of locomotion by the brainstem. Annual Report, 1988, of the Research Committee of the Ministry of Health and Welfare of Japan on Medical, Psychological and Social Studies of the Development, Maturation and the Effects of the Raising Condition of Children.] Tokyo: Ministry of Health and Welfare of Japan, pp. 289–92 (Japanese).

Mori S, Matsuyama K, Kohyama J, Kobayashi Y, Takakusaki K (1992) Neuronal constituents of postural and locomotor control systems and their interactions in cats. *Brain Dev* 14: S109–20.

Mori S, Matsui T, Mori F, Nakajima K, Matsuyama K (2000) Instigation and control of treadmill locomotion in high decerebrate cats by stimulation of the hook bundle of Russell in the cerebellum. *Can J Physiol Pharmacol* 78: 945–57.

Ornitz EM (1972) Development of sleep patterns in autistic children. In: Clement CD, Purpura DP, Mayer FE, eds. *Sleep and the Maturing Nervous System.* New York: Academic Press, pp. 368–81.

Ornitz EM (1983) The functional neuroanatomy of infantile autism. *Int J Neurosci* 19: 85–124.

Pace-Schott EF, Hobson JA (2002) The neurobiology of sleep: genetics, cellular physiology and subcortical networks. *Nat Rev Neurosci* 3: 591–605.

Parmelee AH, Stern E (1972) Development of states in infants. In: Clement CD, Purpura DP, Mayer FE, eds. *Sleep and the Maturing Nervous System.* New York: Academic Press, pp. 199–228.

Parmelee AH, Wenner WH, Schulz HR (1964) Infant sleep patterns: from birth to 16 weeks of age. *J Pediatr* 65: 576–82.

Patzold LM, Richdale AL, Tonge BJ (1998) An investigation into sleep characteristics of children with autism and Asperger's disorder. *J Paediatr Child Health* 34: 528–33.

Quine L (1991) Sleep problems in children with mental handicap. *J Ment Defic Res* 35: 269–90.

Rapin I, Katzman R (1998) Neurobiology of autism. *Ann Neurol* 43: 7–14.

Richdale AL, Prior MR (1995) The sleep/wake rhythm in children with autism. *Eur Child Adolesc Psychiatry* 4: 175–86.

Role LW, Kelly JP (1991) The brain stem: Cranial nerve nuclei and the monoaminergic systems. In: Kandel ER, Schwartz JH, Jessell TM, eds. *Principles of Neural Science, 3rd edn.* Norwalk, CT: Appleton & Lance, pp. 683–99.

Sakai K (1985) Anatomical and physiological basis of paradoxical sleep. In: McGinty DJ, Drucker-Colin R, Morrison AR, Parmeggiani PL, eds. *Brain Mechanism of Sleep.* New York: Raven Press, pp. 111–37.

Segawa M (1982) [Neurological approach on infantile autism – Based on the pathophysiology of sleep disturbances.] *Jpn J Dev Disabil* 4: 184–97 (Japanese).

Segawa M (1985) [Circadian rhythm in early infantile autism.] *Adv Neurol Sci* 29: 140–53 (Japanese).

Segawa M (1998) [Neurological model of autism.] *Brain Sci* 20: 169–71 (Japanese).

Segawa M (1999a) [Development of locomotion; its failure and higher cortical function (I).] *Rinsho Noha* 41: 385–91 (Japanese).

Segawa M (1999b) [Modulation of sleep in early childhood.] In: Torii S, ed. *Sleep Ecology.* Tokyo: Asakura, pp. 110–23 (Japanese).

Segawa M (1999c) Ontogenesis of REM sleep in rapid eye movement sleep. In: Mallich BW, Inoué S, eds. *Rapid Eye Movement Sleep.* New Delhi: Narosa, pp. 39–50.

Segawa M (2001a) Pathophysiology of Rett syndrome from the stand point of clinical characteristics. *Brain Dev* 23 Suppl 1: S94–8.

Segawa M (2001b) Discussant—Pathophysiologies of Rett syndrome. *Brain Dev* 23 Suppl 1: S218–23.

Segawa M (2002) [Development of sleep and biological rhythm.] *Pharma Medica* 20 (suppl): 26–32 (Japanese).

Segawa M, Nomura Y (1991) Pathophysiology of human locomotion: studies on clinical cases. In: Shimamura M, Grillner S, Engerton VR, eds. *Neurobiological Basis of Human Locomotion.* Tokyo: Japan Scientific Societies Press, pp. 317–28.

Segawa M, Katoh J, Nomura Y (1992a) Neurology: as a window to brainstem dysfunction. In: Naruse H, Ornitz EM, eds. *Neurobiology of Infantile Autism.* Amsterdam: Elsevier Science, pp. 187–200.

Segawa M, Katoh M, Katoh J, Nomura Y (1992b) Early modulation of sleep parameters and its importance in later behavior. *Brain Dysfunc* 5: 211–23.

Segawa M, Nomura Y, Hikosaka O, Soda M, Usui S, Kase M (1987) Roles of the basal ganglia and related structure in symptoms of dystonia. In: Carpenter BM, Jayaraman A, eds. *The Basal Ganglia II*. New York: Plenum, pp. 489–504.

Segawa M, Nomura Y, Tanaka S, Hakamada S, Nagata E, Soda M, Kase M (1988) Hereditary progressive dystonia with marked diurnal fluctuation-consideration on its pathophysiology based on the characteristics of clinical and polysomnographical findings. *Adv Neurol* 50: 367–76.

Sherman GF, Garbanati JA, Rosen GD, Yutzey DA, Denenberg VH (1980) Brain and behavioral asymmetries for spatial preference in rats. *Brain Res* 192: 61–7.

Taira M, Takase M, Sasaki H (1998) Sleep disorder in children with autism. *Psychiatry Clin Neurosci* 52: 182–3.

Takahashi K, Shimoda K, Yamada N, Sasaki Y, Hayashi S (1986) Effect of dorsal midbrain lesion in infants rats on development of circadian rhythm. *Brain Dev* 8: 373–81.

Tanaka S, Miyagawa F, Imai H, Hidano T (1987) [Learning abilities of rats with lesions in the dorsal noradrenergic bundle.] *Juntendo Med J* 33: 271–27 (Japanese).

Tanaka S, Nomura Y, Segawa M (1989) [Rotational seizures in tuberous sclerosis.] *Juntendo Med J* 34: 520–7 (Japanese).

Tanguay PE, Ornitz EM, Forsythe AB, Ritvo ER (1976) Rapid eye movement (REM) activity in normal and autistic children during REM sleep. *J Autism Child Schizophr* 6: 275–88.

Thirumalai SS, Shubin RA, Robinson R (2002) Rapid eye movement sleep behavior disorder in children with autism. *J Child Neurol* 17: 173–8.

Ueda S, Nakadate K, Noda AT, Sakakibara S (2004) Prelude to aggression: Animal research for abuse and violence. *Jpn J Pediatr* 57: 1257–64.

Ungerstedt U (1971) Striatal dopamine release after amphetamine or nerve degeneration revealed by rotational behaviour. *Acta Physiol Scand Suppl* 367: 49–68.

Valzelli L (1978) Affective behavior and serotonin. In: Essman WB, ed. *Serotonin in Health and Disease. Vol. 3. The Central Nervous System*. New York, London: Spectrum, pp. 145–201.

Valzelli L, Garattini S (1972) Biochemical and behavioural changes induced by isolation in rats. *Neuropharmacology* 11: 17–22.

Webb WB (1971) Sleep behaviour as a biorhythm. In: Colquhoun WP, ed. *Biological Rhythms and Human Performance*. London: Academic Press, pp. 149–77.

Wiggs L, Stores G (1996) Severe sleep disturbance and daytime challenging behaviour in children with severe learning disabilities. *J Intellect Disabil Res* 40: 518–28.

Wiggs L, Stores G (2004) Sleep patterns and sleep disorders in children with autistic spectrum disorders: insights using parent report and actigraphy. *Dev Med Child Neurol* 46: 372–80.

16
NEUROPSYCHOLOGICAL ASSESSMENT: BASIC CONCEPTS AND CLINICAL UTILITY

Susan K Klein

The role of the neurologist in the evaluation of a child suspected of a developmental disorder, and specifically of a child at risk for an autism spectrum disorder (ASD), is two-fold: first to decide whether there is sufficient evidence for the existence of a disorder, and second to determine, if possible, the biological (or social) cause(s) of the disorder. What to do about the disorder if found will depend on these two parts of the evaluation. Deciding whether or not there is evidence for a disorder is of course crucial because it will determine both what further testing is needed and what to do about the disorder. In the USA in 2005, the diagnostic label the physician gives the child often determines what services will be made available to the child and who pays for them. Parents also seek advice to understand what will happen in the future of this child whose development is not typical.

In order to evaluate a child with suspected ASD, the neurologist must elicit detailed developmental, past medical, and family and social histories, evaluate the child's functional behavior in an interactive context appropriate to the child's age (this is the mental status part of the neurologic evaluation), perform a physical and neurologic (i.e. largely sensorimotor) examination, and review any material from other professionals the parents may have brought to the consultation. Based on a synthesis of all this information, the neurologist can then decide what medical tests or further consultations are indicated.

This chapter reviews the information from educational assessments and neuropsychological evaluations that may be available in this process. It will not cover specific instruments and their psychometric validity. That information is available from many other sources, including Baron's (2004) elegant monograph on neuropsychological assessment of children. This chapter is meant to be a framework for a clinician to evaluate neuropsychological and psychoeducational data that may be available for diagnosis and management of a child with ASD.

WHAT INFORMATION IS USUALLY AVAILABLE?
PSYCHOEDUCATIONAL EVALUATION
In the USA, if the child is less than 3 years old and falls under the federal law that

mandates early intervention for all infants and toddlers at risk for developmental disorders, behavioral and cognitive testing will be provided by the local Early Intervention Center which decides on the need for intervention and its intensity. At 3 years, children with developmental disorders become the responsibility of local departments of education and may be eligible for educational services provided by a specialized preschool program. In preschool and especially school-age children, when the diagnosis and the severity of the deficits are likely to have been clarified, the main issue is to define specific deficits in as much detail as possible, as this will assist the educators and therapists to select the most appropriate way to attempt remediation. In the USA, school districts must evaluate children in need of special services prior to entry into preschool at age 3, prior to entry into kindergarten at age 5, and every three years thereafter or earlier if there has been a significant change in the child or if there is lack of progress suggesting inappropriate intervention. As one might expect, the thoroughness of the evaluation and the appropriateness and extent of the educational services made available to children vary. As a result, a neurologist or (developmental) pediatrician needs to follow the child and may have to recommend to the parents testing outside the school in order to get an independent opinion regarding the child's needs. Of necessity, this chapter focuses on how evaluations are carried out in the USA, because a survey of other countries' procedures would far exceed the resources of the chapter. What is described is therefore not prescriptive and does not claim to provide the ideal approach to evaluation or services.

The purpose of educational evaluations in preschool and school-age children with ASD (autism) is to develop an understanding of each child's strengths and weaknesses as a learner. Most of the time, this can be accomplished with a psychoeducational evaluation. The first place to start is with the evaluations done by school districts that are mandated by special education law. In the USA, psychoeducational evaluations are usually carried out by child or school psychologists who are licensed by the state in which they practice. These child psychologists have specialized training in educational assessment; not all licensed child psychologists do this type of evaluation.

The importance of beginning the psychoeducational assessment with the evaluation carried out by the school district cannot be overemphasized. Even if the parents are frustrated with the lack of responsiveness of their individual school district, or have been advised by other families in their district that getting support from their particular district will be a struggle, they should begin with the school evaluation. The school district will ultimately decide how the recommendations of the psychoeducational assessors will be implemented. District personnel have a strong commitment to bringing out the best in each child, and individuals in the district may be frustrated by political and financial restrictions on what can be proposed for each child. Thus, it is vital that district personnel feel that they are part of the process. School professionals have specialized training in assessing and serving children with special needs, and their contributions should be weighted appropriately. Many districts have such skilled evaluators that a complete picture of the child's strengths and weaknesses can be developed from the school evaluation alone, at no cost to families. Most districts have multiple levels of assessment available: those done at the individual district level, and extended evaluations that are done at consortium levels or subcontracted to private evaluators by the district, again at no cost to families. Families need to become familiar with their state's interpretation of federal law so that they are aware of the type of specialized assessment that can be obtained through public education services.

A private psychoeducational evaluation, paid for by families themselves, is another alternative. Educational assessments obtained privately are often not covered by medical insurance plans, thus adding an additional burden on families who are financially and emotionally stressed. Families may choose private assessments because they need results on a faster timetable than a district can provide, or because they disagree with the district's findings on a psychoeducational assessment (e.g. a child does not qualify for special educational services and the appeals process has been exhausted). Does a private psychoeducational evaluation always need to be carried out by a neuropsychologist? The choice should be guided by the questions about the child. If attention, language or behavioral issues are major concerns, a psychoeducational evaluation will be more than adequate to help develop interventions.

NEUROPSYCHOLOGICAL EVALUATION

A neuropsychological evaluation differs from a psychoeducational evaluation in several respects. A neuropsychological evaluation is usually carried out by a neuropsychologist who is a child psychologist who has had additional training in brain–behavior relationships as well as in educational assessment. In the USA, child neuropsychologists have a separate certifying Board, and many practicing neuropsychologists hold this certification. Neuropsychological evaluations typically extend the psychoeducational evaluation to explore memory and executive function skills. If medical issues such as head injury, remote meningitis, Tourette syndrome or regression of cognitive skills are concerns, a neuropsychological evaluation, which will be longer and more expensive, will probably be indicated.

A private psychoeducational or neuropsychological evaluation may not include an in-depth evaluation of language or communicative skills (see Chapter 4). Depending on the evaluator, it may or may not include detailed behavioral assessments (for example, of disruptive, stereotypic or attention-seeking behaviors), or detailed evaluation of fine motor deficits. Families need to ask the private evaluators what will be included in the assessment at the time they make the appointment or at the intake meeting if these are specific concerns. Supplementation of psychoeducational assessments with in-depth speech and language or occupational therapy assessments add to the cost for families.

The aim of neuropsychological assessment in children with autism – and in all children, for that matter – is to identify areas of learning strengths and weaknesses so that adults can provide academic and behavioral support. Assessment is directed by the needs of the child and the power of the standardized instruments available to test the child.

TABLE 16.1
Core domains for psychological assessment

Medical and social history
Behavior
　　Historical observation
　　Observations during testing
General intelligence
Academic achievement
Executive functions
Attention/concentration/orientation
Memory
Language
　　Phonology
　　Syntax
　　Semantics
　　Discourse
Sensory/perceptual skills
Motor skills
　　Fine motor skills
　　Gross motor skills
Visuomotor and visuoperceptual skills

COMPONENTS OF THE PSYCHOEDUCATIONAL OR NEUROPSYCHOLOGICAL EVALUATION

At every age, the clinician will want to know about each of the core domains of psychological assessment (Table 16.1).

Rather than rely on a standardized battery of testing (such as the Halsted–Reitan; Reitan and Wolfson 1993), Baron (2004) recommends a convergence profile analysis, in which the examiner decides where to focus the psychological testing based on historical information, the questions that are to be answered by the psychological evaluation, and behavioral observations by the psychologist. Thus, the battery of tests selected for a preschool child with suspected ASD might focus more on language capabilities and behavioral observations, as contrasted to the tests given to a preadolescent, which might explore cognitive and metacognitive skills to a greater extent.

PRESCHOOLERS (AGES 2–5 YEARS)

The importance of language testing in preschoolers

Assessment in preschool children usually focuses on diagnosis of ASD in a language disordered child. In ideal circumstances, the child has already been evaluated by Early Intervention services and some standardized assessment of language skills has already been administered (Table 16.2).

TABLE 16.2
Selected standardized language batteries*

Infant and toddler

• Preschool Language Scale	Zimmerman et al. (1997)
• Test of Early Language Development	Hresko et al. (1999)
• Receptive–Expressive Emergent Language Test	Bzoch et al. (2003)

Preschooler

• Preschool Language Scale	Zimmerman et al. (1997)
• Clinical Evaluation of Language Fundamentals	Semel et al. (2006)
• Goldman–Fristoe–Woodcock Test of Auditory Discrimination	Goldman et al. (1970)
• Goldman–Fristoe Test of Articulation	Goldman and Fristoe (2000)
• Children's Communication Checklist	Bishop (2003)

School-age

• Clinical Evaluation of Language Fundamentals	Semel et al. (2006)
• Test of Language Development (Primary, Intermediate)	Hammill and Newcomer (1997)
• Goldman–Fristoe Test of Articulation	Goldman and Fristoe (2000)
• Token Test for Children	See Baron (2004)
• Test of Pragmatic Language	Phelps-Terasaki and Phelps-Gunn (1992)
• Children's Communication Checklist	Bishop (2003)

*See also Chapter 4.

Starting a preschool assessment with language testing is very important, because the psychologist will have difficulty assessing other psychological domains in children with severely delayed language skills. Language assessment is an important part of the psychoeducational assessment because language and cognition are interdependent (Green et al. 1995). It is crucial not to limit language assessment to reporting of verbal utterances but to carefully assess comprehension, as it is always impaired to some degree in preschoolers on the autism spectrum, even in those who may be producing phrases and sentences. Some autistic children will produce a mixture of immediate and delayed echolalia that may seem to be appropriate until it is tested in a situation that stresses language comprehension. In nonverbal children, visual–manual language as well as speech must be evaluated. Does the child point to draw attention or request, use evocative gestures or head nods to get his or her point across, understand that communication is power? As discussed in Chapter 4 there are children with autism who have such profound inability to decode oral language (speech) that they cannot understand or produce it, yet their nonverbal skills may be much less impaired. In these children, attributing lack of language either to severe mental retardation or lack of the will to communicate may not be warranted.

TABLE 16.3
Selected tests of adaptive behavior and behavioral issues

Tests of adaptive behavior	
• Vineland Adaptive Behavior Scales	Sparrow et al. (2005)
• American Association of Mental Retardation Adaptive Behavior Scales–School	Lambert et al. (1993)
Tests of general psychopathology	
• Achenbach System of Empirically Based Measurements (formerly known as the Child Behavior Checklist; many forms including preschool, school-aged, teacher report, self-report)	See Baron (2004)
• Behavior Assessment System for Children	Reynolds and Kamphaus (2004)
Tests of attention	
• Attention Deficit Disorders Evaluation Scale	McCarney and Bauer (2004)
• Conners' Rating Scales	Conners (1996)
• Disruptive Behavior Rating Scale	Erford (1998)
• NICHQ Vanderbilt Assessment Scales	AAP/NICHQ (2002)
• Brown Attention Deficit Disorder Scales	Brown (2001)
• Attention Deficit Hyperactivity Disorder Rating Scale–IV	DuPaul et al. (1998)

Assessing other psychological domains in preschoolers

The skill of the neuropsychologist plays a large part in the reliability of testing preschoolers in other domains (Baron 2004). Even typical preschoolers have limited attention spans, and those on the autism spectrum are likely to not yet have learned to pay attention to stimuli introduced by an adult and that compliance with requests is expected. Therefore obtaining even limited quantitative test results on a few judiciously chosen tests in other psychological domains will require creativity and flexibility on the part of the psychologist who may have to use unorthodox testing approaches.

• *Behavior and social cognition.* Standardized assessments of behavior are also extremely important in diagnosis of ASD in preschoolers. These include the instruments developed to support diagnosis of ASD (see Chapter 17), but should also include more general instruments of adaptive behavior, attention and psychopathology (Table 16.3).

General measures of adaptive behavior organize historical information about daily living skills (for a review, see Deisinger 2001). Behavioral measures in preschoolers will help to identify comorbid disorders of attention and begin to characterize whether disruptive behavior comes from the child's attempt to communicate with others or has other sources (such as abuse) that might require further evaluation by a child psychiatrist.

There are no standardized measures to evaluate representational play. Assessment of

TABLE 16.4
Selected tests of cognition

Infant
- Bayley Scales of Intelligence — Bayley (2005)
- Mullen Scales of Early Learning — Mullen (1995)

Preschool
- Wechsler intelligence tests (many forms, brief, preschool, school-age, adolescent) — See Baron (2004)
- Merrill Palmer Scale of Mental Tests — Roid and Sampers (2005)
- Differential Ability Scales — Elliott (1990)
- Kaufman intelligence tests (many forms, brief, preschool, school-age, adolescent) — See Baron (2004)
- Stanford–Binet Intelligence Scale — Roid (2003)
- McCarthy Scales of Children's Abilities — McCarthy (1972)

School-age
- Wechsler intelligence tests (many forms, brief, preschool, school-age, adolescent) — See Baron (2004)
- Stanford–Binet Intelligence Scale — Roid (2003)
- Kaufman intelligence tests (many forms, brief, preschool, school-age, adolescent) — See Baron (2004)
- Comprehensive Test of Nonberbal Intelligence — Hammill et al. (1996)
- Leiter International Performance Scales — Roid and Miller (1997)
- Differential Ability Scales — Elliott (1990)

Adolescent
- Wechsler intelligence tests (many forms, brief, preschool, school-age, adolescent) — See Baron (2004)
- Stanford–Binet Intelligence Scale — Roid (2003)
- Raven Progressive Matrices — Raven et al. (1998)
- Kaufman intelligence tests (many forms, brief, preschool, school-age, adolescent) — See Baron (2004)

play is critical in diagnosis of ASD. Direct observation is the only means of assessing this at present, but should always be included in the preschool psychological assessment.

• *Cognition.* Psychologists appear to be split on whether cognitive assessment of preschoolers is helpful in diagnosis of ASD at this age. Fombonne (2005) reported that in 21 epidemiologic studies with data, 34% of subjects on average had a "normal" IQ. It is very difficult to test cognition in a preschooler (Rapin 2003). Standardized tests of cognition (Table 16.4) provide only comparisons of the child being tested to age-matched norms.

Parents in particular may be concerned about the IQ score. It is important to remember and to remind parents and others that many factors contribute to the overall predictive value of tests of intelligence in young children (Turkheimer et al. 2003).

Tests of intelligence can be helpful in looking at strengths and weaknesses at every age. Intelligence testing compares a child with special needs to his or her chronological age peers; this was Binet's original purpose in developing his test of intelligence in 1922 (see Madge and Tizard 1981). In preschoolers, intelligence tests are helpful as a check on language skills (picture naming subtests), spatial skills (puzzle subtests), attention (timed subtests, matching subtests), and fine motor skills (matching subtests with manipulatives). Preschool tests of intelligence rarely have delayed recall tests (looking at memory), and are not particularly useful in assessing abstract reasoning, since these skills are limited even in typical children at this age.

A child with ASD will usually have one of two IQ test profiles on the Wechsler series: (1) low verbal scores (especially on the subtests of Comprehension, Similarities, and Vocabulary) with relatively preserved visuospatial abilities (Object Assembly, Block Design) (Green et al. 1995); or (2) near age-level verbal scores, with lower scores on tests of spatial ability (Puzzle Completion, Pattern Recognition, etc.); this conforms to the nonverbal learning disability profile seen in some individuals with Asperger syndrome (Klin et al. 1995, Miller and Ozonoff 2000) and other neurological conditions like hydrocephalus. Neither pattern is associated with a better or worse prognosis; the profiles merely reflect the strengths and weaknesses of the individual, and will likely hold true in subsequent assessments (Freeman et al. 1991).

Another way to look at cognitive skills is by an assessment of "fluid" and "crystallized" intelligence, that is, second order factors derived from raw data by factor analysis (Brody 1992). Fluid intelligence refers to the innate capacity of an individual to acquire new knowledge; crystallized intelligence refers to the ability to use educational and cultural exposure (prior learning) to acquire new knowledge (Cattell 1963). Children with autism show relative deficits in crystallized intelligence, as measured by lower sequential (rule-based) processing on the Kaufman Assessment Battery for Children (Allen et al. 1991). Even in preschoolers, it is possible to observe the deficit in abstract reasoning that is one of the hallmarks of autism (Rutter 1983).

In my opinion, intelligence testing in preschoolers is most helpful in assessing children with suspected ASD when the child has a splinter skill, such as hyperlexia, that suggests advanced skills to parents and teachers. In these situations, cognitive testing can begin to explore how much understanding supports the advanced skill.

• *Motor skills.* Testing of gross and fine motor skills is usually carried out in a preschool psychological assessment, often by other members of an assessment team such as a physical or occupational therapist. These tests will not be reviewed here. For the clinician evaluating the possible presence of ASD, the major importance of these tests lies in identifying a child with global developmental delays. If gross motor skills are delayed on the standardized assessment measures used in preschoolers beyond clumsiness in alternating gait and pedaling skills, the clinician should consider a work-up for autism in the setting of global developmental delay (Shevell et al. 2003). Many children with developmental language disorders and autism will have some fine motor skill delays and motor stereo-typies (see Chapters 5 and 14) (Rapin 1997). For those ASD children who have great difficulty with handwriting, the teaching of keyboard skills, which will ensure that the children are able to produce neat homework, is an option to explore. Many of them have long been interested in computers and may be willing to learn to type reasonably proficiently, perhaps using a keyboard with larger keys.

• *Perceptual and sensory skills.* Sensory assessments are often included in occupational therapy batteries, and sensory supports can be valuable in extinguishing unwanted behaviors (such as self-injurious behaviors). These are notoriously difficult to treat (see Chapters 5 and 17). Skilled occupational therapists can be extremely helpful in helping children acquire such skills as dressing, tying, writing and other activities of daily life. The biologic basis of recommended therapies, such as brushing and vestibular exercises, is poorly understood. Whether these therapies will have a sustained impact on the developing nervous system is unproven and unknown.

• *Achievement.* Some assessment of kindergarten readiness skills is essential for a child with ASD, as they can have reading disabilities that are probably not linked to their diagnosis of autism, but which will significantly impact their education, and possibly their employ-ment. Some examples are tests of phonemic awareness (e.g. rhyming), sequencing (not just sounds but words, telling a short story, etc.), understanding the one-to-one relation of numerals to objects, at least up to 10 (counting in order without skipping), holding a pencil and copying simple geometric shapes (e.g. Beery 1997), and ability to imitate, to sit, to attend and to comply.

ELEMENTARY SCHOOL AGED CHILDREN – GRADES K–3 (AGES 5–9 YEARS)
Language
Every element of language (articulation, fluency, prosody, syntax, semantics, and dis-course) needs to be considered in an evaluation (see Chapter 4). Before the school-age years, all children with autism should have some assessment of pragmatic language, even if they are dependent on an assisted communication device and have no spontaneous spoken language. How children attempt to communicate what they want impacts behavior so profoundly that some understanding of their communication skill level is essential. Use of social skill groups and/or scenarios should be an integral part of language remediation for all children with autism.

Cognition
Cognitive assessments can be much more sophisticated beginning at this level. An examination of subtest score profiles can yield interesting information that can then be pursued by referral to appropriate professionals. Consider, for example, the WISC-IV scores (Wechsler 2005). Four indices, verbal, nonverbal, working memory and processing

speed, are derived from the subtests given. Children who have problems processing spatial information, such as those with nonverbal learning disabilities, will have normal or even above average verbal factor scores (with comprehension closer to the mean than the other scores comprising the factor), a low nonverbal score, and average to slightly below average working memory and processing speed scores. These children can benefit from organizational support as well as recasting spatial information in different ways for learning. A child with attention issues may have low working memory and processing speed scores, which can then be followed up by a standardized measure of attention. Children with reading or language based learning disorders (see below) might have low verbal scores with lower working memory and processing speed scores (reflecting the additional effort they need to understand classroom material). These children might have lower scores on the receptive language subtests of standardized language tests, so it is worth considering language reassessment in children with IQ score profiles that are not "flat", i.e. the same across all subtests.

Achievement

There are no special disorders in academic achievement that are unique to children with autism. Because children with autism have problems with abstract thinking and language skills, clinicians need to be aware of how these deficits might impact academic achievement and, ultimately, vocational skills. School districts, in the current USA era of "No Child Left Behind" (http://www.ed.gov/nclb/landing.jhtml) usually do a reasonable job of standardized academic assessment. Happily, early reading skills are now more commonly being assessed with standardized measures of phonological processing, but this is still variable across districts. Advanced assessment of reading disorders (beyond phonological processing, including measures of fluency, orthographic recognition, comprehension and the like) is not consistently available in school assessments. The clinician should look at achievement scores for reading, math and written expression. Pennington et al. (1993) and Nigg et al. (1998) have developed a formula for identifying reading disability using only IQ and achievement measures that can help identify a child with a reading disability. They define a reading disability by a reading quotient (RQ; derived by RQ = Woodcock–Johnson [Woodcock and Johnson 1977] total reading standardized age score/verbal IQ score) below 0.85 if the reading level is also below the 25th percentile. If children can acquire rote math skills, then attention needs to be directed at whether they can identify and understand money, and abstract math problems (word problems, geometry, etc.). Problems with written expression are probably the most ubiquitous of academic deficits. A problem with reading, abstract thinking, handwriting or attention can result in low scores on tests of written expression.

Gross and fine motor skills

These continue to require support in the school-age years but rarely require specialized assessment or intervention beyond what is available in the schools.

Social cognition

Schools face two behavioral issues in this age group: inattentive/hyperactive behavior, and aggressive behavior. Standardized ratings, as mentioned in the preschool section, can be invaluable in sorting out the sources of each and making appropriate referrals as needed.

MIDDLE SCHOOL AGED CHILDREN – GRADES 4–8 (AGES 10–14 YEARS)

Language, cognition and achievement

The same issues discussed in the school-age section apply here. Higher functioning individuals with autism may struggle more as they are required to integrate what they have learned in various settings, rather than merely focusing on skill building as in earlier years. Review of school-based assessments by supervising educational psychologists within the district, or by (private) neuropsychologists or speech–language consultants, can be helpful in refining teaching goals for children who seem stalled in their academic progress. These specialists evaluate how memory skills, executive functions, organizational strategies and language processing skills affect academic achievement.

A neuropsychologist will explore other dimensions of cognition beyond what is typically carried out in a school evaluation. Schopler and Mesibov (1995) edited an elegant review of components of such a neuropsychological evaluation for children with autism that, with the exception of recent interest in executive function in autism, has not been significantly improved upon in the subsequent decade. Green et al. (1995) discuss theoretical underpinnings behind observations of overselective attention (nonfunctional attention to detail), short term memory and rote memory strengths, and poorer performance on delayed match-to-sample tasks. Lincoln et al. (1995) review the performance of subjects with autism on a host of memory tasks. Individuals with autism have shown normal performance on "short term" memory tasks tapping the primacy/recency effect, echoic memory, visual recognition memory, short term auditory memory and serial memory. "Long-term" memory tasks tend to be somewhat more problematic for subjects with autism. Lincoln et al. (1995) summarize several reports showing autistic children performing more poorly on tasks tapping retention, forced recognition, recall of recent activities, and recall of spoken directions or questions.

Executive functions have been described in many ways. Baddeley (1986) has defined them as "the residual area of ignorance about working memory which we are consistently attempting to reduce . . . [which includes] attentional capacities and is capable of selecting and operating control processes." The components include planning, responding to information learned to shift to the next response, and cognitive flexibility. Executive functions, as Ozonoff (1995) comments, involve holding a mental representation of something in one's head and then making a response based on rules.

Executive functions are measured by neuropsychologists using tests with shifting rules, mazes, production of drawings after the visual stimulus is removed, and verbal fluency (see Baron 2004). Standardized batteries of executive function tests have been developed for use in children. These are used to make educational recommendations to strengthen planning and organizational skills. Children with autism have difficulty shifting set, and their responses to stimuli can be perseverative (for a review, see Ozonoff 1995). Because of their difficulties in formulating concepts, individuals with autism may show cognitive inflexibility on abstract reasoning tasks (Minshew et al. 1992, 2002; Meyer and Minshew 2002). However, as Dawson et al. (2002) point out, "there is no autism-specific pattern of executive dysfunction." Although executive functions, like those governing theory of mind, are believed to originate in frontal lobe regions (Norman and Shallice 1986), clinical neuropsychologists do not usually administer tests of social cognition to assess theory of mind or joint attention.

Lower functioning children with autism continue to focus on discrete goals (e.g. one digit subtraction) without recognition that their failure to acquire basic reading and math skills by this point already restricts their vocational choices. For the latter, vocational planning should begin at this age, but it rarely does. Typically, specialized vocational assessment is not available in the private sector either.

Gross and fine motor skills
Assessment and interventions are the same as for the previous age group.

Social cognition
Behavior problems identified at this point will probably require specialized assessment beyond the resources available to the school district (by child neurologists, clinical psychologists and child psychiatrists). They include attention and aggressive behavior problems. Specialized teams of psychologists and counselors skilled in behavioral techniques are available to schools in wealthier and more urban districts and may be extremely helpful (e.g. Dunn 2005). Examination of language, cognitive and achievement skills can aid in the management of behavior problems, because it can tell you how much the child will understand.

HIGH SCHOOLERS AND BEYOND (14+ YEARS)
Language, cognition, academic achievement and vocational skill development
Assessment of these issues is intimately connected to the assessment of behavior, as planning will be influenced significantly by whether an adolescent behaves appropriately in social settings. In the USA, school districts are responsible for the education of young people with significant disabilities until age 21 years, and for assisting them to discover what skills they can realistically bring to the market place, based on their tastes as well as their abilities.

Vocational planning should guide assessment and intervention of these areas for adolescents and young adults with autism. Higher functioning adolescents need to be assessed for "common sense life skills" to determine whether they will be capable of living independently. Monitoring of social skills in forming relationships is important in order to avoid the isolation of these adolescents from peers. Typically, a school district does not have the resources to provide this behavioral support for skill development, and families must seek it privately.

Lower functioning individuals need active and creative planning for even semi-independent living. Vocational services vary widely across districts, and there appears to be no specific standardized assessment that helps in planning for individuals with autism. Parents often may need to obtain legal as well as behavioral advice as they attempt to design adult living situations for their family members with autism.

Gross and fine motor skills
Assessment and interventions are the same as for the previous age group.

Social cognition
Assessment and interventions are the same as for the previous age group.

NEUROPSYCHOLOGICAL ASSESSMENT AND PROGNOSIS
An average or above average IQ does not of itself guarantee an excellent prognosis for a child with autism. The diagnosis of Asperger syndrome does not guarantee a better prognosis for a child with an ASD than the diagnosis of autistic disorder without significant mental retardation (high functioning autism) or of pervasive developmental disorder not otherwise specified (PDD-NOS) (Meyer and Minshew, 2002). Only a small minority of adults with autism live entirely independently without family or community supports (Ballaban-Gil et al. 1996; Howlin et al. 2000, 2004; Howlin 2003). There are four benchmarks that may yield a better prognosis for independent functioning in adult life: (1) control over significantly disruptive or aggressive behavior; (2) ability to speak in full sentences and produce spontaneous information without reliance on scripts; (3) ability to function at or above a (US) fifth grade level with respect to reading and math skills; and (4) recognition of situations in which others might expose an individual to financial or personal risk. As clinicians we have some control over how the first three can be achieved; the fourth benchmark is intangible. Predicting how much "common sense" a given child with autism will have as an adult is very difficult to determine, and is a challenge to all who work in this field.

REFERENCES
Achenbach TM, Edelbrock CS (1983) *Manual for the Child Behavior Checklist and Revised Profile.* Burlington, VT: University of Vermont, Department of Psychiatry.
Allen MH, Lincoln AJ, Kaufman AS (1991) Sequential and simultaneous processing abilities of high functioning autistic and language impaired children. *J Autism Dev Disord* 21: 483–502.
Baddeley A (1986) *Working Memory.* New York: Oxford University Press.
Ballaban-Gil K, Rapin I, Tuchman RF, Shinnar S (1996) Longitudinal examination of the behavioral, language, and social changes in a population of adolescents and young adults with autistic disorder. *Pediatr Neurol* 15: 217–23.
Baron IS (2004) *Neuropsychological Evaluation of the Child.* New York: Oxford University Press.

Bayley N (2005) *Bayley Scales of Infant and Toddler Development, 3rd edn (Bayley-III).* San Antonio: Harcourt.

Beery K (1997) *Beery–Buktenica Test of Visual–Motor Integration, 4th edn.* Parsippany, NJ: Modern Curriculum Press.

Brody N (1992) *Intelligence, 2nd edn.* New York: Academic Press.

Cattell RB (1963) Theory of fluid and crystallized intelligence: A critical experiment. *J Educ Psychol* 54: 1–22.

Dawson G, Munson J, Estes A, Osterling J, McPartland J, Toth K, Carver L, Abbott R (2002) Neurocognitive function and joint attention ability in young children with autism spectrum disorder versus developmental delay. *Child Dev* 73: 345–58.

Deisinger JA (2001) Diagnosis and assessment of autistic spectrum disorders. In: Wahlberg T, Obiakor F, Burkhardt S, Rotatori AD, eds. *Autistic Spectrum Disorders: Educational and Clinical Interventions.* New York: JAI Elsevier Science, pp. 181–209.

Dunn M (2005) *S.O.S.: Social Skills in our Schools (A Social Skills Program for Children with Pervasive Developmental Disorders and their Typical Peers.* Shawnee Mission, KS: Autism & Asperger Publishing.

Fombonne E. (2005) Epidemiologic studies of the pervasive developmental disorders. In: Volkmar FR, Paul R, Klin A, Cohen D, eds. *Handbook of Autism and Pervasive Developmental Disorders, 3rd edn.* New York, John Wiley, pp. 42–69.

Freeman B, Rahbar B, Ritvo E, Bice T, Yokota A, Ritvo R (1991) The stability of cognitive and behavioral parameters in autism: A twelve-year prospective study. *J Am Acad Child Adolesc Psychiatry* 30: 479–92.

Green L, Fein D, Joy S, Waterhouse L (1995) Cognitive functioning in autism: an overview. In: Schopler E, Mesibov GB, eds. *Learning and Cognition in Autism.* New York: Plenum Press, pp. 13–30.

Howlin P (2003) Outcome in high-functioning adults with autism with and without early language delays: implications for the differentiation between autism and Asperger syndrome. *J Autism Dev Disord* 33: 3–13.

Howlin P, Mawhood L, Rutter M (2000) Autism and developmental receptive language disorder—a follow-up comparison in early adult life. II: Social, behavioural, and psychiatric outcomes. *J Child Psychol Psychiatry* 41: 561–78.

Howlin P, Goode S, Hutton J, Rutter M (2004) Adult outcome for children with autism. *J Child Psychol Psychiatry* 45: 212–29.

Klin A, Volkmar FR, Sparrow SS, Cicchetti DV, Rourke BP (1995) Validity and neuropsychological characterization of Asperger syndrome: convergence with nonverbal learning disabilities syndrome. *J Child Psychol Psychiatry* 36: 1127–40.

Lincoln AJ, Allen MH, Kilman A (1995) The assessment and interpretation of intellectual abilities in people with autism. In: Schopler E, Mesibov GB, eds. *Learning and Cognition in Autism.* New York: Plenum Press, pp. 89–117.

Madge N, Tizard J (1981) Intelligence. In: Rutter M, ed. *Scientific Foundations of Developmental Psychiatry.* Baltimore: University Park Press, pp. 245–66.

Meyer JA, Minshew NJ (2002) An update on neurocognitive profiles in Asperger syndrome and high functioning autism. *Focus Autism Dev Disabil* 17: 152–60.

Miller JN, Ozonoff S (2000) The external validity of Asperger disorder: Lack of evidence from the domain of neuropsychology. *J Abnorm Psychol* 109: 227–38.

Minshew NJ, Goldstein G, Muenz LR, Payton JB (1992) Neuropsychologic functioning in non-mentally retarded autistic individuals. *J Clin Exp Neuropsychol* 14: 740–61.

Minshew NJ, Meyer JA, Goldstein G (2002) Abstract reasoning in autism: A dissociation between concept formation and concept identification. *Neuropsychology* 16: 327–34.

Mullen EM (2005) *Mullen Scales of Early Learning.* Circle Pines, MN: American Guidance Services.

Nigg JT, Carte E, Hinshaw SP, Treuting J (1998) Neuropsychological correlates of antisocial behavior and comorbid disruptive behavior disorders in children with ADHD. *J Abnorm Psychol* 107: 468–80.

Norman DA, Shallice T (1986) Attention to action: Willed and automatic control of behavior. In: Davidson RJ, Schwartz GE, Shapiro D, eds. *Consciousness and Self-regulation: Advances in Research and Theory.* New York: Plenum Press, pp. 1–18.

Ozonoff S (1995) Executive functions in autism. In: Schopler E, Mesibov GB, eds. *Learning and Cognition in Autism.* New York: Plenum Press, pp. 199–219.

Pennington BF, Grossier D, Welsh MC (1993) Contrasting cognitive deficits in attention deficit hyperactivity disorder versus reading disability. *Dev Psychol* 29: 511–23.

Rapin I (1997) Autism. *N Engl J Med* 337: 97–104.

Rapin I (2003) Value and limitations of preschool cognitive tests, with an emphasis on longitudinal study of children on the autistic spectrum. *Brain Dev* 25: 327–34.

Reitan R, Wolfson D (1993) *The Halstead–Reitan Neuropsychological Test Battery: Theory and Clinical Interpretation.* Tuscon, AZ: Neuropsychology Press.

Rutter M (1983) Cognitive deficits in the pathogenesis of autism. *J Child Psychol Psychiatry* 24: 513–31.

Schopler E, Mesibov GB (1995) *Learning and Cognition in Autism.* New York: Plenum Press.

Shevell M, Ashwal S, Donley D, Flint J, Gingold M, Hirtz D, Majnemer A, Noetzel M, Sheth RD; Quality Standards Subcommittee of the American Academy of Neurology; Practice Committee of the Child Neurology Society (2003) Practice parameter: evaluation of the child with global developmental delay: report of the Quality Standards Subcommittee of the American Academy of Neurology and The Practice Committee of the Child Neurology Society. *Neurology* 60: 367–80.

Turkheimer E, Haley A, Waldron M, D'Onofrio B, Gottesman II (2003) Socioeconomic status modifies heritability of IQ in young children. *Psychol Sci* 14: 623–8.

Wechsler D (2005) *Wechsler Intelligence Scale for Children-IV (WISC-IV Integrated), 4th edn.* San Antonio, TX: Harcourt.

Woodcock RW, Johnson MB (1977) *Woodcock–Johnson Psychoeducational Battery.* Allen, TX: Teaching Resources Corporation.

TEST REFERENCES

(See also http://buros.unl.edu for up-to-date information on published psychometric tests.)

AAP/NICHQ (2002) *NICHQ Vanderbilt Attention Deficit Hyperactivity Disorder Rating Scales* (in ADHD Toolkit; download at http://www.nichq.org/nichq).

Bayley N (2005) *Bayley Scales of Infant and Toddler Development, 3rd edn.* San Antonio, TX: Harcourt.

Bishop DVM (2003) *Children's Communication Checklist, 2nd edn.* San Antonio, TX: Harcourt.

Brown TE (2001) *Brown Attention-Deficit Scales.* San Antonio, TX: Harcourt.

Bzoch KR, League R, Brown VL (2003) *Receptive–Expressive Emergent Language Test, 3rd edn.* Austin, TX: Pro-Ed.

Conners CK (1996) *Conners' Rating Scales–Revised.* San Antonio, TX: Harcourt.

DuPaul GJ, Power TJ, Anastopoulos AD, Reid R (1998) *Attention Deficit Hyperactivity Disorder Rating Scale–IV.* New York: Guilford Press.

Elliott CD (1990) *Differential Ability Scales.* San Antonio, TX: Harcourt.

Erford BT (1998) *Disruptive Behavior Rating Scales.* East Aurora, NY: Slosson.

Goldman R, Fristoe M (2000) *Goldman–Fristoe Test of Articulation, 2nd edn.* Circle Pines, MN: American Guidance Service.

Goldman R, Fristoe M, Woodcock RW (1970) *Goldman–Fristoe–Woodcock Test of Auditory Discrimination.* Circle Pines, MN: American Guidance Service.

Hammill DD, Newcomer PL (1997) *Test of Language Development – Intermediate, Primary.* Austin, TX: Pro-Ed.

Hammill DD, Pearson NA, Wiederholt JL (1996) *Comprehensive Test of Nonverbal Intelligence.* Austin, TX: Pro-Ed.

Hresko WP, Reid DK, Hammill DD (1999) *Test of Early Language Development, 3rd edn.* Austin, TX: Pro-Ed.

Lambert N, Nihira K, Leland H (1993) *American Association on Mental Retardation Adaptive Behavior Scales, School. 2nd edn.* Austin, TX: Pro-Ed.

McCarney SB, Bauer AM (2004) *Attention Deficit Disorders Evaluation Scale, 3rd edn.* Columbia, MO: Hawthorne Educational Services.

McCarthy D (1972) *McCarthy Scales of Children's Abilities.* San Antonio, TX: Harcourt.

Mullen EM (1995) *Mullen Scales of Early Learning.* Los Angeles, CA: Western Psychological Services.

Phelps-Terasaki D, Phelps-Gunn T (1992) *Test of Pragmatic Language.* Austin, TX: Pro-Ed.

Raven JC, et al. (1998) *Raven Progressive Matrices and Vocabulary Scales.* San Antonio, TX: Harcourt.

Reynolds CR, Kamphaus RW (2004) *Behavior Assessment System for Children, 2nd edn.* Circle Pines, MN: American Guidance Service.

Roid GH (2003) *Stanford–Binet Intelligence Scale, 5th edn.* Chicago: Riverside.

Roid GH, Miller LJ (1997) *Leiter International Performance Scales–Revised.* Wood Dale, IL: Stoelting.

Roid GH, Sampers JL (2005) *Merrill Palmer Scale of Mental Tests–Revised.* Wood Dale, IL: Stoelting.

Semel E, Wiig EH, Secord W (2006) *Clinical Evaluation of Language Fundamentals, 4th edn.* San Antonio, TX: Harcourt.

Sparrow SS, Balla DA, Cicchetti DV, Harrison PL (2005) *Vineland Adaptive Behavior Scales–II.* Circle Pines, MN: American Guidance Service.

Zimmerman JL, Steiner VG, Pond RE (1997) *Preschool Language Scale,4th edn.* San Antonio, TX: Harcourt.

17

TREATMENT APPROACHES FOR THE AUTISM SPECTRUM DISORDERS

Mark Mintz, Michael Alessandri and Paolo Curatolo

There is no known cure for autism. Despite a wealth of anecdotal reports and testimonies of efficacy, the vast array of interventions being offered as treatments for autism have not been shown in long term controlled studies to alter its core social-communication deficits. The current consensus is that intensive, targeted, behaviorally based early educational interventions, together with an array of ancillary rehabilitative therapies, are the most effective treatments devised to date. Pharmacological intervention is at best an adjunctive therapy that can ameliorate specific behaviors and, when successful, can enable children to participate in and profit from their family and school environments. Advances in the psychopharmacology of autism have been hindered by the absence of reliable instruments to measure the effects of medications, by the lack of double-blind studies (particularly for newer agents), and by the short term duration of pharmacologic trials. The significant gaps in our understanding of the pathophysiology of autism spectrum disorders (ASDs) have limited our ability to develop more effective interventions for children with autism.

When choosing interventions for individuals with ASDs, it is imperative that clinicians rely on evidence-based practices that document efficacy and benefits that outweigh potential risks. Unfortunately many commonly prescribed "therapies" in use today are based on anecdotal, word-of-mouth rather than empirical evidence. This state of affairs is not unique to the ASDs but is particularly prominent within the autism community. The unfortunate consequence for the affected individuals and their families, as well as for the providers who serve them, has been a confusing array of therapeutic options, many of which lack a solid scientific foundation or even plausible basis.

The best types of interventions for ASDs should be designed to achieve two goals: (1) to assist individuals with ASDs to acquire functional skills and realize their optimal potential; and (2) to reduce the array of maladaptive behaviors that are likely to interfere with adaptive functioning. As might be expected, these two objectives are typically addressed in concert. In this chapter we attempt to summarize our working knowledge of the behavioral, educational and pharmacological treatment approaches and discuss how these interventions can be integrated to provide a comprehensive management plan for individuals with autism.

BEHAVIORAL AND EDUCATIONAL INTERVENTIONS

As a direct result of the wide range and heterogeneity of its symptoms, a truly individualized, multimodal, multidisciplinary treatment plan is usually required in order to ensure remediation of skill deficits, enhanced behavioral control, and an optimal long term outcome. Unfortunately, the range and intensity of educational and behavioral services needed for children with ASDs to attempt to achieve the most favorable outcomes often exceed available resources. Because of the ubiquitous challenges in language, learning, social-communication and behavioral control, children with autism are often perceived as minimally educable. This assumption is ill-informed because all children with ASD have a capacity, albeit challenging, to learn at least some important skills when the appropriate therapeutic services, supports and strategies are provided.

Strategies to Promote Skill Acquisition

The major goal of intervention is to achieve functional behavioral changes that generalize across settings and are maintained over time - with the optimal outcome being full inclusion in all aspects of community life. Although children with ASDs are guaranteed an education by law in many countries, there remains considerable controversy over where such children should be educated and supported, what specific instructional strategies should be adopted, and how intensive the educational and related services and supports need to be. Coordinating and managing services for children who have both special educational and health needs is complex. It proves to be particularly challenging for children with ASDs because the underlying communication and social deficits are regularly coupled with cognitive deficiencies (not necessarily mental retardation!) and aberrant behavioral patterns. Therefore it is essential that clinicians aim to make sure the child receives carefully coordinated medical and educational services so that children with ASDs have the opportunity to achieve a favorable outcome. Success for these children in the real world of home, school and community requires comprehensive and interdisciplinary assessment, case management and coordinated planning for medical, psychological, ancillary therapeutic and special education services. Utilizing an interdisciplinary team care coordinated model that wraps services around children and their families on a long term basis will allow medical, clinical and educational professionals to provide cost-effective services and optimal support for the children and their families and to enhance their overall quality of life.

Numerous specific intervention methods have been devised for individuals with ASDs over the years, but few have been well researched and validated. The primary treatments for ASDs continue to be "psycho-educational interventions" (Lord and McGee 2001). There is a growing body of evidence supporting the utility of conceptually sound, well-structured, engaging, intensive, individualized treatments for those affected by autism (Howlin 1998). Yet there are typically large individual differences in response to treatment, and little is known about which intervention methods are best suited to specific individuals with ASDs. Until we become better informed about specific clinical subgroups and their underlying biologic basis, this question is likely to remain unanswered.

Many specific intervention strategies have been proposed, but most can be classified as belonging to one of three basic conceptual approaches to treatment. These three approaches include models grounded in applied behavior analysis, developmental theory and structured teaching. While these approaches are typically presented as distinct, there is in fact considerable overlap in their clinical application in educational and therapeutic settings. Dawson and Osterling (1997) have identified several critical programmatic elements they have in common; these may ultimately prove more important than any fundamental difference in underlying "philosophy". These elements include first, the scope and sequence of the curriculum; second, a supportive teaching environment with strategies and opportunities for generalization of skills, predictability and routines; third, a functional approach to problem behaviors; and fourth, transition planning and family involvement.

Applied Behavior Analysis (ABA) is the application of the fundamental principles of learning theory based on operant conditioning to enhance socially significant behaviors and reduce interfering or undesirable behaviors. Essential elements of this approach include an emphasis on functional relationships between behavior and environments, direct observation and measurement, contextual/environmental factors, and principles of reinforcement (Skinner 1938). The primary assumption guiding ABA is that altering these essential elements will result in behavioral change. Behavior analysis provides a more detailed understanding of the functions of particular behaviors, and the application of behavior analytic principles enables the educator to establish a set of conditions that are likely to foster positive behavioral changes. Several specific instructional methods fall under the ABA umbrella. Three among a number of ABA methods include Discrete Trial Teaching, Analysis of Verbal Behavior, and Pivotal Response Training. They share the targeting of acquisition of specific skills and concepts, together with the reduction of undesirable behaviors. Each is based on the principles of learning theory but differs somewhat in its manner of application.

Discrete Trial Teaching (DTT) emphasizes early and intensive intervention, task analysis, discrete units of learning, systematic instruction, discrimination training, repetitive practice, and generalization and maintenance programming (Lovaas et al. 1974, Lovaas and Smith 1989, McEachin et al. 1993). DTT programs are quite comprehensive, targeting all skill areas such as communication, cognition, motor, social and self-help. Lovaas and colleagues reported that nearly half of their clinical population reached levels of functioning that were indistinguishable from normal controls on standardized measures of intelligence, language and adaptive functioning (McEachin et al. 1993). While a finding of this magnitude has only just been replicated (Sallows and Graupner 2005) and has not been without criticism (e.g. Shea 2004), there can be no doubt that DTT often yields significant remediation of skill deficits and improvements in behavioral control (Sheinkopf and Siegel 1998, Alessandri et al. 2002).

Analysis of Verbal Behavior (VB) has emerged as an essential element of ABA (Skinner 1957). In this application of ABA, particular attention is paid to the various functional elements of language as targets for intervention (Sundberg and Michael 2001, Lopez Ornat and Gallo 2004). Specifically, intervention plans primarily address the following aspects of language: echoics, or verbal imitation skills; mands, or verbal behavior whose form is controlled by states of deprivation and aversion, such as a request for food; tacts, or verbal behavior that is under the control of the nonverbal environment, such as random naming/labeling of an object; and intraverbals, or verbal behavior that is under the control of other verbal behaviors and is strengthened by social reinforcement. Imitation is viewed as essential to all learning, and the early emphasis on teaching a repertoire of echoic (i.e. verbal imitation) responses in VB programs reflects this view. It emphasizes that an echoic repertoire is a prerequisite for the development of the other verbal skills such as requests, labels and reciprocal/conversational language. The systematic assessment and instruction of these verbal aspects of language is a well-validated component of instruction for children with ASDs (Sundberg and Michael 2001), enabling such children to acquire a range of verbal abilities that serve to enhance learning and social-communication.

Pivotal Response Training (PRT), a naturalistic intervention based on the principles of applied behavior analysis and developmental approaches, identifies certain "pivotal" behaviors, such as motivation, self-initiation and responsivity to multiple cues to target in treatment. Pivotal behaviors are considered central to many areas of functioning, and the theory is that positive changes in these behaviors have widespread effects on many other behaviors. PRT taps into a child's motivation for objects or activities with the goal of increasing important skills, typically language acquisition, social interaction and play. Essential aspects of training include turn-taking, reinforcing attempts at correct responding, frequent task variation, allowing the child a choice of activities, interspersing maintenance tasks, and using natural consequences to foster desired behaviors. PRT was specifically designed to be integrated into everyday life so as to facilitate generalization and the maintenance of behavioral change. PRT has been shown to be effective in increasing social, communication and play skills, although most of the research is limited to single-subject multiple baseline designs or small treatment designs (Koegel and Frea 1993, Koegel et al. 1998, Schreibman 2000, Koegel et al. 2001).

INTERVENTIONS BASED ON DEVELOPMENTAL STRATEGIES

In contrast to a traditional behavioral focus on isolated skills or behaviors, developmental interventionists focus on fundamental developmental processes (e.g. social referencing, self-regulation) that underlie particular symptoms and serve as the foundations for future cognitive, social and emotional growth. Supporters of developmental therapies are often critical of the overly structured and mechanical nature of some behavioral strategies, which they argue may intensify, rather than remediate, the child's difficulties acquiring spontaneous and flexible social, emotional and cognitive skills.

The best known developmental therapy is the *Developmental Individual-Difference, Relationship-Based Model* (commonly referred to as *"Floor Time"*). Floor Time is a child-led, parent-implemented model that utilizes developmental principles to help children build social, communication and emotional skills (Wieder and Greenspan 2003). Floor Time is based on the theory that children with ASDs have a biological processing deficit that impairs connections between affect and intent with motor planning and sequencing abilities, and auditory processing and language capacities (Wieder and Greenspan 2003). Floor Time mobilizes children's affect and intent in order to help them progress through six developmental milestones: self-regulation, intimacy, two-way communication, complex communication, emotional ideas, and emotional thinking. To date there have been no peer-reviewed, published studies on the efficacy of Floor Time. Due to their emphasis on spontaneous and flexible social, communication and cognitive skills, these treatments can be a useful complement to traditional behavior therapy. Moreover, by focusing on a child's current level of functioning, developmental therapies allow caretakers to set appropriate treatment objectives that can be realistically attained, thereby instilling in both parent and child a sense of competence.

A second developmental strategy is *Structured Teaching*, the principles of which can be credited to Division TEACCH. TEACCH (Treatment and Education of Autistic and related Communication handicapped CHildren), a statewide model of service delivery in North Carolina, provides coordinated support, outreach, assessment and intervention services (Mesibov and Schopler 1983; Panerai et al. 1997, 2002; Erba 2000; Van Bourgondien et al. 2003). The TEACCH approach has a clear appreciation for learning theory and developmental processes; central to their philosophy are the concepts of "culture" and "structure". TEACCH proponents support the notion that there is a "culture of autism" and that within this culture the need for structure is paramount.

While TEACCH proponents attend to the remediation of skill deficits, they also emphasize the importance of understanding and reinforcing the strengths of individuals with autism. Strategies to promote independent functioning are tailored to those strengths, taking account of the individual's unique needs. Central to TEACCH is the appreciation of an autistic learner's visual aptitude, attention to detail, impressive memory, and reliance on routine. TEACCH is credited with a number of significant clinical contributions, including the development of diagnostic tools, assessment measures, curricula and intervention methods, as well as with the provision of visual systems and supports for behavior, social skills and communication (Bondy and Frost 1998, Ozonoff and Cathcart 1998, Charlop-Christy et al. 2002, Magiati and Howlin 2003).

SPEECH AND LANGUAGE, OCCUPATIONAL, AND SOCIAL SKILL THERAPIES

Numerous ancillary treatments, including speech and language therapies, occupational and physical therapies, as well as music and art therapies are widely provided for children with ASDs. These specific therapies should be driven by symptom presentation and client need, and should be an integral part of a more comprehensive therapeutic support plan. Generally speaking, speech and language therapy, along with occupational therapy represent essential components of the treatment plan for children with ASDs.

In the education and treatment of children with ASDs it is paramount to enhance communication. *Speech and language therapy (SLT)*, in concert with the educational approaches discussed earlier, can help achieve this goal for both verbal and nonverbal children with ASDs at any level of functioning (Prizant et al. 1997). Specific targets for intervention typically include both verbal and nonverbal aspects of communication, and need to focus training on the receptive, expressive and social–pragmatic deficiencies discussed in Chapter 4. SLT can also help with speech disorders such as articulation or fluency disorders, or resonance/voice disorders. For many children with ASDs, there is great utility in introducing adjunctive *augmentative and alternative communication* (AAC), including the use of sign language, visual symbol systems (e.g. the Picture Exchange Communication System which allows the child to exchange visual symbols for social-communication; Frost and Bondy 1994), and voice output communication aides (VOCAs; Lord and McGee 2001).

Given the frequent sensory and motor issues in children with ASDs, as well as the deficits in adaptive functioning, the provision of *occupational therapy* is also likely to benefit a child with ASD. Occupational therapists, working as part of a multidisciplinary treatment team, can develop sensory and instructional activities that are designed to address related symptoms and deficits in children with sensorimotor problems (Schaaf and Miller 2005). The training of specific motor skills such as buttoning, tying and handwriting may help build clumsy apraxic children's self-image and feeling of mastery. The provision of shoes with Velcro fasteners rather than laces and teaching keyboard skills rather than insisting on written homework may go a long way toward decreasing frustration and defusing some behavioral eruptions.

Social skills training programs are important facets of a comprehensive treatment program whose goal is integration of the child into the community. Traditional programs rely upon role modeling and interaction with typical peers, and there are innovative programs that utilize play bricks as the centerpiece of a cooperative team approach (LeGoff 2004, LeGoff and Sherman 2006). A new curriculum uses visual organizers to symbolize some of the complexities of communication and social situations and help children learn to deal more efficiently with them. Teachers and parents can be trained to apply this curriculum to the classroom, the home and the community (Dunn 2005). This approach provides a more economically realistic way than the provision of individual training for the many children who do not learn on their own how to navigate the complexities of societal demands.

PHARMACOTHERAPY

Pharmacological therapies are best considered adjunctive treatments, not remedies or

TABLE 17.1
Rational drug therapy

Use proper titration rate
  – Start low, go slow

Ensure adequate dose
  – Target: minimum effective dose

Ensure adequate duration of medication trial
  – 2–8 weeks for neuroleptics, AEDs, SNRIs/SSRIs
  – If partial response, allow for longer duration of observation

Evaluate for compliance/side-effects
  – Utilize blood levels if applicable
  – Assess for typical responses
  – Monitor for side-effects
    • Physical/neurological examination
    • Laboratory testing

Ensure proper diagnosis
  – Determine if there are comorbid diagnoses
  – Evaluate whether proper therapeutic targets have been chosen

Evaluate whether there is an underlying systemic trigger for the maladaptive behavior, such as pain or underlying medical condition

Ensure that non-pharmacological interventions are maximized

Attempt to secure objectve or quantitative outcome measures

Avoid polypharmacy
  – If necessary, use it rationally with compatible drugs

Periodic review of regimen
  – Consider medical reversals
    • Tapering/discontinuing medication to see if it is still exerting a benefit, while monitoring behavior for stability or worsening

cures. When a medication is to be utilized, there should be a predetermined plan to measure the drug's effect, ideally utilizing standardized and reliable outcome measures. There should be a reassessment of the medication at various points in time to determine the need for its continued use so as to avoid unnecessary chronic drug therapy (Table 17.1).

The decision to add a medication to a child's treatment regimen depends on a number of factors, but should be considered when the child's behavior represents a clear danger to self or others, or is significantly interfering with an ability to learn or socialize, provided there are identifiable target behaviors that may be medication responsive, and have failed behavioral interventions. In addition, medications may play an important role when coexisting neurobehavioral disinhibition or dysregulation impairs the individual's educational or work potential. There are multiple and specific behavioral targets for which adjunctive pharmacological therapy may be beneficial (Table 17.2).

TABLE 17.2
Behavioral targets of adjunctive pharmacological therapy*

	AEDs	Stimulants	SNRIs	NLPs, ANLPs	Anx	Beta-blockers	Alpha-agonists	SSRIs	Nalt	ACI/ NMDA	Anti-histamines
Inattention		++	+++				+				
Hyperactivity, impulsiveness	++	+++	+++	++			++				
Aggressiveness, explosiveness	+++			+++	+	++	++	++			
Self-injurious behaviors	++			+++	+	++		+++	+++		
OCD, perseverations				++	+			+++			
Mood dysregulation, affective instability	+++			+++	++						
Depression	++				+			+++			
Anxiety			+		+++						
Overarousal, agitation	+++			+++	+++	++					
Social inappropriateness				+	++						
Language								+		+	
Sensory issues, language				++	++						
Sleep disturbance				++	+		++	++			++
Stereotypies				++			+	++			
Social relatedness				++				++			

*Strength of recommendations based upon benefits reported in the clinical literature and/or the authors' clinical experience. There may be significant variation of different medications within a given class. Note that the use of listed medications for these neurobehavioral problems should be considered "off label". All medications may cause "atypical" responses.

+ Rare reports of efficacy or minimal clinical experience.
++ Modest reports of efficacy or moderate clinical experience.
+++ Broad reports of efficacy or extensive clinical experience.

Abbreviations: AEDs = antiepileptic drugs; SNRI = selective norepinephrine reuptake inhibitor; (A)NLP = (atypical) neuroleptics; Anx = anxiolytics; SSRI = selective serotonin reuptake inhibitor; Nalt = naltrexone; ACI/NMDA = acetylcholine esterase inhibitor/N-methyl-D-aspartate receptor agonist; OCD = obsessive–compulsive disorder.

TABLE 17.3
Side-effects of neuroleptics and antiepileptics used in autism*

Medication class	Side-effects	References
Neuroleptics/ antipsychotics	Involuntary movements, dystonic reactions, dyskinesias, tardive dyskinesia, neuroleptic malignant syndrome, sedation, weight gain, alteration of lipid profiles, induction of a diabetic state, hepatotoxicity, prolactinemia, reduction in bone density, prolongation of the QT interval, induction of arrhythmias, orthostatic hypertension	Malone et al. (1991), Campbell et al. (1997), Goodnick et al. (2002), Kipps et al. (2005)
Antiepileptics	Teratogenic risk, chemical hepatitis, hepatic failure, pancreatitis, aplastic anemia, agranulocytosis, skin rashes, Stevens–Johnson reaction, diplopia, eye pain or blurry vision, dizziness, ataxia, alopecia, weight gain or loss, gingival hyperplasia, gastrointestinal disturbances, kidney stones, metabolic acidosis	Arroyo and de la Morena (2001), Mintz (2001), French et al. (2004), Kaplan (2004)

*Side-effects vary greatly depending on the agent.

The use of medications in complex heterogenous developmental disorders such as autism is challenging. The most significant problem with medications is the potential side-effect profiles of the varied pharmacological agents used in autism (Table 17.3). The most significant include the risk of organ toxicities, cardiac arrhythmias, adverse metabolic or hormonal changes, excessive weight loss or gain, induction of movement disorders, sleep disruption, cognitive impairment and, in some cases, worsening of baseline behaviors (Gutgesell et al. 1999, Palermo and Curatolo 2004, Curatolo et al. 2004). Medications should not be used as a substitute for behavioral and educational interventions but rather to facilitate them. Prescribing medications as a "knee jerk" response to control certain difficult behaviors without sufficient exploration of treatable underlying causes or alternative non-pharmacological courses of treatment is inappropriate.

In the developmental disorders as in other disorders in medicine the gold standard for evidence-based use of particular pharmacological agents is double blind, placebo controlled clinical trials (McClellan and Werry 2003). Such studies yield a statistical comparison of the effectiveness of medication to placebo, yet the results may in some cases have limited clinical utility compared to the blinded comparison of one medication over another. Unfortunately the evidence for significant effects in medication studies of children with autism is limited due to small numbers of patients, the lack of consistent replication, and the short duration of all the studies reported to date (a few months, often less). In addition, the magnitude of the improvement investigators report is modest at best and only exceptionally reflects significant improvement in the core autistic symptoms

TABLE 17.4
Atypical neuroleptics: proposed mechanisms of action and neurobehavioral targets

	RIS	OLZ	ZIP	APZ	QTP	CLZ**
			Mechanism of action			
D-antagonist	D2	D1,2,4	D2	—	D2	D4>D1,2,3
D-agonist	—	—	—	D2	—	—
Serotonin antagonist	5HT2A	5HT2a,c	5HT2	5HT2a	5HT2	5HT
Serotonin agonist	—	—	—	5HT1a	—	—
Adrenergic antagonist	A-1,2	A-1	A-1	A-1	A-1	+++
Cholinergic antagonist	—	M1-5	—	—	—	+++
Histamine antagonist	H1	H1	H1	—	H1	+++
			Symptom target*			
Psychoses	+++	+++	+++	+++	+++	+++
Bipolar disorder	++	+++	++	+++	++	++
Aggressive behavior	+++	++	+	++	++	++
Self-injurious behavior	+++	++	+	++	+	++
Disruptive behavior	+++	++	+	+	+	+
Hyperactivity	++	++	+	+	+	+

+ Rare reports of efficacy or minimal clinical experience.
++ Modest reports of efficacy or moderate clinical experience.
+++ Broad reports of efficacy or extensive clinical experience.
Abbreviations: RIS = risperidone; OLZ = olanzapine; ZIP = ziprasidone; APZ = apriprazole; QTP = quetiapine; CLZ = clozapine; D = dopamine; 5HT = 5-hydroxytryptophan.
*Strength of recommendations is based upon benefits reported in the clinical literature and/or the authors' clinical experience.
**Clozapine should be used only for treatment resistant cases.

such as social-communicative abilities. Therefore the clinician must often depend upon other, less reliable sources of evidence, including open label trials, retrospective analyses, case reports and peers' clinical experiences. The family's participation in the decision making process is often complicated by unsupported testimonials or false expectations. All of these challenges make the use of medications in autism more of an art than a science.

NEUROLEPTICS/ANTIPSYCHOTICS
The proposed mechanisms of action of both the traditional neuroleptics and the newer generation "atypicals" are listed in (Table 17.4). These compounds derive their pharmacological properties primarily from their ability to modulate dopamine activity, the same properties responsible for their undesirable side-effects (Palermo and Curatolo 2004). This group of medications has always played a prominent role in the treatment of developmental disabilities, specifically for treating such aberrant behaviors as aggression, self-injury, explosive outbursts, agitation, mood dysregulation ("bipolar phenomena") and severe hyperactivity/impulsiveness (Aman and Madrid 1999).

Haloperidol is the classic example of the "older" generation of typical neuroleptics that have been used in autism. Clinical trials suggest that haloperidol may ameliorate the "core" symptoms of social withdrawal and abnormal "object relations", as well as irritability, hyperactivity, mood dysregulation, stereotypies and impaired performance on cognitive tasks (Anderson et al. 1989, Perry et al. 1989). Other traditional neuroleptics that have been used in autism include pimozide and thioridazine, which have been reported to be useful in controlling and reducing a number of maladaptive and problematic behaviors and stereotypies (Naruse et al. 1982, Fulop et al. 1987, Ernst et al. 1992). Risperidone is the best researched of the atypical neuroleptics for the ASDs that were developed in the USA for autism and related developmental disorders. Risperidone was the original medication studied by the Research Units on Pediatric Psychopharmacology (RUPP) (Arnold et al. 2000). Numerous open label trials, closely monitoring for side-effects, as well as short and intermediate length multisite, randomized double-blind, placebo-controlled trials report efficacy for tantrums, aggression, irritability and self-injurious behaviors, with good medication tolerability (Purdon et al. 1994; Mandoki 1995; McDougle et al. 1997, 1998b; Nicolson et al. 1998; Szigethy et al. 1999; Krebs et al. 2001; McCracken et al. 2002; Arnold et al. 2003; Gagliano et al. 2004; Martin et al. 2004; Research Units on Pediatric Psychopharmacology Autism Network 2005). There have been small, uncontrolled studies and case reports suggesting that aripiprazole, quetiapine, ziprasidone and olanzapine may be of benefit for controlling various maladaptive behaviours (Horrigan et al. 1997, Martin et al. 1999, Potenza et al. 1999, McDougle et al. 2002, Stigler et al. 2004). Other neuroleptics are less useful in autism, particularly clozapine which, although is a very powerful and effective atypical neuroleptic for schizophrenia, has limited use in autism because of the risk of agranulocytosis and seizures, and of the need for weekly or bimonthly blood draws (Zuddas et al. 1996).

Despite the now well documented benefits of the neuroleptics for children and adults with autism, we emphasize that their use is limited by their unfavorable side-effect profiles (Table 17.3). For those children who need typical/atypical neuroleptics, the decision to prescribe them must be limited to specific indications; the goal should be short term focused use. Diligent observation and close monitoring for side-effects are in order; we strongly recommend re-evaluation for continued need on a monthly basis. Contrary to what some believe, we stress that these medications, clinically useful as they are for some children, are not panaceas and that they must be used judiciously.

ANTIEPILEPTICS

The role of antiepileptic drugs (AEDs) for the treatment of seizures in autism is well established and usually straightforward. The role of AEDs to manage behavioral issues in children with autism who do not have clinical seizures is controversial; it is discussed in Chapters 10 and 11. There are several reasons why the role of AEDs in children with autism with or without seizures is not only controversial but a conundrum that is difficult to resolve. It is unclear whether identifiable baseline EEG abnormalities can predict

TABLE 17.5
Antiepileptic drugs: proposed mechanisms of action and potential side-effects*

	GBP	LTG	TPM	TGB	OXC	ZNS	LEV	CBZ	VPA	BZP
Mechanism of action										
Sodium channel		✓	✓		✓	✓		✓	✓	
Potassium channel										
Calcium channel	✓	✓	✓		✓	✓	✓		✓	
Glutamate antagonist			✓							
GABA potentiation	✓		✓	✓		✓			✓	✓
Carbonic anhydrase			✓			✓				
Side-effects										
Hepatotoxicity/pancreatitis								✓	✓	
Hematologic								✓	✓	
Glaucoma			✓							
Allergic dermatitis/rash	✓	✓**				✓**		✓**		
Metabolic acidosis/renal stones			✓			✓				
Hyponatremia					✓			✓		
Weight gain									✓	
Weight loss			✓			✓				
Ataxia	✓	✓	✓		✓	✓		✓	✓	✓
Blurred vision		✓			✓			✓	✓	
Cognitive effects			✓	✓	✓	✓		✓	✓	✓
Dizziness	✓	✓	✓	✓	✓	✓	✓	✓	✓	✓
Drowsiness/fatigue	✓	✓		✓	✓	✓	✓	✓	✓	✓
Headache	✓	✓		✓	✓	✓		✓	✓	

Abbreviations: GBP = gabapentin; LTG = lamotrigine; TPM = topiramate; TGB = tiagabine; OXC = oxcarbazepine; ZNS = zonisamide; LEV = levetiracetam; CBZ = carbamazepine; VPA = valproic acid; BZP = benzodiazepine.

Phenobarbital and *phenytoin* may be used for treating seizures in ASDs but are not recommended for behavioral control. *Felbamate* is often effective for intractable epilepsy, but its use is limited by potentially severe liver or bone marrow toxicity. *Vigabatrin* is an effective AED but has the risk of retinal toxicity and has not been widely reported as a mood stabilizer. *Ethosuximide* is most commonly utilized for absence epilepsy. *Primidone* can cause significant adverse behaviors. *Levetiracetam* is occasionally associated with the onset or exacerbation of behavioral difficulties, which in some cases are reportedly ameliorated with pyridoxine. AED side-effects may be related to dosage or serum level, but can also be idiosyncratic, particularly hepatotoxicity, pancreatitis, aplastic anemia, agranulocytosis, allergic reactions and glaucoma.
**Stevens–Johnson syndrome also reported.

behavioral responsiveness to AEDs (Akanuma et al. 2005). In addition it can be difficult to substantiate that it is through the suppression of clinical seizures or subclinical spike activity (Deonna and Roulet-Perez 2005) that AEDs affect behavior. Further complicating the use of AEDs is the phenomenon of "forced normalization", i.e. better seizure control or spike suppression may be associated with psychosis or worsening behaviors (Krishnamoorthy et al. 2002). Besides their antiepileptic effects, AEDs have potential benefits as "mood-stabilizers", and as such they may have a positive effect on behavior independent of their effects on seizures or epileptiform activity (Di Martino and Tuchman 2001). Close monitoring for side-effects, although challenging in autism, especially in those with seizures, is essential (Table 17.3).

Some of the broader therapeutic effects of AEDs include mood stabilization, particularly in individuals with bipolar disorder, and this potential effect has been of interest to clinicians treating individuals with autism. These mood stabilization effects, like AEDs' effects on seizures, are believed to be related to their control of neuronal excitation and their modulation of neurotransmitter activity. AEDs exert their multiple effects via inhibition or potentiation of ionic channels; disruption of neurotransmitter metabolism; impact on neurotransmitter or other receptor function by their antagonism to excitatory neurotransmitters or potentiation of inhibitory neurotransmitters; and inhibition of carbonic anhydrase (Table 17.5) (Brunton et al. 2005). Evidence for the ability of AEDs to exert mood stabilization comes primarily from the psychiatric literature on bipolar disorder (Muzina et al. 2002). Studies involving children with autism have generally involved small numbers of children in poorly controlled or open label studies (Aman et al. 1995).

Valproic acid has been used by clinicians in the management of agitation, aggression and temper outbursts in adults with autism (Sovner 1989). Unfortunately, published clinical studies in children and adults consist of single case reports or open label, non-replicated series of patients with no long term data (Childs and Blair 1997, Plioplys 1994, Nass and Petrucha 1990, Hollander et al. 2001). In one study of lamotrigine in 50 children with intractable epilepsy, 8 of them experienced a decrease in "autism symptoms" without a concomitant decrease in seizures, suggesting a specific benefit of lamotrigine in autism (Uvebrant and Bauziene 1994). This study has not been replicated, and a double-blind placebo controlled trial of lamotrigine in 28 children with autism without seizures indicated no significant benefit (Belsito et al. 2001). The only other AED studied in autism is levetiracetam which, in an open label study of 10 children, was found to have positive effects on hyperactivity, impulsivity, mood instability and aggression (Rugino and Samsock 2002).

SEROTONERGIC DRUGS

Evidence of abnormal brain serotonin synthesis in autism provides a theoretical justification for the use of serotonin reuptake inhibitors (SRIs) in autism (Chugani et al. 1999, Whitaker-Azmitia 2001, Chugani 2002, Palermo and Curatolo 2004). Interest was stirred by reports of high levels of serotonin in the platelets of a significant fraction of children with ASDs, and by behavioral changes induced by tryptophan-free diets and favorable clinical responses to SRIs. The association of anxiety and affective disorders with 5HT-TLPR, a serotonin transporter polymorphism considered a putative but controversial marker for autism, provides another rationale for the use of drugs affecting the serotonin system, despite lack of understanding of the role of serotonin or the reason for abnormalities of its level in autism (Cook et al. 1997; Klauck et al. 1997; Lesch and Mossner 1998; McBride et al. 1998; Persico et al. 2000, 2002).

With the exception of fenfluramine, which has proven to be ineffective and has unacceptable side-effects, the literature suggests that SRIs, both selective SRIs (SSRIs) (e.g. fluoxetine, sertraline, fluvoxamine, paroxetine); and non-selective SRIs (e.g. the tricyclic antidepressants clomipramine, imipramine, desipramine), may have a role in the treatment of "interfering behaviors", specifically those that are repetitive; they may even ameliorate social relatedness, possibly through anxiolytic mechanisms, especially when there is a family history of affective illness (Gordon et al. 1993, Connolly et al. 1997, Branford et al. 1998, Aman et al. 1999, McDougle et al. 2000, Remington et al. 2001, DeLong et al. 2002). A double-blind, placebo-controlled study of fluvoxamine in autistic adults found good tolerability and clinical superiority with respect to placebo in ameliorating repetitive behaviors and aggression, as well as improvement in social relatedness and language (McDougle et al. 1996). However, the majority of published studies of SSRIs have been uncontrolled (Snead et al. 1994, Steingard et al. 1997, Fatemi et al. 1998, McDougle et al. 1998a, Alcami Pertejo et al. 2000). DeLong et al. (1998, 2002) reported dramatic improvement in language in children in open label observation of fluoxetine, again observations flawed by inadequate measurement techniques, short length of study and lack of replication.

The SRIs appear to be generally safe and well tolerated in children, especially for the treatment of mood and obsessive-compulsive disorders. Unfortunately, induction of manic behaviors has been described in children with obsessive–compulsive disorder and bipolar-like syndromes, which represents a challenge in the treatment of the ASDs (Go et al. 1998). In addition, there has been a recent worldwide concern that SRIs specifically, and antidepressants in general, may promote suicidal ideation in adolescents, which is another source of concern that requires careful monitoring (FDA 2004.) The primary drawbacks of tricyclic compounds include the potential for such ECG changes as prolonged QT interval, tachycardia, seizures, sedation, sleep disturbances, and negative behavioral changes (Gordon et al. 1993). Given the high frequency of seizures in patients with autistic disorder and the young age of many of the patients undergoing treatment, caution must be exercised in the use of these compounds.

OTHER MEDICATIONS

Numerous other medications have been tried to target specific autistic symptoms such as anxiety, overarousal, inattention, impulsivity and self-injurious behaviors (Tables 16.2,

TABLE 17.6
Other medications used in autism

Medication	Target symptoms	Comments	References
Buspirone	Generalized anxiety	Partial serotonin receptor agonist and possible D2 receptor antagonist	Realmoto et al. (1989), Hillbrand and Scott (1995)
Clonidine Guanfacine	Overarousal/ hyperactivity, sleep problems	Alpha-adrenergic agonists. Use cautiously in children because of cardiovascular side-effects	Fankhauser et al. (1992), Jaselskis et al. (1992)
Methylphenidate Amphetamine salts	Inattentiveness, hyperactivity, impulsivity	May have atypical responses like mania/activation and irritability, and side-effects such as sleep disturbances, reduction of appetite, tics, increase in stereotypies, and blunting of personality	Quintana et al. (1995), Aman and Langworthy (2000), Handen et al. (2000), Scahill et al. (2004), Stingler et al. (2004)
Propranolol	Aggression, self-injurious behaviors	Beta-blocker; counteracts a systemic adrenergic reflex	Ratey et al. (1987), Luiselli et al. (2000)
Naltrexone	Self-injurious behaviors	Opioid antagonist; early reports were encouraging, but later results have not been so robust	Campbell et al. (1993), Willemsen-Swinkels (1995, 1996)
Donepezil Rivastigmine Galantamine	Cognitive and language problems	Cholinesterase inhibitors; studies have yielded mixed and difficult to interpret results	Chez et al. (2003, 2004), Herztman (2003)

16.6) (Posey and McDougle 2000, Aman 2004). Treatment approaches for commonly associated disorders of autism such as epilepsy and sleep disorders are covered in Chapters 10, 11, 12 and 15. As emphasized in the discussion on the three major groups of medications used in autism, the antipsychotics, antiepileptics and SSRIs, there is a significant gap in our knowledge in regards to the mechanisms of action and clinical effects of all the medications used in autism. The best use of all medications in autism is to target specific symptoms for short periods of time in order to open "windows of opportunity" for educational and behavioral interventions.

ALTERNATIVE/COMPLEMENTARY THERAPIES
A complete review of the vast array of alternative/complementary therapies proposed for the ASDs is beyond the scope of this chapter. Despite the wide publicity garnered by a number of alternative/complementary therapies, evidence for efficacy is mostly limited to anecdotal reports or to the testimonials of parents who swear to their effectiveness

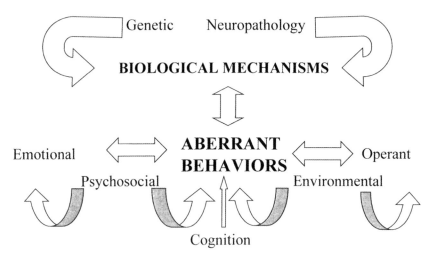

Fig. 17.1. Determinants of aberrant behavior.

(often after having spent a great deal of money providing them for their children). Occupational therapists address some children's aversive responses to tactile stimuli by brushing them, giving them the experience of firm pressure rather than light touch, and rocking, swinging and other ways to enhance "vestibular stimulation". Another popular therapy termed "auditory integration" claims to desensitize aversions to certain auditory stimuli by presenting filtered sounds through headphones. The effectiveness of auditory integration has yet to be shown despite its continued popularity among certain professionals and the lay public (Mudford et al. 2000, Sinha et al. 2004).

Alternative/complementary approaches are not all inherently benign. Some have involved the administration of biological products (secretin/IVIG), toxic dosages of cofactors (megavitamin therapy), or substances of unknown potency or purity purchased in health food stores or from special vendors (Singh et al. 1988, Findling et al. 1997, Gupta 1999, Dunn-Geier et al. 2000, Plioplys 2000, Sandler and Bodfish 2000, Chez et al. 2002, Sponheim et al. 2002, Unis et al. 2002, Coplan et al. 2003, Levy et al. 2003). Often, the "rationale" for utilizing such substances is based upon inaccurate and unproven laboratory testing, such as hair or urine analysis of minerals or neurotransmitters. Even dietary manipulation, benign as it may seem, may distract from better supported therapies (Sandler et al. 2000, Horvath and Perman 2002, Sponheim 2002, Arnold GL et al. 2003).

All clinicians working with children and families with autism must be well informed about all the types of behavioral and medical interventions being offered to children with autism. They must be strong advocates for their patients and as such must discuss the scientific validity of treatment approaches in an unbiased manner, always maintaining a trusting relationship with families (Committee on Children with Disabilities 2001).

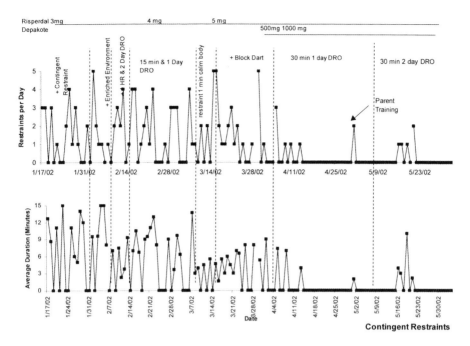

Fig. 17.2. 16-year-old autistic, nonverbal boy with severe aggressive behaviors that presented a risk of harm to himself and others, necessitating the use of protective holds ("restraints"). Use of risperidone up to 5 mg/day, along with changes in the behavioral management plan, did not make an appreciable difference in the frequency and intensity of aggressive behaviors. Valproic acid was added as an alternative mood stabilizer and titrated to 1000 mg/day, which resulted in a significant reduction in aggressive behaviors and a marked reduction in the need for protective holds.

DRO = differential reinforcement of other behavior.

INTEGRATING EDUCATIONAL, BEHAVIORAL AND PHARMACOLOGICAL TREATMENT APPROACHES

Children with ASD often manifest very challenging behaviors. These behaviors can interfere with therapeutic and educational interventions and impact upon the children's quality of life. The determinants maintaining aberrant behaviors can arise from a variety of sources: biologically based mechanisms, learning/conditioning, emotional confounds and cognitive ability (Fig. 17.1). In order to determine the appropriate intervention for a maladaptive behavior, it is important to define it operationally, quantify its occurrence, determine the degree of impairment it confers, and analyze whether it has identifiable antecedents, consequences and functions, or whether it appears to be occurring in an "automatic" manner (Lord and McGee 2001). Defining and quantifying behavioral occurrences over given time intervals or across situational contexts is helpful for assessing whether or not a prescribed therapeutic intervention is yielding the expected behavioral outcome (Fig. 17.2).

Conducting a functional behavior analysis (FBA) is an essential prerequisite to the introduction of any therapeutic intervention (Pelios et al. 1999). The FBA process enables clinicians/therapists to define the function(s) (e.g. attention seeking, escape/avoidance from tasks or demands, communication) of the behavior. The FBA may identify the functional mechanisms that underlie a behavior that is apparently triggered by antecedent "sensory" or nonvolitional mechanisms or maintained by consequent events. If this is the case one is in a position to devise a behavioral intervention plan to reshape the behavior, utilizing procedures to weaken the maintaining contingency or to reinforce alternative replacement behaviors. If the FBA is inconclusive and the behavior seems random ("automatic"), it may be more biologically driven, not fully within a child's volitional control (see Chapter 5), and behavioral interventions may not be adequately successful in reducing the target behavior. Whether or not the behavior seems to be contingent, but particularly if it is not, adjunctive pharmacological therapies may be necessary for achieving a desirable level of behavioral control. Overall, understanding the function of a maladaptive behavior is required for devising an appropriate and effective treatment plan. Applied behavioral analysis can also guide medical management. Measuring the circumstances, frequency and character of the targeted maladaptive behavior provides a record of the effectiveness of a prescribed intervention (Fig. 17.2).

SUMMARY

It is important that a treatment plan for a child with ASD be built upon a firm and justifiable foundation. A complete medical and neurological evaluation is necessary to identify any potential, admittedly infrequent, underlying and identifiable medical disorder that needs to be the primary target of treatment. A thorough assessment of a child's cognitive abilities and social-communication skills, and a functional analysis of aberrant behaviors will allow the formulation of a comprehensive and effective therapy plan. Successful treatment approaches are multimodal and interdisciplinary, tapping *when required* by the individual child into the expertise of pediatric neurology and psychiatry, developmental pediatrics, neuropsychology, behavioral psychology, speech and language, physical and occupational therapies, and education. It is critical that clinicians utilize therapeutic interventions that are individualized and tailored to the needs of each child, rather than more global, nonspecific practices. No child needs every available intervention! Medications are best considered ancillary treatments and their advantages considered in the light of potential undesirable side-effects and toxicities. Child neurologists need to be well informed of the alternative and complementary approaches advocated for the treatment of autism and need to discuss the limitations and potential economic and human costs of these interventions with families. Parents need to hear from child neurologists that there are well established behavioral, educational and pharmacological interventions that do work and that do make a positive difference in all children with autism. In addition, a fair and scientific discussion of the cost–benefit ratio of all interventions should be undertaken and child neurologists should educate the family on the limitations of our knowledge regarding treatment approaches for autism.

There are countless lessons in the history of the ASDs that have taught us that the widespread practice of utilizing unproven therapies based upon testimonials and anecdotal evidence is fraught with failure and disappointment. There is a tremendous need for methodologically sound research aimed at determining the relative efficacy of the various behavioral and educational treatment approaches, as well as the efficacy and safety of pharmacological treatments, based on appropriate and relevant outcome measures. Furthermore, evidence is mounting that earlier interventions result in more favorable long term outcomes. It is therefore incumbent upon the medical and professional community to be knowledgable about the earliest signs and symptoms of ASDs to ensure that evidence-based interventions are initiated as quickly as possible following early identification.

REFERENCES

Akanuma N, Kanemoto K, Adachi N, Kawasaki J, Ito M, Onuma T (2005) Prolonged postictal psychosis with forced normalization (Landolt) in temporal lobe epilepsy. *Epilepsia* 6: 456–9.

Alcami Pertejo M, Peral Guerra M, Gilaberte I (2000) Open study of fluoxetine in children with autism. *Actas Esp Psiquiatr* 28: 353–6.

Alessandri M, Bomba C, Holmes A, Van Driesen D, Holmes DL (2002) [Changes in developmental rates in young children with autism spectrum disorders.] *Persona* 5: 11–25 (Spanish).

Aman MG (1999) Atypical antipsychotics in persons with developmental disabilities. *Ment Retard Dev Disabil Res Rev* 5: 253–63.

Aman MG (2004) Management of hyperactivity and other acting-out problems in patients with autism spectrum disorder. *Semin Pediatr Neurol* 11: 225–8.

Aman MG, Langworthy KS (2000) Pharmacotherapy for hyperactivity in children with autism and other pervasive developmental disorders. *J Autism Dev Disord* 30: 451–9.

Aman MG, Madrid A (1999) Atypical antipsychotics in persons with developmental disabilities. *Ment Retard Dev Disabil Res Rev* 5: 253-263.

Aman MG, Van Bourgondien ME, Wolford PL, Sarphare G (1995) Psychotropic and anticonvulsant drugs in subjects with autism: prevalence and patterns of use. *J Am Acad Child Adolesc Psychiatry* 34: 1672–81.

Aman MG, Arnold LE, Armstrong SC (1999) Review of serotonergic agents and perseverative behavior in patients with developmental disabilities. *Ment Retard Dev Disabil Res Rev* 5: 279–89.

Anderson LT, Campbell M, Adams P, Small AM, Perry R, Shell J (1989) The effects of haloperidol on discrimination learning and behavioral symptoms in autistic children. *J Autism Dev Disord* 19: 227–39.

Arnold GL, Hyman SL, Mooney RA, Kirby RS (2003) Plasma amino acids profiles in children with autism: Potential risk of nutritional deficiencies. *J Autism Dev Disord* 33: 449-454.

Arnold LE, Aman MG, Martin A, Collier-Crespin A, Vitiello B, Tierney E, Asarnow R, Bell-Bradshaw F, Freeman BJ, Gates-Ulanet P, Klin A, McCracken JT, McDougle CJ, McGough JJ, Posey DJ, Scahill L, Swiezy NB, Ritz L, Volkmar F (2000) Assessment in multi-site randomized clinical trials of patients with autistic disorder: the Autism RUPP Network. Research Units on Pediatric Psychopharmacology. *J Autism Dev Disord* 30: 99–111.

Arnold LE, Vitiello B, McDougle C, Scahill L, Shah B, Gonzalez NM, Chuang S, Davies M, Hollway J, Aman MG, Cronin P, Koenig K, Kohn AE, McMahon DJ, Tierney E (2003) Parent-defined target symptoms respond to risperidone in RUPP autism study: customer approach to clinical trials. *J Am Acad Child Adolesc Psychiatry* 42: 1443–50.

Arroyo S, de la Morena A (2001) Life-threatening adverse events of antiepileptic drugs. *Epilepsy Res* 47: 155–74.

Belsito KM, Law PA, Kirk KS, Landa RJ, Zimmerman AW (2001) Lamotrigine therapy for autistic disorder: a randomized, double-blind, placebo-controlled trial. *J Autism Dev Disord* 31: 175–81.

Bondy AS, Frost LA (1998) The picture exchange communication system. *Semin Speech Lang* 19: 373–88.

Branford D, Bhaumik S, Naik B (1998) Selective serotonin re-uptake inhibitors for the treatment of perseverative and maladaptive behaviours of people with intellectual disability. *J Intellect Disabil Res* 42: 301–6.

Brunton L, Lazo J, Parker K, eds. (2005) *Goodman and Gilman's the Pharmacological Basis of Therapeutics, 11th edn.* New York: McGraw-Hill.

Campbell M, Anderson LT, Small AM, Adams P, Gonzalez NM, Ernst M (1993) Naltrexone in autistic children: behavioral symptoms and attentional learning. *J Am Acad Child Adolesc Psychiatry* 32: 1283–91.

Campbell M, Armenteros JL, Malone RP, Adams PB, Eisenberg ZW, Overall JE (1997) Neuroleptic-related dyskinesias in autistic children: a prospective, longitudinal study. *J Am Acad Child Adolesc Psychiatry* 36: 835–43.

Charlop-Christy MH, Carpenter M, Le L, LeBlanc LA, Kellet K (2002) Using the picture exchange communication system (PECS) with children with autism: assessment of PECS acquisition, speech, social-communicative behavior, and problem behavior. *J Appl Behav Anal* 35: 213–31.

Chez MG, Buchanan CP, Aimonovitch MC, Becker M, Schaefer K, Black C, Komen J (2002) Double-blind, placebo-controlled study of L-carnosine supplementation in children with autistic spectrum disorders. *J Child Neurol* 17: 833–7.

Chez MG, Buchanan T, Becker M (2003) Donepezil hydrochloride: a double-blind study in autistic children. *J Pediatr Neurol* 1: 83–8.

Chez MG, Aimonovitch M, Buchanan T, Mrazek S, Tremb RJ (2004) Treating autistic spectrum disorders in children: utility of the cholinesterase inhibitor rivastigmine tartrate. *J Child Neurol* 19: 165–9.

Childs JA, Blair JL (1997) Valproic acid treatment of epilepsy in autistic twins. *J Neurosci Nurs* 29: 244–8.

Chugani DC (2002) Role of altered brain serotonin mechanisms in autism. *Mol Psychiatry* 7: 16–7.

Chugani DC, Muzik O, Behen M, Rothermel R, Janisse JJ, Lee J, Chugani HT (1999) Developmental changes in brain serotonin synthesis capacity in autistic and nonautistic children. *Ann Neurol* 45: 287–95.

Committee on Children with Disabilities (2001) American Academy of Pediatrics: Counseling families who choose complementary and alternative medicine for their child with chronic illness or disability. Committee on Children with Disabilities. *Pediatrics* 107: 598–601; erratum in *Pediatrics* 2001, 108: 507.

Connolly HM, Crary JL, McGoon MD, Hensrud DD, Edwards BS, Edwards WD, Schaff HV (1997) Valvular heart disease associated with fenfluramine-phentermine. *N Engl J Med* 337: 581–8; erratum 1783.

Cook EH, Courchesne R, Lord C, Cox NJ, Yan S, Lincoln A, Haas R, Courchesne E, Leventhal BL (1997) Evidence of linkage between the serotonin transporter and autistic disorder. *Mol Psychiatry* 2: 247–250.

Coplan J, Souders MC, Mulberg AE, Belchic JK, Wray J, Jawad AF, Gallagher PR, Mitchell R,

Gerdes M, Levy SE (2003) Children with autistic spectrum disorders. II: Parents are unable to distinguish secretin from placebo under double-blind conditions. *Arch Dis Child* 88: 737–9.

Curatolo P, Porfirio MC, Manzi B, Seri S (2004) Autism in tuberous sclerosis. *Eur J Paediatr Neurol* 8: 327–32.

Dawson G, Osterling J (1997) Early intervention in autism. In: Guralnick MJ, ed. *The Effectiveness of Early Intervention.* Baltimore: Paul H Brookes, pp. 302–26.

DeLong GR, Teague LA, McSwain Kamran M (1998) Effects of fluoxetine treatment in young children with idiopathic autism. *Dev Med Child Neurol* 40: 551–62.

DeLong GR, Ritch CR, Burch S (2002) Fluoxetine response in children with autistic spectrum disorders: correlation with familial major affective disorder and intellectual achievement. *Dev Med Child Neurol* 44: 652–9.

Deonna T, Roulet-Perez E, eds. (2005) *Cognitive and Behavioural Disorders of Epileptic Origin in Children. Clinics in Developmental Medicine No. 168.* London: Mac Keith Press.

Di Martino A, Tuchman RF (2001) Antiepileptic drugs: affective use in autism spectrum disorders. *Pediatr Neurol* 25: 199–207.

Dunn M (2005) *S.O.S.: Social Skills in our Schools (A Social Skills Program for Children with Pervasive Developmental Disorders and their Typical Peers).* Shawnee Mission, KS: Autism & Asperger Publishing.

Dunn-Geier J, Ho HH, Auersperg E, Doyle D, Eaves L, Matsuba C, Orrbine E, Pham B, Whiting S (2000) Effect of secretin on children with autism: a randomized controlled trial. *Dev Med Child Neurol* 42: 796–802.

Erba HW (2000) Early intervention programs for children with autism: conceptual frameworks for implementation. *Am J Orthopsychiatry* 70: 82–94.

Ernst M, Magee HJ, Gonzalez NM, Locascio JJ, Rosenberg CR, Campbell M (1992) Pimozide in autistic children. *Psychopharmacol Bull* 28: 187–91.

Fankhauser MP, Karumanchi VC, German ML, Yates A, Karumanchi SD (1992) A double-blind, placebo-controlled study of the efficacy of transdermal clonidine in autism. *J Clin Psychiatry* 53: 77–82.

Fatemi SH, Realmuto GM, Khan L, Thuras P (1998) Fluoxetine in treatment of adolescent patients with autism: a longitudinal open trial. *J Autism Dev Disord* 28: 303–7.

FDA (2004) Public Health Advisory: Suicidality in children and adolescents being treated with antidepressant medications (online publication: www.fda.gov/cder/drug/antidepressants/SSRIPHA200410.htm).

Findling RL, Maxwell K, Scotese-Wojtila L, Huang J, Yamashita T, Wiznitzer M (1997) High-dose pyridoxine and magnesium administration in children with autistic disorder: an absence of salutary effects in a double-blind, placebo-controlled study. *J Autism Dev Disord* 27: 467–78.

French JA, Kanner AM, Bautista J, Abou-Khalil B, Browne T, Harden CL, Theodore WH, Bazil C, Stern J, Schachter SC, Bergen D, Hirtz D, Montouris GD, Nespeca M, Gidal B, Marks WJ, Turk WR, Fischer JH, Bourgeois B, Wilner A, Faught RE, Sachdeo RC, Beydoun A, Glauser TA; Therapeutics and Technology Assessment Subcommittee of the American Academy of Neurology; Quality Standards Subcommittee of the American Academy of Neurology; American Epilepsy Society (2004) Efficacy and tolerability of the new antiepileptic drugs. II: Treatment of refractory epilepsy: report of the Therapeutics and Technology Assessment Subcommittee and Quality Standards Subcommittee of the American Academy of Neurology and the American Epilepsy Society. *Neurology* 62: 1261–73.

Frost L, Bondy A (1994) *PECS: The Picture Exchange Communication System Training Manual.* Cherry Hill, NJ: Pyramid Educational Consultants.

Fulop G, Phillips RA, Shapiro AK, Gomes JA, Shapiro E, Nordlie JW (1987) ECG changes during haloperidol and pimozide treatment of Tourette's disorder. *Am J Psychiatry* 144: 673–5.

Gagliano A, Germano E, Pustorino G, Impallomeni C, D'Arrigo C, Calamoneri F, Spina E (2004) Risperidone treatment of children with autistic disorder: effectiveness, tolerability, and pharmacokinetic implications. *J Child Adolesc Psychopharmacol* 14: 39–47.

Go FS, Malley EE, Birmaher B, Rosenberg DR (1998) Manic behaviors associated with fluoxetine in three 12 to 18 year olds with obsessive–compulsive disorder. *J Child Adolesc Psychopharmacol* 8: 73–80.

Goodnick PJ, Jerry J, Parra F (2002) Psychotropic drugs and the ECG: focus on the QTc interval. *Expert Opin Pharmacother* 3: 479–98.

Gordon CT, State RC, Nelson JE, Hamburger SD, Rapoport JL (1993) A double-blind comparison of clomipramine, desipramine, and placebo in the treatment of autistic disorder. *Arch Gen Psychiatry* 50: 441–7.

Gupta S (1999) Treatment of children with autism with intravenous immunoglobulin. J Child Neurol 14: 203-205.

Gutgesell H, Atkins D, Barst R, Buck M, Franklin W, Humes R, Ringel R, Shaddy R, Taubert KA (1999) AHA Scientific Statement: Cardiovascular monitoring of children and adolescents receiving psychotropic drugs. *Circulation* 99: 979–82; reprinted in *J Am Acad Child Adolesc Psychiatry* 1999, 38: 1047–50.

Handen BL, Johnson CR, Lubetsky M (2000) Efficacy of methylphenidate among children with autism and symptoms of attention-deficit hyperactivity disorder. *J Autism Dev Disord* 30: 245–55.

Hertzman M (2003) Galantamine in the treatment of adult autism: a report of three clinical cases. *Int J Psychiatry Med* 33: 395–8.

Hillbrand M, Scott K (1995) The use of buspirone with aggressive behavior. *J Autism Dev Disord* 25: 663–4.

Hollander E, Dolgoff-Kaspar R, Cartwright C, Rawitt R, Novotny S (2001) An open trial of divalproex sodium in the autism spectrum disorders. *J Clin Psychiatry* 62: 530–4.

Horrigan JP, Barnhill LJ, Courvoisie HE (1997) Olanzapine in PDD. *J Am Acad Child Adolesc Psychiatry* 36: 1166–7.

Horvath K, Perman JA (2002) Autism and gastrointestinal symptoms. *Curr Gastroenterol Rep* 4: 251–8.

Howlin P (1998) Practitioner review: psychological and educational treatments for autism. *J Child Psychol Psychiatry* 39: 307–22.

Jaselskis CA, Cook EH, Fletcher KE, Leventhal BL (1992) Clonidine treatment of hyperactive and impulsive children with autistic disorder. *J Clin Psychopharmacol* 12: 322–7.

Kaplan PW (2004) Reproductive health effects and teratogenicity of antiepileptic drugs. *Neurology* 63: 13–23.

Kipps CM, Fung VS, Grattan-Smith P, de Moore GM, Morris JG (2005) Movement disorder emergencies. *Mov Disord* 20: 322–34.

Klauck SM, Poustka F, Benner A, Lesch KP, Poustka A (1997) Serotonin transporter (5-HTT) gene variants associated with autism? *Hum Mol Genet* 6: 2233–8.

Koegel LK, Koegel RL, Carter CM (1998) Pivotal responses and the natural language teaching paradigm. *Semin Speech Lang* 19: 355–71.

Koegel RL, Frea WD (1993) Treatment of social behavior in autism through the modification of pivotal social skills. *J Appl Behav Anal* 26: 369–77.

Koegel RL, Koegel LK, McNerney EK (2001) Pivotal areas in intervention for autism. *J Clin Child*

Psychol 30: 19–32.

Krebs S, Dormann H, Muth-Selbach U, Hahn EG, Brune K, Schneider HT (2001) Risperidone-induced cholestatic hepatitis. *Eur J Gastroenterol Hepatol* 13: 67–9.

Krishnamoorthy ES, Trimble MR, Sander JW, Kanner AM (2002) Forced normalization at the interface between epilepsy and psychiatry. *Epilepsy Behav* 3: 303–8.

LeGoff DB (2004) Use of LEGO as a therapeutic medium for improving social competence. *J Autism Dev Disord* 34: 557–71.

LeGoff D, Sherman M (2006) Long-term outcome of social skills intervention based on interactive LEGO play. *Autism* 10: 1–13.

Lesch KP, Mossner R (1998) Genetically driven variation in serotonin uptake: is there a link to affective spectrum, neurodevelopmental, and neurodegenerative disorders? *Biol Psychiatry* 44: 179–92.

Levy SE, Souders MC, Wray J, Jawad AF, Gallagher PR, Coplan J, Belchic JK, Gerdes M, Mitchell R, Mulberg AE (2003) Children with autistic spectrum disorders. I: Comparison of placebo and single dose of human synthetic secretin. *Arch Dis Child* 88: 731–6.

Lopez Ornat S, Gallo P (2004) Acquisition, learning, or development of language? Skinner's "Verbal Behavior" revisited. *Span J Psychol* 7: 161–70.

Lord C, McGee JP, eds. (2001) *Educating Children with Autism. Committee on Educational Interventions for Children with Autism, Division of Behavior and Social Sciences and Education.* Washington, DC: National Academy Press.

Lovaas OI, Schreibman L, Koegel RL (1974) A behavior modification approach to the treatment of autistic children. *J Autism Child Schizophr* 4: 111–29.

Lovaas OI, Smith T (1989) A comprehensive behavioral theory of autistic children: paradigm for research and treatment. *J Behav Ther Exp Psychiatry* 20: 17–29.

Luiselli JK, Blew P, Keane J, Thibadeau S, Holzman T (2000) Pharmacotherapy for severe aggression in a child with autism: "open label" evaluation of multiple medications on response frequency and intensity of behavioral intervention. *J Behav Ther Exp Psychiatry* 31: 219–30.

Magiati I, Howlin P (2003) A pilot evaluation study of the Picture Exchange Communication System (PECS) for children with autistic spectrum disorders. *Autism* 7: 297–320.

Malone RP, Ernst M, Godfrey KA, Locascio JJ, Campbell M (1991) Repeated episodes of neuroleptic-related dyskinesias in autistic children. *Psychopharmacol Bull* 27: 113–7.

Mandoki MW (1995) Risperidone treatment of children and adolescents: Increased risk of extrapyramidal side-effects? *J Child Adolesc Psychopharmacol* 5: 49–67.

Martin A, Koenig K, Scahill L, Bregman J (1999) Open-label quetiapine in the treatment of children and adolescents with autistic disorder. *J Child Adolesc Psychopharmacol* 9: 99–107.

Martin A, Scahill L, Anderson GM, Aman M, Arnold LE, McCracken J, McDougle CJ, Tierney E, Chuang S, Vitiello B (2004) Weight and leptin changes among risperidone-treated youths with autism: 6-month prospective data. *Am J Psychiatry* 161: 1125–7.

McBride PA, Anderson GM, Hertzig ME, Snow ME, Thompson SM, Khait VD, Shapiro T, Cohen DJ (1998) Effects of diagnosis, race, and puberty on platelet serotonin levels in autism and mental retardation. *J Am Acad Child Adolesc Psychiatry* 37: 767–76.

McClellan JM, Werry JS (2003) Evidence-based treatments in child and adolescent psychiatry: an inventory. *J Am Acad Child Adolesc Psychiatry* 42: 1388–400.

McCracken JT, McGough J, Shah B, Cronin P, Hong D, Aman MG, Arnold LE, Lindsay R, Nash P, Hollway J, McDougle CJ, Posey D, Swiezy N, Kohn A, Scahill L, Martin A, Koenig K, Volkmar F, Carroll D, Lancor A, Tierney E, Ghuman J, Gonzalez NM, Grados M, Vitiello B, Ritz L, Davies M, Robinson J, McMahon D; Research Units on Pediatric Psychopharmacology

Autism Network (2002) Risperidone in children with autism and serious behavioral problems. *N Engl J Med* 347: 314–21.

McDougle CJ, Naylor ST, Cohen DJ, Volkmar FR, Heninger GR, Price LH (1996) A double-blind, placebo-controlled study of fluvoxamine in adults with autistic disorder. *Arch Gen Psychiatry* 53: 1001–8.

McDougle CJ, Holmes JP, Bronson MR, Anderson GM, Volkmar FR, Price LH, Cohen DJ (1997) Risperidone treatment of children and adolescents with pervasive developmental disorders: a prospective open-label study. *J Am Acad Child Adolesc Psychiatry* 36: 685–93.

McDougle CJ, Brodkin ES, Naylor ST, Carlson DC, Cohen DJ, Price LH (1998a) Sertraline in adults with pervasive developmental disorders: A prospective open-label investigation. *J Clin Psychopharmacol* 18: 62–6.

McDougle CJ, Holmes JP, Carlson DC, Pelton GH, Cohen DJ, Price LH (1998b) A double-blind, placebo-controlled study of risperidone in adults with autistic disorder and other pervasive developmental disorders. *Arch Gen Psychiatry* 55: 633–41.

McDougle CJ, Kresch LE, Posey DJ (2000) Repetitive thoughts and behavior in pervasive developmental disorders: Treatment with serotonin reuptake inhibitors. *J Autism Dev Disord* 30: 427–35.

McDougle CJ, Kem DL, Posey DJ (2002) Case series: use of ziprasidone for maladaptive symptoms in youths with autism. *J Am Acad Child Adolesc Psychiatry* 41: 921–7.

McEachin JJ, Smith T, Lovaas OI (1993) Long-term outcome for children with autism who received early intensive behavioral treatment. *Am J Ment Retard* 97: 359–91.

Mesibov GB, Schopler E (1983) The development of community-based programs for autistic adolescents. *Child Health Care* 12: 20–4.

Mintz M (2001) Metabolic acidosis induced by topiramate: response to bicarbonate supplementation. *Adv Stud Med* 1: 277–8.

Mudford OC, Cross BA, Breen S, Cullen C, Reeves D, Gould J, Douglas J (2000) Auditory integration training for children with autism: no behavioral benefits detected. *Am J Ment Retard* 105: 118–29.

Muzina DJ, El-Sayegh S, Calabrese JR (2002) Antiepileptic drugs in psychiatry—focus on randomized controlled trial. *Epilepsy Res* 50: 195–202.

Naruse H, Nagahata M, Nakane Y, Shirahashi K, Takesada M, Yamazaki K (1982) A multi-center double-blind trial of pimozide (Orap), haloperidol and placebo in children with behavioral disorders, using crossover design. *Acta Paedopsychiatr* 48: 173–84.

Nass R, Petrucha D (1990) Acquired aphasia with convulsive disorder: a pervasive developmental disorder variant. *J Child Neurol* 5: 327–8.

Nicolson R, Awad G, Sloman L (1998) An open trial of risperidone in young autistic children. *J Am Acad Child Adolesc Psychiatry* 37: 372–6.

Ozonoff S, Cathcart K (1998) Effectiveness of a home program intervention for young children with autism. *J Autism Dev Disord* 28: 25–32.

Palermo MT, Curatolo P (2004) Pharmacologic treatment of autism. *J Child Neurol* 9: 155–64.

Panerai S, Ferrante L, Caputo V (1997) The TEACCH strategy in mentally retarded children with autism: a multidimensional assessment. Pilot study. Treatment and Education of Autistic and Communication Handicapped children. *J Autism Dev Disord* 27: 345–7.

Panerai S, Ferrante L, Zingale M (2002) Benefits of the Treatment and Education of Autistic and Communication Handicapped Children (TEACCH) programme as compared with a non-specific approach. *J Intellect Disabil Res* 46: 318–27.

Pelios L, Morren J, Tesch D, Axelrod S (1999) The impact of functional analysis methodology on treatment choice for self-injurious and aggressive behavior. *J Appl Behav Anal* 32: 185–95.

Perry R, Campbell M, Adams P, Lynch N, Spencer EK, Curren EL, Overall JE (1989) Long-term efficacy of haloperidol in autistic children: continuous versus discontinuous drug administration. *J Am Acad Child Adolesc Psychiatry* 28: 87–92.

Persico AM, Militerni R, Bravaccio C, Schneider C, Melmed R, Conciatori M, Damiani V, Baldi A, Keller F (2000) Lack of association between serotonin transporter gene promoter variants and autistic disorder in two ethnically distinct samples. *Am J Med Genet* 96: 123–7.

Persico AM, Pascucci T, Puglisi-Allegra S, Militerni R, Bravaccio C, Schneider C, Melmed R, Trillo S, Montecchi F, Palermo M, Rabinowitz D, Reichelt KL, Conciatori M, Marino R, Keller F (2002) Serotonin transporter gene promoter variants do not explain the hyperserotoninemia in autistic children. *Mol Psychiatry* 7: 795–800.

Plioplys AV (1994) Autism: electroencephalogram abnormalities and clinical improvement with valproic acid. *Arch Pediatr Adolesc Med* 148: 220–2.

Plioplys AV (2000) Intravenous immunoglobulin treatment in autism. *J Autism Dev Disord* 30: 73–4.

Posey DJ, McDougle CJ (2000) The pharmacotherapy of target symptoms associated with autistic disorder and other pervasive developmental disorders. *Harv Rev Psychiatry* 2: 45–63.

Posey D, Puntney J, Sasher TM, Kem DL, McDougle CJ (2004) Guanfacine treatment of hyperactivity and inattention in autism: a retrospective analysis of 80 cases. *J Child Adolesc Psychopharmacol* 14: 233–41.

Potenza MN, Holmes JP, Kanes SJ, McDougle CJ (1999) Olanzapine treatment of children, adolescents, and adults with pervasive developmental disorders: an open-label pilot study. *J Clin Psychopharmacol* 19: 37–44.

Prizant BM, Schuler AL, Wetherby AM, Rydell P (1997) Enhancing language and communication: language approaches. In: Cohen D, Volkmar FR, eds. *Handbook of Autism and Pervasive Developmental Disorders.* New York: John Wiley, pp. 572–605.

Purdon SE, Lit W, Labelle A, Jones BD (1994) Risperidone in the treatment of pervasive developmental disorder. *Can J Psychiatry* 39: 400–5.

Quintana H, Birmaher B, Stedge D, Lennon S, Freed J, Bridge J, Greenhill L (1995) Use of methylphenidate in the treatment of children with autistic disorder. *J Autism Dev Disord* 25: 283–94.

Ratey JJ, Bemporad J, Sorgi P, Bick P, Polakoff S, O'Driscoll G, Mikkelsen E (1987) Open trial effects of beta-blockers on speech and social behaviors in 8 autistic adults. *J Autism Dev Disord* 17: 439–46.

Realmuto GM, August GJ, Garfinkel BD (1989) Clinical effect of buspirone in autistic children. *J Clin Psychopharmacol* 9: 122–5.

Remington G, Sloman L, Konstantareas M, Parker K, Gow R (2001) Clomipramine versus haloperidol in the treatment of autistic disorder: a double-blind, placebo-controlled, crossover study. *J Clin Psychopharmacol* 21: 440–4.

Research Units on Pediatric Psychopharmacology Autism Network (2005) Risperidone treatment of autistic disorder: longer-term benefits and blinded discontinuation after 6 months. *Am J Psychiatry* 162: 1361–9.

Rugino TA, Samsock TC. (2002) Levetiracetam in autistic children: an open-label study. *J Dev Behav Pediatr* 23: 225–30.

Sandler AD, Bodfish JW (2000) Placebo effects in autism: lessons from secretin. *J Dev Behav Pediatr* 21: 247–350.

Sandler RH, Finegold SM, Bolte ER, Buchanan CP, Maxwell AP, Vaisanen ML, Nelson MN,

Wexler HM (2000) Short-term benefit from oral vancomycin treatment of regressive-onset autism. *J Child Neurol* 15: 429–35.

Sallows GO, Graupner TD (2005) Intensive behavioral treatment for children with autism: four-year outcome and predictors. *Am J Ment Retard* 110: 417–38.

Scahill L, Vitiello B, Aman MG, McCracken J, McDougle C, Tierney E, Davies M, and the Autism Network (2004) Methylphenidate in autism: Results from the RUPP Autism Network Paper presented at the New Clinical Drug Evaluation Unit (NCDEU) Conference, May 2004, Phoenix, AZ.

Schaaf RC, Miller LJ (2005) Occupational therapy using a sensory integrative approach for children with developmental disabilities. *Ment Retard Dev Disabil Res Rev* 11: 143–8.

Schreibman L (2000) Intensive behavioral/psychoeducational treatments for autism: research needs and future directions. *J Autism Dev Disord* 30: 373–8.

Shea V (2004) A perspective on the research literature related to early intensive behavioral intervention (Lovaas) for young children with autism. *Autism* 8: 349–67.

Sheinkopf SJ, Siegel B (1998) Home-based behavioral treatment of young children with autism. *J Autism Dev Disord* 28: 15–23.

Sinha Y, Silove N, Wheeler D, Williams K (2004) Auditory integration training and other sound therapies for autism spectrum disorders. Cochrane Database Syst Rev, CD003681.

Singh VK, Fudenberg HH, Emerson D, Coleman M (1988) Immunodiagnosis and immunotherapy in autistic children. *Ann NY Acad Sci* 540: 602–4.

Skinner BF (1938) *The Behavior of Organisms: An Experimental Analysis.* New York: Appleton-Century.

Skinner BF (1957) *Verbal Behavior.* New York: Appleton-Century-Crofts.

Snead RW, Boon F, Presberg J (1994) Paroxetine for self-injurious behavior. *J Am Acad Child Adolesc Psychiatry* 33: 909–10.

Sovner R (1989) The use of valproate in the treatment of mentally retarded persons with typical and atypical bipolar disorders. *J Clin Psychiatry* 50: 40–3.

Sponheim E (2002) Gluten-free diet in infantile autism: A study of the effects on food choice and nutrition. *J Hum Nutr Diet* 15: 261–9.

Sponheim E, Oftedal G, Helverschou SB (2002) Multiple doses of secretin in the treatment of autism: a controlled study. *Acta Paediatr* 91: 540–5.

Steingard RJ, Zimnitzky B, DeMaso DR, Bauman ML, Bucci JP (1997) Sertraline treatment of transition-associated anxiety and agitation in children with autistic disorder. *J Child Adolesc Psychopharmacol* 7: 9–15.

Stigler KA, Desmond LA, Posey DJ, Wiegand RE, McDougle CJ (2004a) A naturalistic retrospective analysis of psychostimulants in pervasive developmental disorders. *J Child Adolesc Psychpharmacol* 14: 49-56.

Stigler KA, Posey DJ, McDougle CJ (2004b) Aripiprazole for maladaptive behavior in pervasive developmental disorders. *J Child Adolesc Psychopharmacol* 14: 455–63.

Sundberg ML, Michael J (2001) The benefits of Skinner's analysis of verbal behavior for children with autism. *Behav Modif* 25: 698–724.

Szigethy E, Wiznitzer M, Branicky LA, Maxwell K, Findling RL (1999) Risperidone-induced hepatotoxicity in children and adolescents? A chart review study. *J Child Adolesc Psychopharmacol* 9: 93–8.

Unis AS, Munson JA, Rogers SJ, Goldson E, Osterling J, Gabriels R, Abbott RD, Dawson G (2002) A randomized, double-blind, placebo-controlled trial of porcine versus synthetic secretin for reducing symptoms of autism. *J Am Acad Child Adolesc Psychiatry* 41: 1315–21.

Uvebrant P, Bauziene R (1994) Intractable epilepsy in children. The efficacy of lamotrigine treatment, including non-seizure-related benefits. *Neuropediatrics* 6: 284–9.

Van Bourgondien ME, Reichle NC, Schopler E (2003) Effects of a model treatment approach on adults with autism. *J Autism Dev Disord* 33: 131–40.

Wieder S, Greenspan SI (2003) Climbing the symbolic ladder in the DIR model through floor time/interactive play. *Autism* 7: 425–35.

Willemsen-Swinkels SH, Buitelaar JK, Nijhof GJ, van Engeland H (1995) Failure of naltrexone hydrochloride to reduce self-injurious and autistic behavior in mentally retarded adults: a double-blind placebo-controlled study. *Arch Gen Psychiatry* 52: 766–73.

Willemsen-Swinkels SH, Buitelaar JK, van Engeland H (1996) The effects of chronic naltrexone treatment in young autistic children: a double-blind placebo-controlled crossover study. *Biol Psychiatry* 39: 1023–31.

Whitaker-Azmitia PM (2001) Serotonin and brain development: role in human developmental diseases. *Brain Res Bull* 56: 479–85.

Zuddas A, Ledda MG, Fratta A, Muglia P, Cianchetti C (1996) Clinical effects of clozapine on autistic disorder. *Am J Psychiatry* 153: 738.

18
OUTCOMES OF CHILDREN WITH AUTISM

Evdokia Anagnostou and Michael Shevell

Autism is a devastating neurodevelopmental disorder that causes lifelong functional impairment and severely impacts both affected individuals and their families. The ability to prognosticate accurately empowers families to plan for the future of their children and to develop reasonable expectations. In addition, information on outcome fosters adaptation to disability and enables the development of effective ways of coping for families faced with the prospect of long term care for their child with autism. Outcome knowledge also modifies health care and educational and social networks, which allows appropriate planning to meet the ongoing needs of these children as they transition into adolescence and adulthood. In addition, documenting the natural history of this disorder is necessary for the evaluation of possible new interventions, since ultimately the markers of success of such treatments will depend to a degree on their ability to improve longer term adaptive and functional outcomes.

Outcome research in autism is plagued with potential methodological difficulties. The diagnostic criteria for autism have undergone serial changes as our diagnostic construct has evolved, making comparisons at different time points problematic. Diagnostic criteria employed in North America are somewhat different from those used in Europe, further limiting our ability to compare studies. Autism itself is a very heterogeneous disorder, and as such, outcome studies have included subjects with a wide spectrum of cognitive, language, social and behavioral levels of functioning (Howlin et al. 2004).

The majority of the outcome studies have utilized sample sizes that are too small to reach definitive conclusions with confidence or to examine the effect of contributing or confounding factors adequately. Studies have used different outcome measures to measure similar behaviors and even within studies to measure similar behavioral issues at different life points. Even with cognitive testing, where measures are theoretically standardized, there are problems comparing scores between earlier and later versions of the same test, as with the WISC for example (Howlin et al. 1998). Often qualitative rather than quantitative judgments about the severity of a particular behavior are utilized, which are susceptible to bias, inconsistency and a range of potentially modifying contextual factors (Nordin and Gillberg 1998). For example, aggressive behavior in a young child may be simply problematic, whereas the same behavior exhibited by an older child or adult may be seen as much more severe, given the individual's acquired size and strength (Seltzer et al. 2004). This may create the illusion of a worsening of symptoms. For that reason direct observation may be necessary to accurately assess severity, but this may be too labor intensive and is often not employed in long term longitudinal studies. Furthermore, long term studies tend to assess individuals at two time points. Although useful information can be gathered using this technique, we often get no information on the intervening processes that have taken place and therefore have limited insight into the factors that have ameliorated or exacerbated a behavior or skill. Finally, patients with "secondary" causes of autism, such as fragile-X syndrome and tuberous sclerosis, have been systematically excluded in some studies but not in others, making comparisons between studies particularly challenging (Seltzer et al. 2004).

An effort has recently been made to agree on common outcome measures for clinical trials in autism. The authors are aware of active work currently being undertaken by multiple autism researchers in collaboration with the NIH to produce a grid of recommended outcome measures to be used in future behavioral studies. A similar effort was the Cure Autism Now (CAN) Foundation's Clinical Trials Task Force that met in 2002 to suggest measures for treatment response for possible use in clinical trials (Aman et al. 2004). The committee concluded that there are no "perfect" measures for core and associated symptoms in autism and strongly recommended specific probing for side-effects in randomized trials. Their recommendations are summarized in Table 18.1. We encourage the reader to look at the full article since only instruments with solid data in this population were included in the table. As a result a variety of instruments assessing social deficits – e.g. the Social Responsiveness Scale (Constantino et al. 2003), Matson Evaluation of Social Skills with Youngsters (MESSY; Matson 1990) and the social subscales of the Autism Diagnostic Observation Schedule (ADOS-G; Lord et al. 2000) – and language – e.g. the Peabody Picture Vocabulary Test (PPVT; Dunn 1970) and the Early Social Communication Scales (ESCS; Mundy and Hogan 1996) – were not included in the table but were discussed in detail in the text.

In this chapter, we attempt to summarize available prospective, retrospective and cross-sectional studies that have reported on the stability of diagnosis, outcomes in the core symptoms of autism, problematic behaviors, cognition and adaptive skills in adolescence and adulthood. One should keep in mind, though, that most of the patients in the cohorts described below have not had the type and intensity of early intervention that most children with autism are receiving now, and as a result, most of the data presented are somewhat reflective of the natural history of autism, although in some cohorts the children did receive various behavioral treatments. It may be difficult to generalize effectively from these studies to the outcomes of the children currently being seen in clinical settings.

OUTCOMES OF CORE AND OTHER SYMPTOMS

Several prospective and retrospective studies have looked at the stability of the diagnosis

TABLE 18.1
Instruments for assessing target symptoms often associated with autism spectrum disorders

Constellation/scale name (subscale) [age groups]	Rec	Reliability	Validity	OS?	Raters	Limitations
Irritability[1]						
Aberrant Behavior Checklist (irritability) [C, TA, Ad]	A	I-R, IC, T-T	Cn, Cr	Yes	Pr, T, O	Few aggression items
Developmental Behaviour Checklist (disruptive, antisocial) [C, TA]	A	I-R, IC, T-T	Cn, Cr	Yes	Pr, T, O	Some tangential items
ECI/CSI/ASI (oppositional defiant disorder, conduct disorder) [P, C, TA]	B	IC	Cn, Cr	No	Pr, T	Devised for typically developing children
Children's Psychiatric Rating Scale (anger/uncooperativeness) [P, C, TA]	B	I-R	Cn	Yes	CL	Only 4 items
NCBRF (conduct problems) [C, TA]	B	I-R, IC, T-T	Cn	Yes	Pr, T	Emphasizes disruptive behaviors
DASH-II (impulse control) [TA, Ad]	B	I-R, IC, T-T	Cn	No	O	Normed with severe/profound MR group. DSM-IV derived
Preschool Behavior Questionnaire (hostile-aggressive) [P]	B	I-R, T-T	Cn	No	T	Teacher only
Hyperactivity/inattention/impulsiveness[2]						
Aberrant Behavior Checklist (hyperactivity) [C, TA, Ad]	A	I-R, IC, T-T	Cn, Cr	Yes	Pr, T, O	N/A
ECI/CSI/ASI (ADHD) [P, C, TA]	B	IC	Cn, Cr	No	Pr, T	Devised for typically developing children
Children's Psychiatric Rating Scale (hyperactivity factor) [P, C, TA]	B	I-R	Cn	Yes	CL	Only 3 items
NCBRF (hyperactive) [C, TA]	A	I-R, IC, T-T	Cn	Yes	Pr, T	N/A
Preschool Behavior Questionnaire (hyperactive–distractible) [P]	B	I-R, T-T	Cn	No	T	Only 4 items; teacher only
Compulsive, Ritualistic, Perseverative[3]						
Repetitive Behavior Scale–Revised (stereotyped; self-injurious; compulsive; ritualistic; sameness; restricted behavior) [C, TA, Ad]	B	I-R, IC, T-T	Cn, Cr	No	O	Psychometric data presented in conference; peer-reviewed data not yet available
C-YBOCS/YBOCS (obsessions, compulsions) [C, TA, Ad]	B	I-R, T-T		Yes	CL	Derived from normal-ability patients; compulsions only in non-verbal patients; sensitivity to mild change may be limited
Stereotypic Behavior Scale [C, TA, Ad]	B	I-R, IC, T-T	Cn	No	O	Confined to stereotypies
Aberrant Behavior Checklist (stereotypic behavior) [C, TA, A]	B	I-R, IC, T-T	Cn, Cr	Yes	Pr, T, O	Confined to stereotypies

Anxiety and Fears[4]

ADAMS (general anxiety) [TA, Ad]	B	I-R, IC, T-T	Cn, Cr	No	Pr, CL, O	Only 7 items
Emotional Disorders Rating Scale (anxiety) [C, TA]	B	I-R, T-T	Cr	No	O	Only 6 items; mediocre T-T reliability; difficult to obtain?
Fear Survey for Children–Revised [C, TA]	B	I-R, T-T	Cn, Cr	No	S	N/A
Preschool Behavior Questionnaire (anxious/fearful) [P]	B	I-R, T-T	Cn	No	T	Designed for preschoolers
ECI/SCI/ASI (generalized anxiety disorder, separation anxiety disorder) [P, C, TA]	B	IT	Cn, Cr	No	Pr, T	Devised for typically developing children

Self-Injury[5]

Behavior Problems Inventory (self-injury) [C, TA, Ad]	A	I-R, IC, T-T	Cn	No	O, Pr	N/A
DASH-II (self-injurious behaviors) [TA, Ad]	B	I-R, IC	Cr	No	O	Primarily developed for subjects with severe mental retardation
Repetitive Behavior Scale-Revised [C, TA, Ad]	B	I-R, IC, T-T	Cn, Cr	No	O	Peer-reviewed data not available yet
Self Injurious Behavior Questionnaire [TA, Ad]	B	Unknown	Unknown	Yes	O	Mixes aggressive and self-injurious behaviors

Other

ECI/CSI/ASI (major depressive disorder, dysthymia, bipolar disorder) [P, C, TA]	B	I-R, IC	Cn, Cr	No	Pr, T	Devised for typically developing children

Summarized from Aman et al. (2004).

[1]Volatile, emotional, sometimes explosive behavior. The following behaviors may be evident: temper tantrums, aggression, mood swings, self-injury, destructiveness, outbursts, screaming.

[2]Physical overactivity, marked difficulty sustaining attention, and impulsiveness. Such patients may be at risk in parking lots or near roads. They may be exceptionally difficult to manage in stimulating environments, such as supermarkets and stores. In some patients, only one or two of the elements may be present.

[3]Preoccupation with repetitive behaviors, expectation of repetitions from others, repeated speech (immediate or delayed), insistence on sameness within environment or routine, excessive precooupation with narrow interests, and physically stereotyped movements.

[4]Excessive worrying, nervousness, avoidance, and/or phobic responses in relation to events or stimuli.

[5]Repetitive mechanical acts, done voluntarily, that cause tissue damage to the person.

Abbreviations: Rec = recommendations; OS = outcome studies; ECI = Early Childhood Inventory; CSI = Child Symptom Inventory; ASI = Adolescent Symptom Inventory; NCBRF = Nisonger Child Behavior Rating Form; DASH-II = Diagnostic Assessment for the Severely Handicapped–Version II; C-YBOCS = Children's Yale–Brown Obsessive–Compulsive Scale; YBOCS = Yale–Brown Obsessive–Compulsive Scale; ADAMS = Anxiety, Depression, and Mood Scale; ADHD = attention deficit hyperactivity disorder; C = children (6–12 years of age); TA = teens/adolescents; Ad = adults; P = preschoolers; A = highly recommended for the target behavior; B = less enthusiasm that measure would be appropriate for the target behavior; I-R = interrater reliability; IC = internal consistency; T-T = test–retest reliability; Cn = construct validity; Cr = criterion group validity; Pr = parent; T = teacher; O = other; CL = clinician; S = self; MR = mentally retarded; DSM-IV = Diagnostic and Statistical Manual of Mental Disorders, 4th edn; N/A = not applicable.

of autism. There is remarkable consistency among most studies irrespective of individual sample characteristics, definitions utilized and design methodologies. Approximately 75–85% of individuals with an autism diagnosis in childhood continue to score within the autism spectrum into adolescence and adulthood (Rutter et al. 1967, Mesibov et al. 1989, Piven et al. 1996, Boelte and Poustka 2000). Children with an original diagnosis of Asperger syndrome (ASP) or a pervasive developmental disorder–not otherwise specified (PDD-NOS) are more likely to "outgrow" their diagnosis in adulthood (Seltzer et al. 2003) than children diagnosed with an autistic disorder.

SOCIAL DEFICITS

The available data suggest that social deficits remain an ongoing significant problem into adolescence and adulthood. In one of the early prospective studies (Rutter et al. 1967), in which social deficits were rated on the basis of observation and informant reports, a third of the autistic adolescents were rated as having "poor" social adjustment, whereas less than 10% were rated as having "good" social adjustment. In later studies, social deficits have been evaluated using the Autism Diagnostic Interview (ADI; Lord et al. 1994), a structured interview with the caregiver that includes detailed information on social and communicative functions, repetitive behaviors, problematic behaviors and unusual sensory interests. Information is gathered about current symptoms, but also symptoms in childhood, to establish the developmental progress of the disorder. The social domain of the Vineland Adaptive Behavior Scale (Sparrow et al. 1984) has been used to corroborate findings from the ADI. In a study by Howlin et al. (2000), only 16.7% of adult patients scored in the average range or better in the social domain of the Vineland. This domain includes information on interpersonal relationships, play and leisure activities, and coping skills. Over half had "none" or "very limited" social contacts based on the ADI and a third were "awkward" in social contact. Only 15% were reported to have any close friendships and only 10% were rated as having normal social relations. Other studies by the same research group have corroborated these initial results (Howlin et al. 2003, 2004).

Some retrospective studies have documented some improvements in social skills over time. Seltzer et al. (2003) reported on a cohort of 400 individuals with autism. Although all of the subjects met criteria for autism spectrum disorders (ASDs) in the social domain of the ADI in childhood, 15% of the sample did not meet these criteria in adolescence. However, only 8% of this sample demonstrated friendships (defined by the ADI as relationships involving reciprocal activities outside of organized settings) (Orsmond et al. 2004). Similarly, in a group of autistic adolescents and adults with performance IQ above 65, Piven et al. (1996) reported improvements in the social domain of the ADI, based on a comparison of current scores to scores reported retrospectively for age 4-5 years, in 80% of autistic adolescents and adults.

The observation that many individuals with autism do not experience loneliness despite being isolated (Howlin et al. 2000) is particularly interesting. The idea that there exist several different phenotypes of social deficits in autism has been put forward. Some authors have described four social sub-phenotypes: aloof, passive, active but odd, and loner (Wing 1997). Aloof autistic people may accept physical affection from familiar people but tend to be indifferent to others, especially their peers. Passive autistic people tend not to interact spontaneously socially but rather to accept approaches from others passively. Loners tend to prefer to be alone but, overall, have subtler social deficits. On the other hand, active but odd autistic individuals attempt to interact socially but are odd and inappropriate. One can see that the first three groups may be less likely to experience loneliness than the fourth group. The groups may also differ in the rates of comorbid social anxiety, but this is an area for future research exploration.

Overall, approximately half of the autistic adolescents and adults studied so far have severe social deficits and, although improvements are noted with age, the extent of these improvements remains modest.

COMMUNICATION

There is some evidence to suggest that communication difficulties in autistic individuals improve into adolescence and adulthood. In one of the first prospective studies after Kanner's original cohort, improvements in language were noted in approximately half of subjects originally diagnosed with an "infantile psychosis" (Rutter et al. 1967). However, repetitive speech, idiosyncratic use of language (pronominal reversal, neologisms), and other persisting inappropriate patterns of language use were still noted in up to 75% of autistic individuals. In prospective studies by the same group 30 years later, moderate improvements were noted in the majority of autistic subjects (Mawhood et al. 2000, Howlin et al. 2004). Still, in the first sample consisting of autistic adults who had a performance IQ above 70 in childhood, approximately two-thirds scored below the 10-year age level in receptive language skills, and half scored below the 10-year age level in expressive language skills. One third of the sample was judged to have 'poor' spoken language that was largely echolalic in character. In the second sample consisting of autistic adults with a performance IQ of above 50 in childhood, approximately half had language below the 6-year age level and only 15% scored above the 15-year age level. In the same sample, 40% still were rated as having a severe language impairment based on the ADI and only 10% were rated as having good language performance. However, in both studies, considerable heterogeneity was noted, with some individuals making significant gains. In addition, in a comparison of subjects with autistic disorder versus Asperger syndrome matched for age and IQ, only a slight superiority in language abilities was documented in the Asperger group, suggesting the existence of significant language difficulties into adulthood for individuals with Asperger syndrome (Howlin 2003).

Retrospective studies support these findings. In a sample of 400 adolescents and adults diagnosed with ASD in childhood (Seltzer et al. 2003), approximately one third of the sample had improved enough so as to not meet current criteria for autistic disorder on the communication domain of the ADI. However, there was considerable variability among subjects and across different communicative behaviors; idiosyncratic language improved the most and gestural language was less likely to improve. In an ADI study of adults with nonverbal IQs above 65, 82% were noted to have improvements in the communication domain (Piven et al. 1996). In a retrospective study involving phone interviews (Ballaban-Gil et al. 1996), the majority of subjects were observed by parents to have made some language improvements in adolescence and adulthood if they were diagnosed before the age of 6 years, but were much less likely to have improved if they were diagnosed after the age of 6. In addition, children with mild mental retardation were less likely to improve than subjects with documented normal IQs.

Cross-sectional data support the notion of a persistence of communication difficulties into adulthood. Janicki and Jacobson (1983) reported that 78% of their sample of adults had expressive or receptive language deficits and one fifth had repetitive speech patterns characterized by echolalia and perseveration.

In summary, available data suggest that language and communication deficits improve to some extent over the lifespan, but clinically significant deficits persist into adulthood in the majority of autistic individuals.

REPETITIVE BEHAVIORS AND RESTRICTIVE INTERESTS

Research on the evolution of repetitive behaviors in autistic adolescents and adults is relatively scant. In the cohort reported by Rutter et al. (1967), some improvements were noted, but all subjects with repetitive behaviors in childhood continued to report difficulties in this domain 10 years later, and unfortunately, the authors observed a tendency for increases in the frequency and complexity of these behaviors in adolescence. In later studies, approximately 90% of autistic adolescents and adults reported continuing difficulties with repetitive behaviors (Seltzer et al. 2003, Howlin et al. 2004). Of interest, unusual preoccupations and complex stereotypies seemed to decrease (Seltzer et al. 2003). In retrospective studies, there was some evidence for improvement with age in this domain (Mesibov et al. 1989, Ballaban-Gil et al. 1996, Piven et al. 1996, Fecteau et al. 2003), but changes were not as prominent as the improvements noted in the social and language domains.

In summary, repetitive behaviors seem to be less likely to show significant improvement with age, although changes in the nature of the repetitive behaviors do seem to occur across the lifespan.

PROBLEMATIC BEHAVIORS

There are unfortunately very few data on the evolution of problematic behaviors in autism. Most of the outcome studies have focused on changes in the core symptom domains. However, often it is the problematic behaviors that bring a child into a physician's office, or prompt placement of an adult into a residential long term care facility or the prescription of heavy doses of psychotropic medications. In the cohort reported by Howlin et al. (2000), approximately half the patients were documented to have a severe behavioral disturbance. No other information regarding the nature and character of this disturbance was provided. In a retrospective study of 99 autistic adolescents and adults (Ballaban-Gil et al. 1996), problematic behaviors were defined to include tantrums, rages, aggression, self injury, and other socially unacceptable behaviors, excluding stereotypies. At the time of the evaluation, problematic behaviors were a continuing problem for two thirds of the autistic adolescents and adults. A third of the adolescents and 40% of the adults were receiving medication to control their behavior. Of the subjects whose parents had reported prior problematic behaviors in childhood, half reported an increased severity, a third were unchanged, and 20% were improved. There was no effect of gender on these behaviors except for self-injury, which was present in 65% of women vs 34% of men. Cognitive abilities did not seem to predict the occurrence of such problematic behaviors.

Overall, we do not have enough data to describe with certainty the developmental course of problematic behaviors in autism but it seems that they continue to remain a serious problem into adulthood.

COGNITION

Early prospective studies documented stability in cognitive function throughout the lifespan, including little change in verbal or performance IQ (Rutter et al. 1967). An interesting pattern emerges in more recent studies. Although the full IQ seems to be stable, there is a decline in the performance IQ accompanied by an increase in the verbal IQ (Mawhood et al. 2000, Howlin et al. 2004). In addition, although the mean changes in both studies were moderate, there was a subset of individuals who demonstrated considerable gains in their verbal IQs. In the first study, almost 50% of the sample showed an increase of more than 15 points (one standard deviation). Subjects who scored above 70 on performance/verbal IQ subscales showed the least change (Howlin et al. 2004). The significance of these changes is not yet known in terms of their ability to predict outcome, but given that early intervention has been the only intervention shown so far to increase IQ, these are of great interest.

ADAPTIVE OUTCOMES IN ADULTHOOD

A number of studies have examined the functional outcomes in adulthood of children with autism. In the first cohort to be reported (Kanner et al. 1973), almost all of the original autistic subjects were living either with their parents, or in supervised settings, state institutions or psychiatric hospitals. Still, 11% had secured employment of some form. Among the group overall, those with better communication skills had more favorable functional outcomes. In a series of systematic studies at about the same time describing a cohort of 63 individuals (Rutter et al. 1967), only 3 subjects were employed and the great majority were again living at home or under daily supervision. Fourteen per cent of this sample were described to have made a "good" social adjustment, defined as a near normal social life and independent functioning, whereas 61% were rated as having made a "poor" social adjustment. Later studies in the 1970s and eighties showed similar results with up to 14% of individuals rated as having made a "good" adjustment and approximately half the sample rated as having made a "poor adjustment" (Lotter 1974a, Gillberg and Steffenburg 1987). Starting in the 1990s, studies from Japan reported better outcomes, although these changes have not been consistently observed in most samples from North America and Europe. In two Japanese studies (Kobayashi et al. 1992, Kobayashi and Murata 1998), a quarter of the sample were judged to have "good" functional outcomes as indicated by employment and independence in daily activity; another 25% were shown to have a "fair" outcome, defined as no employment but relative independence in daily living skills, and approximately 50% had a "poor" outcome. However, in a British cohort (Howlin et al. 2000), reported soon after the second Japanese study, only 5% of individuals with autism were employed and 72% of the sample had little independence in daily living skills. Approximately half the sample lived in residential facilities and another 31% still lived with their parents. In a North American sample investigated by phone interview (Ballaban-Gil et al. 1996), only 11% had regular employment and that was usually in menial entry-level jobs. Another 16% were working in sheltered vocational settings. Approximately half the adults lived in residential placements. In this sample, even among adults with normal or near normal intelligence, 23% were living in supervised settings. Similarly, Venter et al. (1992) described a sample in which only 18% lived relatively independently. In this sample, a third of the subjects were competitively employed but again in menial jobs. Somewhat better outcomes were reported by Szatmari et al. (1989), in a sample of individuals with IQs above 90. In this group, a third had regular employment and half were completely independent. The discrepancies may reflect differences in economies or opportunities for disabled individuals in the respective countries and may not reflect true differences in the abilities of the samples reported.

Few adults with autistic disorder get married or have sexual relationships. Howlin et al. (2000) reported only one heterosexual relationship in a cohort of 19 adults. In a separate sample reported by the same group, three out of 68 individuals married (Howlin et al. 2004). Of the cohort reported by Szatmari et al. (1989), a quarter of the subjects had dated and one was married.

Lastly, in terms of education, the majority of people with autistic disorder spend their school life in the special educational system (Howlin et al. 2000). In a study that compared adults with Asperger syndrome to those with high functioning autism, approximately half of the Asperger individuals went to college as opposed to 24% of people with high functioning autism (Howlin 2003); however, higher education in the Asperger group did not translate into better eventual employment opportunities than those noted for the high functioning autism group.

Although it is very hard to compare these studies given major differences in original sample characteristics and outcome measures used, it is fair to conclude that at least half of the autistic patients studied thus far do not live independently, do not find work in competitive jobs, and few marry or have enduring partner relationships. Those who work tend to be employed at menial jobs, and higher education often does not translate into better job opportunities. However, 15–25% of individuals with autism, depending on the study, live an independent life. Predictors of possible favorable outcomes are discussed later in this chapter.

CRIMINAL BEHAVIOR IN ADULTHOOD

There have been several reports suggesting the presence of antisocial and aggressive behaviors in adults with ASDs (Mawson et al. 1985, Tantam 1988, Wolff 1991, Green et al. 2000). However, there are several methodological difficulties with such studies. The diagnosis of the patients reported is not always clear and ranges from "schizoid" personality to Asperger syndrome with body dysmorphic disorder features and hallucinations. In addition, these are mostly case series and case reports that are plagued by sampling and referral bias. Although some people with ASD do exhibit antisocial behaviors in adulthood, there are no epidemiologic studies to suggest increased rates of such behaviors in ASDs compared to the general population.

MEDICAL AND PSYCHIATRIC COMORBIDITY ISSUES

Until studies of comorbid medical conditions in autism, e.g. immune deficiencies, are carried out, no information will be available on their effects on quality of life and outcome, although it stands to reason that they could only worsen outlook.

The most comprehensive assessment of mortality risk in autism to date has been carried out by Shavelle et al. (2001), looking at patients enrolled in California's neurodevelopmental disabilities service system between 1983 and 1997. Among individuals with autism, mortality was at its highest among 5- to 10-year-olds (Standard Mortality Ratio [SMR] = 5.4) and lowest (SMR = 2.1) among those over 20 years of age. Mental retardation and the presence of seizures seem to place individuals with autism at an increased risk for death. Indeed, seizures were a major risk factor for death in adulthood, although it should be noted that in the general population excess mortality in epilepsy is now well documented (Sander 2003). The discussion of epilepsy in Chapters 10 and 11 does not mention mortality because reliable data are not available, except for anecdotal reports and clinical impressions that epilepsy, as one would expect, contributes significantly to the heightened mortality in autism.

Prevalence estimates for affective and anxiety disorders in this population although available, need to be considered within the scope of the difficulty of making these types of diagnosis in individuals with autism. Rumsey et al. (1985) found evidence for generalized anxiety (50%), separation anxiety (14%), phobia (7%), obsessional thinking (29%) and compulsions (21%) in a group of young adults with a history of autistic disorder. Severe anxiety symptoms are present in up to 85% of children with autism (Muris et al. 1998). Estimates for the prevalence of affective disorders are as high as 64%; for depression specifically, the prevalence estimates are as high as 28% (Ghaziuddin et al. 2002, Howlin 2002). The risk of depression seems to increase with age. Initially, retrospective studies had suggested that the risk of schizophrenia may be increased in autism (Petty et al. 1984), although studies of larger samples (Volkmar and Cohen 1991) and prospective studies (Howlin et al. 2000) have failed to replicate these initial findings.

Overall, it seems that people with autism have higher mortality rates than the general population, and major risk factors include mental retardation and seizure disorder. In addition individuals with autism have an increased prevalence of affective and anxiety disorders, but most likely are not at increased risk for psychotic disorders (Seltzer et al. 2004). Long term prospective studies are required to further characterize these relationships.

FACTORS PREDICTING OUTCOME

The evidence for factors predicting long term outcomes in autism is limited but relatively consistent. Of the variables examined, language and IQ seem to account for most but not all of the variance observed. In one of the original prospective studies (Rutter et al. 1967), the higher the IQ the better the outcomes studied in adolescence. IQs over 50 were predictive of better adaptive skills in a study by Gillberg and Steffenburg (1987), and in a recent study children who had performance IQs above 70 were more likely to be employed and have friends in adulthood (Howlin et al. 2004). However, in a separate cohort studied by the same group, it was verbal and not performance IQ that mostly predicted better adaptive outcomes (Howlin et al. 2000). Early language has long been postulated to be predictive of better outcomes in adulthood. In the original cohort studies by Kanner, better outcomes were observed with adults who had better early language skills. Follow-up studies have repeatedly shown that absent or poor non-social language at age 5–6 years is associated with poor outcomes in adulthood (Rutter et al. 1967, Gillberg and Steffenburg 1987). In a prospective study of 19 high functioning autistic men (Howlin et al. 2000), childhood scores on a test of receptive language (PPVT) accounted for a third of the variability in a composite score of adult functioning that included language and social competence, repetitive behaviors and independence. Other predictor variables such as gender, residential and educational placements, psychiatric and associated medical disorders and social support have been occasionally examined but without showing consistent results.

There are no long term studies to examine the effect of early intervention on adult outcomes. However, data from cohorts reported in the 1990s suggests better academic achievement compared to data from cohorts reported earlier (Venter et al. 1992). Although there may be various explanations for this, such as changes in diagnostic criteria, exposure to structured academic and psychosocial interventions at an early age is also likely associated with such improvements. It should be noted, however, that for these later cohorts the gains seemed to be limited to academic achievement. Prospective studies that account for intensity, duration and type of interventions are necessary to properly examine the impact of early intervention in long-term functional outcomes.

Lastly, there have been some reports based on clinical observations that some people with ASDs manage to use a circumscribed interest in a functional way (Kanner 1973, Howlin and Rutter 1987). However, others seem to have a perfectly usable skill within their circumscribed interests that never becomes functional. More research is required to fully explore the role of potentially functional circumscribed interests in predicting long term functional outcomes.

CONCLUSIONS AND FUTURE RESEARCH

In summary, although the literature is plagued with methodological problems, it is apparent that children with autism improve as a group into adolescence and adulthood. These changes are at best modest and there is great heterogeneity in possible outcomes. Of particular interest is the small group (15–25%) of autistic patients who function in the normal range in adulthood. Study of the possible factors that may have influenced these outcomes will be invaluable for influencing the design of novel interventions in early childhood. Further research of problematic behaviors will also be of great importance given that such behaviors are a major cause of morbidity and do not seem as a whole to improve in adulthood. Given that most children are currently receiving intensive early intervention, we will probably not get any further data on the natural history of the core symptom domains of autism except for the study of possible outcomes in middle adulthood or beyond. Anecdotal reports have suggested that some older adults diagnosed with personality disorders actually meet criteria for Asperger syndrome or high functioning autism, but a detailed and accurate developmental history is rarely obtained in adult psychiatric settings. Prospective studies into late adulthood will be of great interest given that autism is a lifespan disorder with relatively little reduction in life expectancy, but very little is currently known about the phenomenology of the disease at later stages in the lifespan. Additionally, there is increasing evidence for the effectiveness of early intervention in autism. Given the cost and time commitment of these interventions, we urgently need prospective randomized trials and longitudinal long term studies of their effectiveness.

The explosion of research studies reported on autism in the last 10 years is very encouraging. Further effort is required so that large multicenter trials with appropriate sample sizes, appropriate control groups when required (normal controls vs controls with other developmental disabilities), and common outcome measures that address the core deficits and other concerns of autistic individuals can be initiated so that studies can be comparable and meaningful to ongoing care provisions for this population.

REFERENCES

Aman MG, Novotny S, Samango-Sprouse C, Lecavalier L, Leonard E, Gadow KD, King BH, Pearson DA, Gernsbacher MA, Chez M (2004) Outcome measures for clinical drug trials in autism. *CNS Spectr* 9: 36–47.

Ballaban-Gil K, Rapin I, Tuchman R, Shinnar S (1996) Longitudinal examination of the behavioral, language, and social changes in a population of adolescents and young adults with autistic disorder. *Pediatr Neurol* 15: 217–23.

Boelte S, Poustka F (2000) Diagnosis of autism: the connection between current and historical information. *Autism* 4: 38290.

Constantino JN, Davis SA, Todd RD, Schindler MK, Gross MM, Brophy SL, Metzger LM,

Shoushtari CS, Splinter R, Reich W (2003) Validation of a brief quantitative measure of autistic traits: comparison of the Social Responsiveness Scale with the Autism Diagnostic Interview Revised. *J Autism Dev Disord* 33: 427–33.

Dunn LM (1970) *Peabody Picture Vocabulary Test – Revised.* Circle Pines, MN: American Guidance Service.

Fecteau S, Mottron L, Bertiaume C, Burack JA (2003) Developmental changes of autistic symptoms. *Autism* 7: 255–68.

Ghaziuddin M, Ghaziuddin N, Greden J (2002) Depression in persons with autism: implications for research and clinical care. *J Autism Dev Disord* 32: 299–306.

Gilberg C, Steffenburg S (1987) Outcome and prognostic factors in infantile autism and similar conditions: a population-based study of 46 cases followed through puberty. *J Autism Dev Disord* 17: 273–87.

Green J, Gilchrest A, Burton D, Cox A (2000) Social and psychiatric functioning in adolescents with Asperger's syndrome compared with conduct disorder. *J Autism Dev Disord* 30: 279–93.

Howlin P (2002) Autistic disorders. In: Howlin P, Udwin O, eds. *Outcomes in Neurodevelopmental and Genetic Disorders.* Cambridge: Cambridge University Press, pp.136–68.

Howlin P (2003) Outcome in high-functioning adults with autism with and without language delays: Implications for the differentiation between autism and Asperger syndrome. *J Autism Dev Disord* 33: 3–13.

Howlin P, Rutter M (1987) *Treatment of Autistic Children.* Chichester, W Sussex: Wiley.

Howlin P, Udwin O, Davies M (1998) Cognitive functioning in adults with Williams syndrome. *J Child Psychol Psychiatry* 35: 183–90.

Howlin P, Mawhood L, Rutter M (2000) Autism and developmental receptive language disorder – a follow up comparison in early adult life. II: Social, behavioral, and psychiatric outcomes. *J Child Psychol Psychiatry* 41: 561–78.

Howlin P, Goode S, Hutton J, Rutter M (2004) Adult outcome in children with autism. *J Child Psychol Psychiatry* 45: 212–29.

Janicki M, Jacobson J (1983) Selected clinical features and service characteristics of autistic adults. *Psychol Rep* 52: 387–90.

Kanner L (1973) *Childhood Psychosis: Initial Studies and New Insights.* New York: Plenum Press.

Kobayashi R, Murata T (1998) Behavioral characteristics of 187 young adults with autism. *Psychiatry Clin Neurosci* 52: 383–90.

Kobayashi R, Murata T, Yoshiga K (1992) A follow-up study of 201 children with autism in Hyushu and Yamaguchi areas, Japan. *J Autism Dev Disord* 22: 395–411.

Lotter V (1974) Social adjustment and placement of autistic children in Middlesex: a follow-up study. *J Autism Child Schizophr* 4: 11–32.

Lord C, Rutter M, Le Couteur A (1994) Autism Diagnostic Interview-Revised: A revised version of a diagnostic interview for caregivers of individuals with possible pervasive developmental disorders. *J Autism Dev Disord* 24: 659–85.

Lord C, Risi S, Lambrecht L, Cook EH, Leventhal BL, DiLavore PC, Pickles A, Rutter M (2000) The Autism Observation Schedule–Generic: A standard measure of social and communication deficits associated with the spectrum of autism. *J Autism Dev Disord* 30: 205–23.

Matson JL (1990) *Matson Evaluation of Social Skills with Youngsters (MESSY).* Worthington, OH: IDS Publishing.

Mawhood L, Howlin P, Rutter M (2000) Autism and developmental receptive language disorder— a comparative follow-up in early adult life. I: Cognitive and language outcomes. *J Child Psychol Psychiatry* 41: 547–59.

Mawson D, Grounds A, Tantam D (1985) Violence and Asperger's syndrome: a case study. *Br J Psychiatry* 147: 566–9.

Mesibov GB, Schopler E, Schaffer B, Michal N (1989) Use of the childhood autism rating scale with autistic adolescents and adults. *J Acad Child Adolesc Psychiatry* 28: 538–41.

Mundy P, Hogan A (1996) *A Preliminary Manual for the Abridged Early Social Communication Scales (ESCS).* Coral Gables, FL: University of Miami Press.

Muris P, Steerneman P, Merckelbach H, Holdrinet I, Meesters C (1998) Comorbid anxiety symptoms in children with pervasive developmental disorders. *J Anxiety Disord* 12: 387–93.

Nordin V, Gillberg C (1998) The long term course of autistic disorders: Update on follow up studies. *Acta Psychiatr Scand* 97: 99–108.

Orsmond GI, Krauss MW, Seltzer MM (2004) Peer relationships and social and recreational activities among adolescents and adults with autism. *J Autism Dev Disord* 34: 245–56.

Petty LK, Ornitz EM, Michelman JD, Zimmerman EG (1984) Autistic children who become schizophrenic. *Arch Gen Psychiatry* 41: 129–35.

Piven J, Harper J, Palmer P, Arndt S (1996) Course of behavioral change in autism: a retrospective study of high IQ adolescents and adults. *J Am Acad Child Adolesc Psychiatry* 35: 523–9.

Rumsey JM, Rapoport JL, Sceery WR (1985) Autistic children as adults: psychiatric, social, and behavioral outcomes. *J Am Acad Child Psychiatry* 24: 465–73.

Rutter M, Greenfeld D, Lockyer L (1967) A five to fifteen year follow-up study of infantile psychosis. II. Social and behavioral outcome. *Br J Psychiatry* 113: 1183–99.

Sander JW (2003) The epidemiology of epilepsy revisited. *Curr Opin Neurol* 16: 165–70.

Seltzer MM, Wyngaarden Krauss M, Shattuck PT, Orsmond G, Swe A, Lord C (2003) The symptoms of autism spectrum disorders in adolescence and adulthood. *J Autism Dev Disord* 33: 565–81.

Seltzer MM, Shattuck P, Abbebuto L, Greenberg JS (2004) Trajectory of development in adolescents and adults with autism. *Ment Retard Dev Disabil Res Rev* 10: 234–47.

Shavelle RM, Strauss D, Pickett J (2001) Causes of death in autism. *J Autism Dev Disord* 31: 569–76.

Sparrow SS, Balla DA, Cicchetti DV (1984) *Vineland Adaptive Behavior Scales: A Revision of the Vineland Social Maturity Scale by Edgar Doll.* Circle Pines, MN: American Guidance Service.

Szatmari P, Bartolucci G, Bremner R, Bond S, Rich S (1989) A follow-up study of high-functioning autistic children. *J Autism Dev Disord* 19: 213–25.

Tantam D (1988) Lifelong eccentricity and social isolation. I: Psychiatric, social and forensic aspects. *Br J Psychiatry* 153: 777–82.

Venter A, Lord C, Schopler E (1992) A follow-up study of high-functioning autistic children. *J Child Psychol Psychiatry* 33: 489–507.

Volkmar FR, Cohen DJ (1991) Comorbid association of autism and schizophrenia. *Am J Psychiatry* 148: 1705-1707.

Wing L (1997) The autistic spectrum. *Lancet* 350: 1761–6.

Wolff S (1991) "Schizoid" personality in childhood and adulthood. II: Adult adjustment and the continuity with schizotypal personality disorder. *Br J Psychiatry* 159: 620–9.

19

WHAT WE HAVE LEARNED, WHERE WE NEED TO GO

Roberto F Tuchman and Isabelle Rapin

The preceding chapters provide a clinical and neurobiological panorama of autism in 2006. They show that our current clinical understanding has filled in and refined, but not altered in any fundamental way, the description of this developmental disorder of children that Kanner and Asperger provided six decades ago. Both were aware that the syndrome they were describing varied in its severity and in its surprisingly uneven cognitive and behavioral consequences. Both were impressed with evidence of its familial roots but were uncertain, as we still are, of how much of the familiality might be linked to biologic and how much to more tenuous parental personality factors and their sociologic circumstances. Both were aware that the autism spectrum disorders (ASDs) were persistent, but Asperger especially noted that they were not necessarily completely intractable and that appropriate educational intervention helped some children. The start made in the last two decades toward gaining an understanding of the brain basis of autism required multidisciplinary progress in the neurosciences that no one working six decades ago could have imagined.

Autism has evolved into a powerful clinical and research tool for investigating and highlighting the complexities of brain–behavior relationships, but it also illustrates how very difficult it is to map complex behaviors onto specific brain systems. It shows that it is essential that the clinical and research strategies adopted to advance understanding of autism be both broad and specific. From a clinical perspective, we have become aware that we need to cast a wide net to capture the entire spectrum of individuals with ASDs, while at the same time we must use our growing knowledge about biological systems to generate testable hypotheses to answer specific questions. It is remarkable how much autism and related disorders have become part of the neurosciences in the 21st century. Autism now holds an important place in the practice of neurology and especially of child neurology.

Clinical management of children with ASDs requires a diverse team of professionals that includes not only child neurologists but also experts in communication, neuropharmacology, neuropsychology, psychiatry, education, sensorimotor function and child development. Autism research as well requires the expertise of a broad range of disciplines such as genetics, neuropathology, neuroradiology, neurophysiology, neurochemistry, neuroimmunology and epidemiology. There remain many questions begging for answers as we pursue our understanding of autism.

In concluding this monograph, we would like to highlight three broad questions, each with clinical and research implications, which child neurologists working with children with autism will need to confront over the next decade. The first question that still challenges all clinicians and researchers working with autism is how to go about developing a more precise typology of autism. This question hinges on the prevalence and causes of autism. Answers to the prevalence question are essential first steps toward defining risk factors linked to its development. Defining the typology of autism and its subtypes is essential if we hope to map very specific behaviors to their corresponding neural networks. The second question is how much do we really know about the neurology and, specifically, the etiologies of autism? This question is a central one for child neurologists interested in autism. Despite the recent progress in our understanding of the genetic and acquired etiologies of autism, we need to acknowledge its limitations for illuminating the autism phenotype. Both of these questions lead us to an obvious third question which is: what do we really know about the effectiveness of interventions in children with autism, and can interventions at a critical stage of development have a genuinely positive impact on the outcome of autism? It is evident that devising more effective interventions and understanding their consequences requires a much deeper knowledge of the pathophysiology of autism.

We will discuss these questions within the framework of developmental neurology by addressing specifically the issue of what we know and what still must be learned about the typology, etiology and pathophysiology of autism. We have no doubt that the strategies used to answer these questions, that is, the way we frame testable hypotheses, will determine how much progress we make in our understanding of brain–behavior relationships in autism.

QUESTION 1: IS THERE IN FACT MORE AUTISM? – THE TYPOLOGY OF AUTISM

It is now amply documented and widely accepted that the rate at which autism is diagnosed has escalated over the past two decades. Does this mean that the prevalence of the biologic disorder has increased? The evidence suggests that increased awareness, earlier diagnosis, broadening of the diagnostic criteria, and access to many new educational interventions are factors each of which has contributed to the increase in reported rates of autism. The criteria for a diagnosis of autism are behavioral, have changed over time, and are limited by the lack of biological markers specific to the ASDs. These factors, together with the heterogeneous nature of their phenotypes, make the investigation of whether there is in fact more autism very difficult. Furthermore there is no guarantee that an answer to this question will substantially advance our understanding of autism. From a scientific perspective, the more instructive question is not whether there is a rise in the prevalence of autism but whether we can identify novel causal factors that contribute to the rise.

We now know that the etiologies of autism are complex. A robust research finding is that heredity plays a major causal role by the impact of the many genes that control early fetal brain development. The heightened risk of autism in families with traits such as developmental language disorders, bipolar and obsessive–compulsive disorders, among others, provides clear evidence for multigenetic influences (Larsson et al. 2005). But there is equally compelling evidence that prenatal environmental factors such as viral infections like rubella and cytomegalovirus (CMV), and probably yet to be identified others, are causal in some children with autism. On the other hand, evidence for some other suspected environmental risk factors, notably vaccines or certain toxins, as culprits for the alleged increase in the incidence of autism can now be definitively dismissed. This is not to say that specific as yet unknown environmental risk factors for the development of autism do not exist. We need to focus future epidemiological studies on both genetic and environmental factors that can identify children who will go on to have autism from those who will not, and also from those who will develop other developmental disorders. In addition, it will be equally important for epidemiological research to focus on protective factors that ensure normal neurological development.

Important steps for understanding causal factors related to autism require systematic documentation of the earliest signs of autism and the testing of specific hypotheses regarding their underlying neurodevelopmental substrates. Several investigators are currently engaged in longitudinal studies of high-risk infants, all of whom have an older sibling diagnosed with an ASD. These studies suggest that by 12 months of age some of the siblings who are later diagnosed with autism may be distinguishable from unaffected siblings and from controls with low risk for autism (Zwaigenbaum et al. 2005). Unfortunately, sibs' shared genes and environments limit the prospect of identifying unique causal factors in autism from even this unique population.

It is important to study children with mental retardation with and without autism because, although mental retardation is not a defining feature of autism, it coexists in a substantial proportion of children on the spectrum. Cognitive ability as reflected by the intelligence quotient is predictive of outcome, although outcome is variable even in ASD children with IQ scores above 70 (Howlin et al. 2004). Research indicates that at least 40% of individuals with severe to moderate retardation meet behavioral criteria for autism (Shah et al. 1982). It will be instructive to determine how the 60% of individuals with severe to moderate mental retardation who do not meet behavioral criteria for autism differ neurologically from those who are on the spectrum.

A potentially instructive example of severe mental retardation without autism is Cockayne syndrome, which arises as the consequence of any one of several recessive gene mutations (Rapin et al. 2000). The brains of these children are presumably normal at birth but fail to grow adequately postnatally and later degenerate because of a severe progressive leukodystrophy causing significant motor – including cerebellar – signs that reflect white matter and neuronal pathology (Soffer et al. 1979, Lindenbaum et al. 2001). How can it be, in the face of a disease with such widespread effects on brain development and maintenance that the brain weighs only a third to a half of expectation, that the children remain notoriously cheerful and interactive? Why do these children not have the autism phenotype, given such devastatingly abnormally brains?

Rett syndrome provides another important example of our primitive understanding of the brain conditions associated with autism. Its gene and molecular effects are known but its somatic effects remain poorly understood. For a finite period of time in late infancy and very early childhood, most girls with Rett syndrome meet criteria for autism. In contrast to children with classic autism, many of these girls lose their aloofness and become interactive and sociable despite failure of brain growth, severe mental retardation, lack of speech and unremitting hand stereotypies.

Study of the networks that are spared despite profoundly abnormal brains in individuals with disorders such as Cockayne syndrome, who are conspicuously non-autistic, and Rett syndrome, in whom autistic traits are often transient, may shed light on classic autism by telling us something about the timing of the brain damage or maldevelopment that underlies autism. Better understanding of the interaction between background genes and the specific genes or other brain pathologies causative of autism may also help uncover the neurobiologic basis of its symptomatology (Glaze 2004).

Increased awareness of the breadth of their symptomatology has led to an inevitable expansion of diagnostic criteria for the ASDs. The research community, but not yet most of the public, now understands that autism is not a categorical diagnosis, inasmuch as all of the symptoms in the three behavioral domains that define it are dimensional. Yes, a minority of autism's potential *etiologies*, for example congenital rubella, tuberous sclerosis or fragile-X, are indeed categorical. But it is well established that none of these categorical etiologies is invariably associated with autism, which indicates that what counts phenotypically is not etiology per se. Rather, what does count is what networks in the individual's brain are dysfunctional, whether the dysfunction arises from fortuitous damage, or genetic or nongenetic atypical development. Also, whether an accidental insult like preterm birth or a gene or combination of genes known to influence brain development will cause an autistic phenotype depends on the genetic background of the individual, inasmuch as these background genes modulate the phenotypic consequences of the responsible mutation or acquired brain lesion.

As there is no biological marker for autism, the clinician's role should not end with the diagnosis of autism but should in fact begin there. What are needed are meticulous descriptions of the particular social, language and repetitive behaviors of each diagnosed child. There is not one type of social, language or motor deficit unique to all children with ASDs. It is these differential aspects of autism that will help define specific subgroups and provide discrete behavioral correlates that can be mapped onto brain structure and function. To answer definitively the question of whether there is more autism today, we will need to define the typology of autism so that we can relate the complex behaviors that define this behavioral syndrome to both the risk factors and neurological substrates causally related to the ASDs.

QUESTION 2: WHAT IS THE NEUROLOGY OF AUTISM? – ETIOLOGIES OF AUTISM

The one research finding that all investigators are likely to agree on is that there is no one cause for autism. Autism is not only heterogeneous phenotypically, it is also a developmental disorder that brain maturation changes over time; how it changes varies among children in ways that likely reflect each individual's biology. Although defining valid subgroups of individuals with autism has been an elusive task, it is a crucial next step for advancing our understanding of autism.

Determining which of the now documented neurological findings that occur in autism are specific or unique to autism (or to any one of its many potential etiologies) will require research on specific subgroups and dimensions of autism, using innovative research strategies. For example, there is a suggestion that repetitive behaviors in autism (motor stereotypies) and, perhaps, resistance to change may be linked to specific aspects of the serotonin neurotransmitter system (Coon et al. 2005) and to neuroanatomical abnormalities, specifically volumes of the right caudate and total putamen (Hollander et al. 2005). For these types of studies to advance knowledge requires the inclusion of well matched control groups of normally developed individuals and, equally importantly, the inclusion of non-autistic developmentally impaired subjects who share either the behaviors of interest or similar underlying brain pathologies. This second type of controls may help to show how unique to the broader autism phenotype any findings really are. For example, in one of our studies of the relationship of autism to epilepsy, it became clear that the major risk factor for epilepsy in autism is the degree of cognitive and motor deficit. Unexpectedly, however, including a group of children with language disorders without autism made it clear that language dysfunction was in and of itself a risk factor for epilepsy (Tuchman et al. 1991). More specifically the study suggested that the more severe the receptive language deficit in children with autism without significant cognitive deficit and in those with language disorder, the more likely the child was to have epilepsy.

We need studies that quantify specific aspects of the social deficit in autism and then link these deficits to specific brain regions or neural networks. It is likely that breakthroughs in the genetics and neurobiology of autism will come from identifying and applying quantitative techniques to the assessment of rigorously defined aspects of several dimensions of autism (endophenotypes) (McCauley et al. 2005). Breakthroughs are much less likely to come from studying large heterogeneously affected populations.

We know more about symptoms that coexist with autism than about its etiologies. For example, a disorder like epilepsy is common in certain subgroups of children with autism, even though it is controversial whether or how often epilepsy is the primary cause of their autism (Deonna and Roulet-Perez 2005). Furthermore, although a number of etiologies of autism are known, their pathogenic role in autism or in specific subgroups of individuals with autism is not understood. The most robust neuroanatomical finding in autism is the tendency toward unusually large brains in young autistic children (Woodhouse et al. 1996; Courchesne et al. 2003, 2004), but we do not know whether early brain overgrowth followed by premature slowing of growth is a primary or secondary consequence of the disorder. The same is true of less robust findings such as the changes in neocortical minicolumns (Casanova et al. 2002) and neurotransmitters (Lam et al. 2005), or observations such as neuroinflammatory findings recently described in autistic brains (Vargas et al. 2005).

The case has been made that genetic studies are our best hope for understanding what is the primary cause versus the consequence in autism (Veenstra-Vanderweele et al. 2004). Although there may be some truth to this view, we have stressed repeatedly that, among the many identifiable genetic disorders that are causal in autism, not one is invariably associated with the autistic phenotype. The number of genes of etiological importance in autism is unknown, but we already know that they are many. We are currently learning that the orchestration of brain development is even more complex than heretofore appreciated. In addition, it is the products of the genes and not the genes themselves that are responsible for the behavioral characteristics of autism. Studies will need to be conducted using new techniques such as the proteomic approach for identifying protein abnormalities due to aberrant gene expression or the timing of gene expression in the brains of individuals with autism (Junaid et al. 2004). A further complication is that the effects of the identical protein product of an aberrant (or normal) gene may vary in different biological environments. Despite the fact that so-called idiopathic autism is now known to be a highly heritable disorder associated with an atypical pattern of brain growth, there is also compelling evidence that various biological and environmental factors contribute to the causation of autism. Emotional stresses, if their timing is right, can profoundly influence behavior and even trigger autistic regression in some vulnerable children (Kurita et al. 1992); their expression reflects altered neurotransmission, and it seems they may even disrupt maturational programs responsible for major brain structures (Vermeulen et al. 2005). The inescapable conclusion is that many different types of mechanisms besides single gene modulated perturbations of brain development influence the autism phenotype.

QUESTION 3: WHAT DO WE KNOW ABOUT THE ROLE OF INTERVENTIONS ON THE OUTCOME OF CHILDREN WITH AUTISM? – THE PATHOPHYSIOLOGY OF AUTISM

Information on the effects of interventions in autism is extremely limited. Developing an understanding of the pathophysiology of autism is critical for designing rational medical and educational interventions. The reality is that we know very little about the natural history of specific subgroups of children with autism. From a clinical perspective, there are children with autism who despite little if any intervention have good outcomes, and then there are those who receive intensive intervention whose outcome is dismal. It seems that the biological potential of an individual, as reflected by his or her cognitive status, is the final determinant of outcome.

There is no doubt that appropriate behavioral and educational interventions have a positive impact on the developmental trajectory of *all* children with autism. In addition, medications can ameliorate specific symptoms and are required to enable the integration of some individuals into educational and family settings. Nevertheless, neither pharmacological nor non-pharmacological interventions are a cure for autism. Their impact on the outcome of the majority of children with autism is at best modest, especially with regard to the core symptoms of language and social skills.

Effective medical treatments will require the development of biomarkers linked to specific functions in the brain that can be related to specific aspects of the autistic phenotype. There never will be one treatment for autism. The best we can hope for is to understand the pathophysiology of homogeneous subgroups of children well enough to enable the development of empirically based treatments for each of them. The aim of pharmacological treatment in autism is to ameliorate coexisting symptoms such as anxiety, mood disorders, aggressivity, self-injury, impaired attention and inadequate impulse control. Understanding the pathophysiology of each of these associated disorders will enhance our ability to treat them specifically, but this may not be sufficient when they occur in autistic individuals because they may be differentially influenced by biological factors unique to autism. Future research on the pathophysiology of autism needs to focus not only on whether there is a social deficit or a language deficit in a child on the spectrum, but also on the specific type of social or language deficit, because they are likely to require quite different interventions.

It remains unclear how even unequivocally organic correlates of autism such as large brain and white matter volumes fit into a coherent pathophysiological explanation. Autism is a disorder that affects the processing and integration of multiple simultaneously activated brain circuits (Welsh et al. 2005, Just et al. 2004); but which processing components are dysfunctional and how this leads to the phenotype of autism remains to be elucidated. Specifically testable hypotheses regarding the particular computational disturbances that characterize specific subgroups of children with ASDs must be generated; they need to address discrete neuropsychological deficits in their social and communicative skills. Clever paradigms to map these deficits onto brain structure and function using state of the art imaging and neurophysiological tools will be required. To be fully informative, functional techniques will need to be applied both before and after specific interventions. They will need to be repeated later to determine whether any observed changes attributable to the intervention are transient or permanent and whether they survive the cessation of active intervention. Although this type of study has been carried out in children with dyslexia and attention deficit disorders (Aylward et al. 2003, Shafritz et al. 2004), it has yet to be performed in children with autism.

Complicating this type of research is the likelihood that multiple biological routes may lead to the same behavioral disturbance, inasmuch as all complex behaviors depend on activity in complex distributed neural networks vulnerable to diverse types of pathologies at multiple potential sites. The previously quoted complex interrelationship between genetics, neurodevelopment and epilepsy in the tuberous sclerosis complex (TSC) exemplifies the difficulty in attempting to unravel the pathophysiology of autism. Although seizures and mental retardation are definite risk factors for the development of an autism spectrum disorder in TSC, neither is sufficient or necessary for its development (Asano et al. 2001, Bolton 2004).

Until we have more objective criteria, there will be disagreement among experts as to the appropriate label for children with different deficits pointing to an ASD. The autism label, as is the case for the cerebral palsy, epilepsy and dementia labels, refers to a group of disorders with many distinct etiologies. The utility of the autism label is that it provides a useful social-medical term to refer to children and adults with social deficits (Krageloh-Mann 2005). If we are ever to reduce the current vagueness and disagreements in this field, we cannot overemphasize the importance of using common behavioral diagnostic criteria, and of the need for rigorous biologic, behavioral, and longitudinal multidisciplinary research that crosses institutions and even countries and cultures.

FINAL PERSPECTIVE

This book shows that, although we have made a significant start toward unraveling the causes of autism and their multiple impacts on the developing brain, these advances have yet to be translated into either prevention or specific treatments. As we proceed toward answers to the three broad questions posed in this chapter, we believe it likely that we will identify numerous subgroups that will define the *autisms*, and that we will speak of the autisms in the same manner that we now speak of the epilepsies or the dementias. The approaches we use to identify subgroups within the autisms will probably be similar to those we used to define the epilepsies in that they will rely on both clinical criteria and neurobiologic markers. Among etiologic and neurobiologic markers, some will define proteins that affect axonal guidance, synaptic receptors, neurotransmitters or modulators, and the organization of widespread functional networks; others will shed light on symptomatology and on reasons for the effectiveness of serendipitously discovered useful interventions, be they pharmacological or educational. The creation of homogenous subgroups with specific biological markers and quantification of the different dimensional deficits of autism, such as those of sociability, language and the stereotypies, will at last support the development of rational medical and educational interventions. The role of the neurologist, working hand in hand with other clinicians and educators on the one hand and with a broad cadre of basic scientists and investigators of human brain imaging and neurophysiology on the other, will be to make sure that these empirically guided tools are widely used to continue to delineate the neural underpinnings of autism. We need to make sure to use our new biologic knowledge in ongoing dialogues with scientists of all relevant disciplines in order to help define new testable hypotheses. In this way we can play a role in advancing the understanding of the ASDs and finding new ways to help our patients become optimally functioning adults.

REFERENCES

Asano E, Chugani DC, Muzik O, Behen M, Janisse J, Rothermel R, Mangner TJ, Chakraborty PK, Chugani HT (2001) Autism in tuberous sclerosis complex is related to both cortical and subcortical dysfunction. *Neurology* 57: 1269–77.

Aylward EH, Richards TL, Berninger VW, Nagy WE, Field KM, Grimme AC, Richards AL, Thomson JB, Cramer SC (2003) Instructional treatment associated with changes in brain activation in children with dyslexia. *Neurology* 61: 212–9.

Bolton PF (2004) Neuroepileptic correlates of autistic symptomatology in tuberous sclerosis. *Ment Retard Dev Disabil Res Rev* 10: 126–31.

Casanova MF, Buxhoeveden DP, Switala AE, Roy E (2002) Minicolumnar pathology in autism. *Neurology* 58: 428–32.

Coon H, Dunn D, Lainhart J, Miller J, Hamil C, Battaglia A, Tancredi R, Leppert MF, Weiss R, McMahon W (2005) Possible association between autism and variants in the brain-expressed tryptophan hydroxylase gene (TPH2). *Am J Med Genet B Neuropsychiatr Genet* 135: 42–6.

Courchesne E, Carper R, Akshoomoff N (2003) Evidence of brain overgrowth in the first year of life in autism. *JAMA* 290: 337–44.

Courchesne E, Redcay E, Kennedy DP (2004) The autistic brain: birth through adulthood. *Curr Opin Neurol* 17: 489–96.

Deonna T, Roulet-Perez E (2005) *Cognitive and Behavioural Disorders of Epileptic Origin in Children. Clinics in Developmental Medicine No. 168.* London: Mac Keith Press.

Glaze DG (2004) Rett syndrome: of girls and mice—lessons for regression in autism. *Ment Retard Dev Disabil Res Rev* 10: 154–58.

Hollander E, Anagnostou E, Chaplin W, Esposito K, Haznedar MM, Licalzi E, Wasserman S, Soorya L, Buchsbaum M (2005) Striatal volume on magnetic resonance imaging and repetitive behaviors in autism. *Biol Psychiatry* 58: 226–32.

Howlin P, Goode S, Hutton J, Rutter M (2004) Adult outcome for children with autism. *J Child Psychol Psychiatry* 45: 212–29.

Junaid MA, Kowal D, Barua M, Pullarkat PS, Sklower Brooks S, Pullarkat RK (2004) Proteomic studies identified a single nucleotide polymorphism in glyoxalase I as autism susceptibility factor. *Am J Med Genet A* 131: 11–7.

Just MA, Cherkassky VL, Keller TA, Minshew NJ (2004) Cortical activation and synchronization during sentence comprehension in high-functioning autism: evidence of underconnectivity. *Brain* 127: 1811–21.

Krageloh-Mann I (2005) Cerebral palsy: towards developmental neuroscience. *Dev Med Child Neurol* 47: 435 (editorial).

Kurita H, Kita M, Miyake Y (1992) A comparative study of development and symptoms among disintegrative psychosis and infantile autism with and without speech loss. *J Autism Dev Disord* 22: 175-188.

Lam KS, Aman MG, Arnold LE (2005) Neurochemical correlates of autistic disorder: A review of the literature. *Res Dev Disabil* (epub ahead of print).

Larsson HJ, Eaton WW, Madsen KM, Vestergaard M, Olesen AV, Agerbo E, Schendel D, Thorsen P, Mortensen PB (2005) Risk factors for autism: perinatal factors, parental psychiatric history, and socioeconomic status. *Am J Epidemiol* 161: 916–25; discussion 926–8.

Lindenbaum Y, Dickson D, Rosenbaum P, Kraemer K, Robbins I, Rapin I (2001) Xeroderma pigmentosum/Cockayne syndrome complex: first neuropathological study and review of eight other cases. *Eur J Paediatr Neurol* 5: 225–42.

McCauley JL, Li C, Jiang L, Olson LM, Crockett G, Gainer K, Folstein SE, Haines JL, Sutcliffe

JS (2005) Genome-wide and Ordered-Subset linkage analyses provide support for autism loci on 17q and 19p with evidence of phenotypic and interlocus genetic correlates. *BMC Med Genet* 6: 1.

Rapin I, Lindenbaum Y, Dickson DW, Kraemer KH, Robbins JH (2000) Cockayne syndrome and xeroderma pigmentosum. *Neurology* 55: 1442–9.

Shafritz KM, Marchione KE, Gore JC, Shaywitz SE, Shaywitz BA (2004) The effects of methylphenidate on neural systems of attention in attention deficit hyperactivity disorder. *Am J Psychiatry* 161: 1990–7.

Shah A, Holmes N, Wing L (1982) Prevalence of autism and related conditions in adults in a mental handicap hospital. *Appl Res Ment Retard* 3: 303–17.

Soffer D, Grotsky HW, Rapin I, Suzuki K (1979) Cockayne syndrome: unusual neuropathological findings and review of the literature. *Ann Neurol* 6: 340–8.

Tuchman RF, Rapin I, Shinnar S (1991) Autistic and dysphasic children. II: Epilepsy. *Pediatrics* 88: 1219–25.

Vargas DL, Nascimbene C, Krishnan C, Zimmerman AW, Pardo CA (2005) Neuroglial activation and neuroinflammation in the brain of patients with autism. *Ann Neurol* 57: 67-81.

Veenstra-Vanderweele J, Christian SL, Cook EH (2004) Autism as a paradigmatic complex genetic disorder. *Annu Rev Genomics Hum Genet* 5: 379–405.

Vermeulen G, Seidl R, Mercimek-Mahmutoglu S, Rotteveel JJ, Scheper GC, van der Knaap MS (2005) Fright is a provoking factor in vanishing white matter disease. *Ann Neurol* 57: 560–3.

Welsh JP, Ahn ES, Placantonakis DG (2005) Is autism due to brain desynchronization? *Int J Dev Neurosci* 23: 253-263.

Woodhouse W, Bailey A, Rutter M, Bolton P, Baird G, Le Couteur A (1996) Head circumference in autism and other pervasive developmental disorders. *J Child Psychol Psychiatry* 37: 665–71.

Zwaigenbaum L, Bryson S, Rogers T, Roberts W, Brian J, Szatmari P (2005) Behavioral manifestations of autism in the first year of life. *Int J Dev Neurosci* 23: 143–52.

INDEX

social skills therapy, treatment, 286
sociodemographics, *see* epidemiology
socioeconomics, 28–9
somatosensory system, 216–19
    stimuli, 216
    tactile defensiveness, 216
SPCH1 gene, *see FOXP2* gene
special services, psychoeducational evaluation, 266
speech development, family studies, 96
speech therapy, *see* treatment
SSRIs, *see* selective serotonin reuptake inhibitors (SSRIs)
ST7/RAY1 gene, *102*
standardized motor examinations, motor deficits, 233
Stanford–Binet Intelligence Scale, *271*
status epilepticus
language regression, 61
magnetic resonance imaging, 179
regression, 179
Stereotypic Behavior Scale, *310*
stereotypies, 68–78
    amphetamine-induced, 71
    definition, 68, *69*
    developmental disabilities, 73
        developmental language disorders, 74
        differential diagnosis, 73–4
        mental retardation, 73
Huntington disease, 75
movement disorder vs self-stimulation, 74–5
natural history, 70–1
nervous system development, 75
neurobiology, 71–2
neuroimaging, 72
    Parkinson disease, 75
    rodent models, 71
    sensory disorders, 72–3, 74–5
    social response elicitation, 75
    tics vs, *69*, 70
    without developmental disabilities, 72
    see also repetitive behaviors; *specific behaviors*
stimuli
    sensory/perceptual responsiveness, 205
    somatosensory system, 216
stria medullaris, brainstem, 128

Structured Teaching, 285
study designs, epidemiology, 21–2, 23
subclinical epilepsy, *see* epilepsy
subcortical dysfunction
    auditory system, 209
    motor deficits, 238
    sensory/perceptual responsiveness, 221
subject complexity, sensory/perceptual responsiveness, 205
suboptimal connectivity, brain development, 130
superior olivary cells, brainstem, 129
superior parietal region, motor imitation, 239
superior temporal gyrus, 44
superior temporal sulcus (STS) region, 239
surgery, epilepsy treatment, 184
surveillance epidemiology, 22
symptoms, *see* signs and symptoms (of autism)
synapse development, 88–9
    brain overgrowth, 88
    glutamate abnormalities, 87
syndromic autism
    definition, *2*, 7
    idiopathic autism vs, 7
    see also specific conditions

tactile defensiveness, somatosensory system, 216
task complexity, sensory/perceptual responsiveness, 205
T cells, 142
TEACCH (Treatment and Education of Autistic and related Communication handicapped Children), 285
temporal binding deficits, 162–3
temporal lobe, volume, 118
temporoparietal areas, 59
Test of Early Language Development, *269*
Test of Language Development, *269*
Test of Motor Impairment – Henderson Revision, 238
Test of Pragmatic Language, *269*
thalamus
    serotonin, 124
    sleep disorders, 189
thalidomide, 30, 99
theory of mind (ToM: metacognition)

input pathways, 214
stimuli processing, 214–6
　block design, 214–5
　face vs non-face perception, 215
　functional magnetic resonance imaging
　　(fMRI), 215–6
　neuroanatomy, 215–6
vocational skills, high school children, 276–7
voice output communication aides (VOCAs),
　286

weak central coherence hypothesis
　sensory/perceptual responsiveness, 222
　social deficit, 40

Wernicke's area, language and communica-
　tion, 59
Weschler intelligence tests, *271*, 272
　elementary aged children, 273–4
West syndrome (infantile spasm), 164
white matter
　brain size, 121–2, 130
　frontal lobe, 121
Williams syndrome, 99–100
Wing Subgroup Questionnaire (WSQ), 41
WNT2 gene, *102*, 104
working memory, social deficit, 40

ziprasidone, *290*, 291